Diagnosis and Management of Mental Disorders

Diagnosis and Management of Mental Disorders

Edited by John Dalvi

AMERICAN
MEDICAL PUBLISHERS
www.americanmedicalpublishers.com

American Medical Publishers,
41 Flatbush Avenue,
1st Floor, New York,
NY 11217, USA

Visit us on the World Wide Web at:
www.americanmedicalpublishers.com

ISBN: 978-1-63927-439-0

Cataloging-in-Publication Data

Diagnosis and management of mental disorders / edited by John Dalvi.
p. cm.
Includes bibliographical references and index.
ISBN 978-1-63927-439-0
1. Psychology, Pathological. 2. Psychiatry. I. Dalvi, John.
RC454.4 .U53 2021
616.89--dc23

Table of Contents

Preface IX

Chapter 1 **Risk behavior in patients with severe mental disorders: a prospective study of 121,830 patients managed in rural households of western China** 1
Yuanyuan Liu, Xiang Liu, Hong Wen, Dan Wang, Xianmei Yang, Weiwei Tang, Yaxi Li, Tao Zhang and Min Yang

Chapter 2 **Diagnosis of somatoform disorders in primary care: diagnostic agreement, predictors, and comaprisons with depression and anxiety** 14
Katharina Piontek, Meike C. Shedden-Mora, Maria Gladigau, Amina Kuby and Bernd Löwe

Chapter 3 **Barriers to effective diabetes management – a survey of people with severe mental illness** 22
Kathleen Mulligan, Hayley McBain, Frederique Lamontagne-Godwin, Jacqui Chapman, Chris Flood, Mark Haddad, Julia Jones and Alan Simpson

Chapter 4 **Treatment results for severe psychiatric illness: which method is best suited to denote the outcome of mental health care?** 37
Edwin de Beurs, Matthijs Blankers, Philippe Delespaul, Erik van Duijn, Niels Mulder, Annet Nugter, Wilma Swildens, Bea G. Tiemens, Jan Theunissen, Arno F. A. van Voorst and Jaap van Weeghel

Chapter 5 **Trajectories of antidepressant medication use in individuals before and after being granted disability pension due to common mental disorders** 47
Syed Rahman, Michael Wiberg, Kristina Alexanderson, Jussi Jokinen, Antti Tanskanen and Ellenor Mittendorfer-Rutz

Chapter 6 **Body image in patients with somatoform disorder** 57
M. Scheffers, H. Kalisvaart, J. T. van Busschbach, R. J. Bosscher, M. A. J. van Duijn, S. A. M. van Broeckhuysen-Kloth, R. A. Schoevers and R. Geenen

Chapter 7 **Predictors of medication adherence among patients with severe psychiatric disorders: findings from the baseline assessment of a randomized controlled trial (Tecla)** 65
Ulrike Stentzel, Neeltje van den Berg, Lara N. Schulze, Thea Schwaneberg, Franziska Radicke, Jens M. Langosch, Harald J. Freyberger, Wolfgang Hoffmann and Hans-Jörgen Grabe

Chapter 8 **Excited catatonia in a patient with fatal pulmonary embolism and a successful treatment strategy** 73
Wei-Ting Tseng and Tiao-Lai Huang

Chapter 9 **A community-based peer support service for persons with severe mental illness** 76
Yunge Fan, Ning Ma, Liang Ma, Wei Xu, J. Steven Lamberti and Eric D. Caine

Chapter 10 **Experiences with the implementation of Individual Placement and Support for people with severe mental illness: a qualitative study among stakeholders** 86
Miljana Vukadin, Frederieke G. Schaafsma, Marjan J. Westerman, Harry W. C. Michon and Johannes R. Anema

Chapter 11 **Psychopathological sequelae of female genital mutilation and their neuroendocrinological associations** 95
Anke Köbach, Martina Ruf-Leuschner and Thomas Elbert

Chapter 12 **The effect of positive psychology interventions on well-being and distress in clinical samples with psychiatric or somatic disorders** 107
Farid Chakhssi, Jannis T. Kraiss, Marion Sommers-Spijkerman and Ernst T. Bohlmeijer

Chapter 13 **Factors associated with health service utilisation for common mental disorders** 124
Tessa Roberts, Georgina Miguel Esponda, Dzmitry Krupchanka, Rahul Shidhaye, Vikram Patel and Sujit Rathod

Chapter 14 **Evaluation of attitudes and knowledge toward mental disorders in a sample of the Chinese population using a web-based approach** 143
Juan Li, Meng-meng Zhang, Lin Zhao, Wen-qiang Li, Jun-lin Mu and Zhao-hui Zhang

Chapter 15 **The prevalence of psychiatric disorders among students aged 6-16 years old in central Hunan** 151
Yan-Mei Shen, Bella Siu Man Chan, Jian-Bo Liu, Yuan-Yue Zhou, Xi-Long Cui, Yu-Qiong He, Yu-min Fang, Yu-Tao Xiang and Xue-Rong Luo

Chapter 16 **Persistent catatonia following epileptic seizures** 160
Ragnar Verbraeken and Jurjen J. Luykx

Chapter 17 **Evaluation of an interaction-skills training for reducing the burden of family caregivers of patients with severe mental illness: a pre-posttest design** 165
Yasmin Gharavi, Barbara Stringer, Adriaan Hoogendoorn, Jan Boogaarts, Bas Van Raaij and Berno Van Meijel

Chapter 18 **Psychosocial stress impairs health behavior in patients with mental disorders** 173
Till Fabian Beutel, Rüdiger Zwerenz and Matthias Michal

Chapter 19 **Prevalence and stability of mental disorders among young adults: findings from a longitudinal study** 186
Kristin Gustavson, Ann Kristin Knudsen, Ragnar Nesvåg, Gun Peggy Knudsen, Stein Emil Vollset and Ted Reichborn-Kjennerud

Chapter 20 **Characteristics, motivations and experiences of volunteer befrienders for people with mental illness** 201
Sarah Toner, Lauren M. Hickling, Mariana Pinto da Costa, Megan Cassidy and Stefan Priebe

Chapter 21 **Preferences for befriending schemes: a survey of patients with severe mental illness....211**
Sarah Toner, Megan Cassidy, Agnes Chevalier, Aida Farreny, Monica Leverton, Mariana Pinto da Costa and Stefan Priebe

Chapter 22 **Perceptions of free will in obsessive-compulsive disorder....219**
Lucas J. B. van Oudheusden, Stasja Draisma, Sandra van der Salm, Danielle Cath, Patricia van Oppen, Anton J. L. M. van Balkom and Gerben Meynen

Permissions

List of Contributors

Index

Preface

I am honored to present to you this unique book which encompasses the most up-to-date data in the field. I was extremely pleased to get this opportunity of editing the work of experts from across the globe. I have also written papers in this field and researched the various aspects revolving around the progress of the discipline. I have tried to unify my knowledge along with that of stalwarts from every corner of the world, to produce a text which not only benefits the readers but also facilitates the growth of the field.

Mental disorder is a psychological syndrome that causes significant distress of personal functioning. These features can be persistent, remitting, and relapsing. The way a person behaves, feels, perceives, or thinks are some factor that defines mental disorders. Some common types of mental disorders are depression, dementia, bipolar disorder and schizophrenia. Mental disorder is associated with distress and disability. It can increase the risk of death and can also cause a significant loss of autonomy. It is generally caused due to environmental and genetic factors, drugs and personal traits. Treatment of mental disorders includes psychotherapy and psychiatric medication. It may also involve lifestyle changes, social interventions, peer support and self-help. This book unravels the recent studies in the field of mental disorders. Some of the diverse topics covered herein address the varied disorders that fall under this category. The extensive content of this book provides the readers with a thorough understanding of the subject.

Finally, I would like to thank all the contributing authors for their valuable time and contributions. This book would not have been possible without their efforts. I would also like to thank my friends and family for their constant support.

Editor

1

Risk behavior in patients with severe mental disorders: a prospective study of 121,830 patients managed in rural households of western China

Yuanyuan Liu[1†], Xiang Liu[2†], Hong Wen[3†], Dan Wang[3], Xianmei Yang[3], Weiwei Tang[1,4], Yaxi Li[1,4], Tao Zhang[1] and Min Yang[1,4*]

Abstract

Background: The management of severe mental disorder (SMD) patients in communities is an important initiative of healthcare reform in China. Yet the effects in terms of risk behavior of patients are unclear, particularly in rural areas. This study aims to examine high risk behaviors, changing trends, and possible associated factors among SMD patients in the rural areas of western China.

Methods: This analysis examined incidence rate (IR) of high risk behavior of 121,830 managed SMD patients in rural area of Sichuan province, based on data from the national system from 2006 to 2013. Register rate, high risk behavior IR, and time distribution and area distribution of high risk behavior were described. Two-level Poisson regression model was used to analyze associates of high risk behavior of patients, which include demographic characteristics at individual level, socio-economic condition and health system indicators at region level.

Results: It was revealed that 6804 (5.58%) of managed patients were involved in 17,220 high risk behavior events, which gave an overall IR of 0.0998 (per person year) on the basis of 172,564 person years of follow-up. The IR varied widely across municipalities, in the range of 0.0305–0.3397. The IR of high risk behavior in the cohort had increased since 2006, and peaked by 2011, at 0.2392. At the individual level, males aged 25 to 44, who were unmarried and in poverty, illiterate or semiliterate, had a family history of mental disorders and antipsychotic treatments, longer duration illnesses, were associated with an increased IR risk. At the regional level, higher psychiatric practitioner visits and the lower annual net income of rural residents per capita, were associated with an increased IR risk.

Conclusions: This is the first large prospective study that revealed the current situation of the register rate, high risk behavior incidence rate in SMD patients in rural area of western China, and examined associates and the differences of high risk behavior of patients among municipalities. The findings may provide evidences that lead to guide prevention and control for risk behavior in SMD patients in rural areas of China, as well as to improve mental health services for this population. It could provide some reference for other developing countries too.

Keywords: Risk behavior, Severe mental disorders, Prospective study, Rural households, China

* Correspondence: yangmin2013@scu.edu.cn
[†]Equal contributors
[1]Department of Epidemiology and Health Statistics, West China School of Public Health, Sichuan University, Chengdu, Sichuan, People's Republic of China
[4]West China Research Center for Rural Health Development, Sichuan University, No.17 Section 3, South Renmin Road, Chengdu, Sichuan 610041, People's Republic of China
Full list of author information is available at the end of the article

Background

In China, severe mental disorders (SMD) include six types: schizophrenia, schizoaffective disorder, delusional disorder, bipolar disorder, psychotic disorder due to epilepsy, and mental retardation with mental disorders [1]. It is estimated that there are about 16 million individuals with SMD in China [2], which translates to serious public health and societal problems associated with high disease burdens [3]. In order to reduce these immense social and economic burdens, as well as to protect the legal rights of patients with serious mental disorders, the Chinese government has undertaken many efforts over the last decade, as part of the reform of China's mental health system [4, 5]. In 2005, the National Continuing Management and Intervention Program for Psychoses (also known as Central Government Support for the Local Management and Treatment of Severe Mental Illnesses Project or "686 Project") [6, 7] was launched to rebuild China's public health infrastructure following the SARS epidemic. The "686 Project" was established using the WHO's recommended strategy for integrating hospital- and community-based mental health services. Following a decade long trial in selected regions, the "686 Project" moved beyond the initial pilot phase toward a process of scaling up community mental health services throughout the country [8]. In 2009, the management of psychoses was included in the National Basic Public Health Services. A guideline of China's National Basic Public Health Services (2011) specified services for the management of psychoses [9]. In 2012, the Ministry of Health (now the National Health and Family Planning Commission, NHFPC) officially issued a government document: Chinese Managerial and Treatment Regulations for Severely Mentally Disordered Patients (also known as the Working Criteria on Management of Psychoses) [1]. Subsequently, China's initial national mental health legislation was adopted by the Standing Committee of the National People's Congress, with the law taking effect in 2013 [10, 11]. The aim of the legislation was to promote mental health, improve health service quality, as well as protect patients with serious mental disorders. One of the most important targets in the management of patients with SMD was to prevent and reduce violent behavior that caused harm to themselves or others [12].

Despite significant political progress with quite comprehensive and instructive nationwide policies in place, the development of mental health service systems and service delivery in China still faces many problems. There exist wide disparities among provinces and regions in terms of socio-economic and developmental levels. In several underdeveloped western areas, the mental health service reform process has been slowed by the poor understanding of public health policies, lack of human health resources, and the required professional skills [4]. Sichuan province possesses the largest population in western China. Its population reached 91.33 million in 2013, with 65 million in the rural areas [13]. It is estimated that there were more than 800,000 patients with SMD in Sichuan province in 2013 [14]. Yet research into the management effects of the system, in terms of risk behaviors in patients with SMD in western China, particularly in rural areas [15],[1] has rarely been reported [16, 17]. There has been little data available with which to assess the quality of the management of psychoses services locally, or on a large scale, or the efficiency of government initiatives for mental health reform in China [18, 19].

To fill the gap, this study aimed to gather evidence to address the following questions: What is the current situation of risk behavior in patients with SMD and received community services in the rural areas of Sichuan province, and are there any areas with differences in risk behaviors? Are there any changes in the trends of risk behavior outcomes of managed patients in recent years? What are the associated factors with the risk behavior of patients? Might regional socioeconomic factors or health system factors be impacting the risk behavior outcomes of patients? The answers to the above questions will likely assist with the enhancement of prevention and control for risk behavior in patients with SMD in the rural areas of western China. Further, it will help to improve mental health care and services for this population through associated health agencies.

Methods

Data sources

The dataset for this study was obtained from the National System of Basic Information Collection and Analysis for Psychoses (abbreviated as **NS**). The NS initiated a pilot trial in 2006, which was scaled up to practically the entire country by 2010. The data system was developed by the NHFPC [1], and managed by professionals at the Centers for Disease Control and Prevention (CDCs) and the Mental Health Centers (MHCs) of China. Primarily, the data system employed two approaches to engage patients. Initially, they identified patients who were referred from psychiatric hospitals or related departments in general hospitals. Secondly, they screened patients for possible psychosis who were referred from the China Disabled Persons' Federation (CDPF), local communities, township health centers, neighborhoods, or village committees. These patients were subsequently examined by psychiatrists, and those who met the diagnostic criteria (ICD-10 or DSM-IV) [20] for psychotic disorders were evaluated for their disease condition by the national working group. This evaluation was focused on a risk assessment of violence, mental symptoms, self consciousness, social functionality, adverse drug reactions, and other serious physiological diseases [4]. The frequency of evaluation in a follow-up was determined by patient's disease condition. Patients whose diseases were stable, or basically stable, were followed at least once every three months. The criteria for stable or basically stable were as follows: low risk score at level 0-2 (see the definitions of risk levels in the next section), no significant mental symptoms, no adverse drug reactions or serious physiological diseases, good self consciousness, and social functionality. Otherwise, patients were classified as being in an unstable condition, who received weekly or monthly follow-ups [1]. Sichuan was one of the first provinces to establish NS in China, which commenced in May 2006. Up to December 2013, 155,478 patients were registered in the provincial system. In the whole follow-up period, patients may enter or leave the cohort at any time. Their follow-up period reached 7. 35 years at the longest, with a mean follow uptime of 1. 40 years (SD: 0.87). Following data integrity checks, we obtained 144,243 valid cases, with the cases having error or missing values in outcome variables excluded. Among them 121,830 (84.5%) patients lived and were managed in rural areas, whereas the remaining 22,413 (15.5%) patients resided in urban areas.

Study measures

We considered the risk behavior of patients as a key measure for the quality of the management of psychoses services. Risk behavior was defined on a scale of from 0 to 5. Level 0 (L0) did not refer to any of the following behaviors indicated in levels 1 to 5. Level 1 (L1) risk behavior included verbal threats and shouts to others, but no physically destructive behavior. Level 2 (L2) included the destruction of property, but was home limited, and with persuasion could be stopped. Level 3 (L3) obviously included the destruction of property regardless of the occasion, which with attempted persuasion could not be stopped. Level 4 (L4) was defined by continuous destructive behavior to individuals or property regardless of the occasion, which with attempted persuasion could not be stopped. Level 5(L5) was defined by any violent behavior against individuals using controlled dangerous weapons, or other dangerous behavior such as arson, blasts, etc., regardless of the occasion. According to Chinese Managerial and Treatment Regulations for Severely Mentally Disordered Patients, the risk level between L0 and L2 was classified as "low risk behavior" and L3 – L5 as "high risk behavior" [1]. In this study, the number of high risk behavior incidents of each patient that were recorded in the follow-up period in the dataset, were defined as outcome variables. The follow-up year of each patient was employed as a denominator to define the incidence of high risk behavior.

To examine potential associated factors with the incidence of risk behavior of patients, we considered several groups of variables. The first group pertained to demographic characteristics at the individual level, which were released by the NS, such as gender, age, family history of mental disorder, marital status, ethnic group, education qualification, economic status, type of diagnosis, duration of illness, antipsychotic treatments, and participation in the "686 Project". The second group of variables involved socioeconomic conditions at the region or municipal level, such as the annual net income of rural residents per capita (ANIPC), employment proportion of rural residents (EP%), and per capita minimal livelihood funds for rural residents under basic provision protection (PCMLF). The above regional variables were collected from the Sichuan Statistical Yearbook (2014), which are the official statistics of 2013 [13]. The third group of variables was related to health system indicators that were collected by the Mental Health Center of Sichuan Province in 2013. These indicators were specific to mental health service for patients with SMD at the regional level. Variables included the number of agencies for severe mental disordered (NASMD), number of inpatient beds for severe mental disordered (NBSMD), number of psychiatric practitioners (including assistant psychiatric practitioners) per one hundred thousand people (NPP/100,000), and the average number of follow-ups for patients in the rural region (AFP).

Statistical analyses

Since the incidence of high risk behavior was infrequent, and hierarchical structure in this dataset is presented with individuals nested within municipalities, multilevel Poisson regression was used to model incident rate ratios (IRRs), and to examine associated factors. At the individual level, demographic characteristic variables assisted with the identification of subgroups for high risk screening and prevention. At the regional level, municipality socioeconomic variables helped to assess the extent to which contextual factors might impact individual behaviors in addition to individual risk factors. Similarly, health system indicators at the municipal level were utilized to examine how health system performance might impact individual risk behaviors, with the aim being that evidence might shed light on the best use of health resources.

Three two-level Poisson models with random intercepts were constructed to examine risk factors at different levels and by variable groups. Model 0 had no variables, but was used to test regional clustering effects and estimate regional variations in high risk behavior incidence as a benchmark. Model 1 included individual-level factors, whereas Model 2 incorporated both individual-level and region-level variables. Model fits, following the addition of each group of variables, was evaluated by pseudo-AIC criteria [21]. The total years of follow-up during the study period, was the offset variable (underlying person-time) for the regression models. The General Ward χ^2 statistic was employed to test significance of random coefficients.

These studies received Institutional Review Board approval for research involving human subjects from Sichuan University and Mental Health Center of Sichuan Province, where the research was conducted. The analysis was conducted using SAS 9.3 and SPSS 19.0.

Results

Registered patients were distributed in 19 out of 21 municipalities in Sichuan province, as shown in Fig. 1a. The missing cases in two municipalities were due to the fact that there were no recognized mental health care agencies in the regions, and the NS system was not mature enough to generate reliable management data at the time when the study data were collected. As these two municipalities accounted for 2.4% of the total population in the province, the analysis in the study represented 97.6% of the population in Sichuan.

The overall registration rate of patients was 1.92 per thousand population, in the range of from 0.54 to 4.05 ‰ across municipalities (see Table 1). Over 8 years, 6804 (5.58%) out of 121,830 managed patients were involved with 17,220 instances of high risk behavior, which gave an overall incidence rate 0.0998 (per person-year) on the basis of 172,564 person years of follow-up. As shown in Table 1 and Fig. 1b, the incidence rate varied significantly across municipalities, in the range of from 0.0305 to 0.3397 (per person-year).

Examining the registration number by year, the results in Table 2 suggest that the NS system was in a pilot period spanning 2006 – 2009, and only a small proportion of

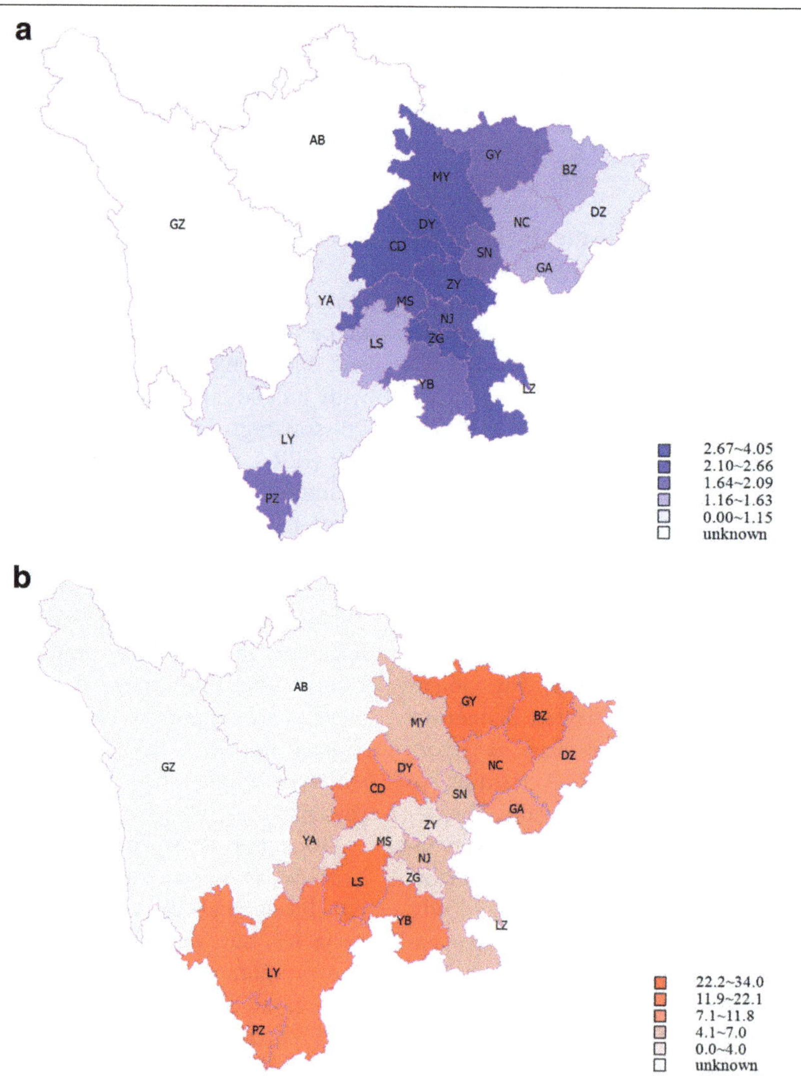

Fig. 1 **a** Distribution of registration rate (‰) of patients with SMD in rural areas in Sichuan province (2006 – 2013). **b** Distribution of incidence rate (%) of high risk behavior in patients with SMD in rural areas in Sichuan (2006 – 2013)

Table 1 Regional distribution of patients with SMD and incidence of high risk behaviors of patients in rural households of Sichuan province in cohort, from 2006 to 2013[a]

Regions	Registered patients			High risk behavior			
	Population (million)	N_1	Registration rate (‰)	N_2	No. of high risk behaviors	Follow-up person years	Incidence rate (%)
1 CD	4.59	18,588	4.05	752	3593	30,118.68	11.93
2 ZG	2.17	8039	3.70	271	508	12,620.50	4.03
3 PZ	0.52	853	1.64	83	138	622.63	22.16
4 LZ	3.56	7490	2.10	355	707	10,013.31	7.06
5 DY	2.75	7883	2.87	617	1225	12,933.39	9.47
6 MY	3.89	8916	2.29	430	901	15,157.51	5.94
7 GY	2.38	3897	1.64	447	1307	4971.04	26.29
8 SN	2.82	4645	1.65	159	279	6745.85	4.14
9 NJ	3.30	7745	2.35	303	652	13,035.34	5.00
10 LS	2.38	3637	1.53	384	994	4217.26	23.57
11 NC	5.82	7174	1.23	536	1362	7429.37	18.33
12 MS	2.53	5651	2.23	119	257	7523.61	3.42
13 YB	4.44	8093	1.82	631	1244	9646.55	12.90
14 GA	3.80	4392	1.16	292	424	5404.53	7.85
15 DZ	5.48	5630	1.03	221	667	7088.68	9.41
16 YA	1.14	1169	1.03	63	85	1382.37	6.15
17 BZ	3.12	4463	1.43	720	2167	6378.79	33.97
18 ZY	4.18	11,143	2.67	289	485	15,888.46	3.05
19 LY	4.46	2422	0.54	132	225	1386.21	16.23
Total	63.35	121,830	1.92	6804	17,220	172,564.09	9.98

[a]Population refers to agricultural population in 2013
N_1: the number of registered patients with SMD
Register rate: the rate of registered patients with SMD in local population. Limited by variable objective conditions, registration rate is lower than the prevalence rate of SMD. *Register rate* = N_1/ Population
N_2: the number of high risk behavior patients in registered patients with SMD. As mentioned in 2.1.1, whether a patient is classified into a high risk group is according to the highest risk level in their follow-up period. If they were once, or more times, evaluated as L3 to L5, they were classified into a high risk group
No. of high risk behaviors: the number of occurrences for high risk behavior in registered patients with SMD. In this study, there were 115,026 patients whose *no. of high risk behaviors* was 0, and the remaining patients with *no. of high risk behaviors* ranged from 1 to 40
Follow-up person years: the sum of the years of follow-up time of registered patients with SMD
Incidence rate: the incidence rate of high risk behavior in registered patients, and the follow-ups in person years were used as the denominator to define the incidence of high risk behavior. *Incidence rate* = *No of high risk behaviors / Follow-up person years*
To avoid the values being too small, all incidence rates in Tables 1, 2, 3 and 4 were multiply by 100%

Table 2 Time distribution of high risk behavior of patients with SMDs in rural households of Sichuan province

Year	N_1	N_2	No. of high risk behaviors	Follow-up person years	Incidence rate (%)
2006	6	0	0	1.27	0.00
2007	40	2	2	20.87	9.58
2008	75	1	1	57.81	1.73
2009	320	16	16	150.99	10.60
2010	6046	254	371	2557.09	14.51
2011	66,549	3852	6045	25,271.64	23.92
2012	97,668	2689	6141	75,017.99	8.19
2013	101,581	1930	4644	69,321.44	6.70

patients were managed in the system. The rapid increase in the number of registered patients following 2009 suggested the positive impact of national policy and investment in the system since 2009. The quality of the data was, at least, improved in terms of coverage and completion.

The temporal trend in the incidence rate of high risk behavior (Table 2), was observed to increase and peak at 0.2392 (per person year) by 2011, followed by a downward trend. This might have been a reflection of the management effects following the development of community mental health services in recent years. The violent behavior of patients comprised one of the management and preventive targets of the services.

A further examination of changing trends in the high risk behavior incidence rate by municipality, from 2011 to 2013 (Table 3), revealed that except for one municipality, an annual downward trend of from between 5 and 77% in the outcome was observed across all municipalities, with an overall annual rate of decrease of 47%.

According to the descriptive analysis results of Table 4, it may be seen that patients with following characteristics were more likely to have high risk behaviors: male, aged 15 to 44, national minority, a family history of mental disorders, unmarried, living in poverty, illiterate/semiliterate, illness duration of 10 to 29 years, no antipsychotic treatment, not participating in "686 Project", and follow-up time of less than 4 years.

As the univariate analysis did not take into consideration of the effects of other variables, multivariate analyses were further carried out to control the potential confounders. A baseline Model 0 that did not include any variables estimated the variance of random effects of the outcome at municipal level as 0.486 ($\chi^2 = 8.922$, $P = 0.003$). This implied that the incidence rates of the high risk behavior were significantly varied among municipalities. Having considered individual level factors, Model 1 in Table 5 shows that several of these factors were significantly associated with high IRR, rather than their reference group: aged between 25 and 44, unmarried, having family history of mental disorders, and on antipsychotic treatment; longer duration of illness increases risk, with an IRR range of from1.125 (10 to 19 years), 1.153 (20 to 29 years), to 1.165 (≧30 years), compared to an illness duration of < 10 years.

Factors that seemly had lower IRR than their comparison groups were: female gender, age ≧60, not in poverty, with elementary education and above; bipolar affective disorder, mental disorders due to epilepsy and mental retardation, with mental disorders having a lower IRR

Table 3 Incidence rate of high risk behavior by region of rural Sichuan province from 2011 to 2013[a]

Region	2011			2012			2013			
	No. of high risk behaviors	Follow-up person years	Incidence rate (%)	No. of high risk behaviors	Follow-up person years	Incidence rate (%)	No. of high risk behaviors	Follow-up person years	Incidence rate (%)	Annual rate of change[a]
1 CD	1109	4031.33	27.51	1418	12,234.69	11.59	1061	13,743.52	7.72	−0.47
2 ZG	254	1691.39	15.02	160	5333.33	3.00	78	5492.96	1.42	−0.69
3 PZ	4	41.07	9.74	11	168.20	6.54	123	409.32	30.05	0.77
4 LZ	337	1280.08	26.33	235	4234.23	5.55	88	4378.11	2.01	−0.72
5 DY	751	2722.03	27.59	115	5066.08	2.27	272	4857.14	5.60	−0.55
6 MY	448	2370.25	18.90	334	6972.86	4.79	81	5625.00	1.44	−0.72
7 GY	468	807.15	57.98	590	2327.42	25.35	244	1788.86	13.64	−0.51
8 SN	123	1470.52	8.36	77	2851.85	2.70	27	1985.29	1.36	−0.60
9 NJ	337	2523.60	13.35	260	5816.55	4.47	44	4313.73	1.02	−0.72
10 LS	244	422.82	57.71	423	1696.07	24.94	327	2070.93	15.79	−0.48
11 NC	572	1460.63	39.16	505	3454.17	14.62	259	2273.92	11.39	−0.46
12 MS	88	1145.18	7.68	92	3076.92	2.99	57	3097.83	1.84	−0.51
13 YB	309	950.19	32.52	655	4428.67	14.79	269	4151.23	6.48	−0.55
14 GA	247	784.79	31.47	85	2537.31	3.35	71	1977.72	3.59	−0.66
15 DZ	172	710.48	24.21	287	3235.63	8.87	205	3005.87	6.82	−0.47
16 YA	52	137.49	37.82	18	640.57	2.81	15	595.24	2.52	−0.74
17 BZ	297	526.01	56.46	496	3167.31	15.66	1369	2669.14	51.29	−0.05
18 ZY	222	1977.65	11.23	183	7093.02	2.58	38	6440.68	0.59	−0.77
19 LY	11	218.03	5.04	197	693.91	28.39	16	465.12	3.44	−0.17
Total	6045	25,270.70	23.92	6141	74,981.68	8.19	4644	69,313.43	6.70	−0.47

[a]Annual rate of change==$\sqrt[n]{a_n/a_0}$-1

Table 4 Distribution of high risk behavior by characteristics of patients with SMDs in rural households of Sichuan province

Characteristic	N_1	N_2	No of high risk behaviors	Follow-up person years	Incidence rate (%)
Gender					
1 = male	59,957	3737	9707	84,164.46	11.53
2 = female	61,873	3067	7513	88,399.63	8.50
Age					
1 = 15 to 24	5932	275	783	7424.24	10.55
2 = 25 to 44	45,022	2859	7232	63,412.73	11.40
3 = 45 to 59	37,632	1952	4969	54,161.07	9.17
4 = ≧60	33,244	1718	4236	47,566.04	8.91
Nationality					
1 = Han	120,428	6739	17,113	171,753.73	9.96
2 = Minority	1402	65	107	810.36	13.20
Family history of mental illness					
0 = no	116,988	6472	16,376	165,982.10	9.87
1 = yes	4842	332	844	6581.99	12.82
Marital status					
1 = married	73,619	3679	8988	105,017.25	8.56
2 = unmarried	46,396	3033	8039	64,914.40	12.38
3 = NK	1815	92	193	2632.44	7.33
Economic status					
1 = poverty[a]	78,932	4867	12,883	113,025.02	11.40
2 = non-poverty	17,134	694	1744	25,198.74	6.92
3 = NK	25,764	1243	2593	34,340.33	7.55
Education degree					
1 = illiteracy/semiliterate	42,697	2404	6309	59,656.04	10.58
2 = elementary education and above	74,325	4130	10,374	106,046.29	9.78
3 = NK	4808	270	537	6861.77	7.83
Diagnosis type					
1 = schizophrenia	103,412	6055	15,362	149,703.01	10.26
2 = schizoaffective disorder	1849	121	256	2143.59	11.94
3 = delusional disorder	480	20	72	673.90	10.68
4 = bipolar disorder	2995	168	415	3918.84	10.59
5 = psychotic disorder due to epilepsy	4980	234	693	6561.95	10.56
6 = mental retardation with mental disorders	8114	206	422	9562.81	4.41
Duration of illness					
1 = < 10 years	46,009	2305	5544	58,635.88	9.45
2 = 10 to 19 years	36,468	2212	5689	54,715.99	10.40
3 = 20 to 29 years	22,381	1333	3533	34,039.29	10.38
4 = ≧30 years	16,972	954	2454	25,172.93	9.75
Antipsychotic treatment					
0 = no	27,489	1549	4193	35,999.18	11.65
1 = yes	94,341	5255	13,027	136,564.91	9.54
Participation in 686 project					
0 = no	14,522	1300	2613	22,780.70	11.47

Table 4 Distribution of high risk behavior by characteristics of patients with SMDs in rural households of Sichuan province *(Continued)*

Characteristic	N_1	N_2	No of high risk behaviors	Follow-up person years	Incidence rate (%)
1 = yes	107,285	5504	14,607	149,752.54	9.75
3 = NK	23	0	0	30.84	0.00
Follow-up time					
1 = < 2 years	84,477	3978	8787	83,345.00	10.54
2 = 2 to 4 years	37,196	2817	8401	88,440.56	9.50
3 = >4 years	157	9	32	778.53	4.11

[a]Poverty refers to the economic status that is below the local poverty line by income level

compared to schizophrenia. Patients participating in the "686 Project" appeared to have lower risk (IRR = 0.767) than otherwise. Model 2 incorporated municipal factors into Model 1, which reduced the municipal level variance for random effects, from 0.502 ($P = 0.003$) in Model 1, down to 0.417($P = 0.011$). Higher numbers of psychiatric practitioners (including assistant psychiatric practitioners) per 100,000 population (NPP/100,000), and the lower annual net income of rural residents per capita (ANIPC), were associated with an increased IRR. They accounted for only about 17% of the difference in the incidence rate of high risk behavior of patients among municipalities. With adjustment for municipality factors, the effects of all individual factors on the incidence rate remained unchanged as in Model 1.

Discussion

The NS is the only mental health themed surveillance system in China [17, 18]. This is the first large prospective study based on the NS of Sichuan province to reveal the current situation of the registration rate, high risk behavior incidence rate in patients with SMD in the rural areas of western China. Individual and regional factors were examined in association with the high risk behavior incidence rates of patients, and the differences of the high risk behavior of patients among municipalities in Sichuan province. These findings may provide useful evidence to guide the prevention and control of risk behaviors in patients with SMD in the rural areas of western China, as well as to improve mental health services for this population.

The registration rate of patients with SMD

A previous large epidemiological survey, spanning 2001 – 2005 in four provinces of China reported an adjusted 1-month prevalence of psychotic disorder at 1.0% (95% CI: 0.8-1.1) [2]. A meta analysis of 2,284,957 Chinese individuals reported a lifetime prevalence of schizophrenia alone as 0.36% in 1990, which increased to 0.83% in 2010 [22]. The Chinese government set the goal for the national detection rate of severe mentally disordered patients for the NS system at 0.35% in 2014 [23].

The registered patients of rural areas with SMD in the NS system in this study was at 0.192%, which was lower than the prevalence rate of patients with SMD in the general population, and lower than the national detection rate target. This was because approximately two thirds of the identified patients were not included in the NS system for community services. They were: (1) patients who were completely cured, and (2) patients who could not be cured; however, at a degenerating stage were harmless to society. This means that the NS system cannot be used to report the true prevalence of SMD in the population. However, from 2006 to 2013, the registration rate gradually rose from almost null to 0.192%, which was particularly the case after the Chinese government launched the Phase 1 NS system at the national scale in 2011. This might reflect a positive effect of system efficiency for the management of more patients in rural areas.

The large variation in the registration rates, from 0. 405% in CD to 0.054% in LY, may reflect the quality of the NS system among municipalities related to multiple regional contextual factors such as socioeconomics, access to health services, health workforce resources, and education. As the capital of Sichuan province, CD had the highest per capita annual net income of rural residents in the province in 2014 [13]; hence, it benefited from 27 mental health agencies, 0.46‰ per capita inpatient psychiatric beds, and 0.037‰ per capita psychiatric practitioners (including assistant psychiatric practitioners). In contrast, the LY Autonomous Prefecture is located in a mountainous area, with the per capita annual net income of rural residents ranked at the bottom third of the province. It has only three mental health agencies, 0.17‰ per capita inpatient psychiatric beds, and 0.007‰ per capita psychiatric practitioners (including assistant psychiatric practitioners). Therefore it is critical to examine, as in this study, how disparities in these municipal level factors might impact patient outcomes, such as high risk behavior.

Table 5 Two-level Poisson regression analyses for associates with high risk behavior of patients with severe mental illness in rural households of Sichuan Province

Variables	Model1		Model2	
Fixed effect	Coefficient	IRR(95% CI)	Coefficient	IRR(95% CI)
Regional Level				
NPP (per 100,000 pop.)	–	–	0.494*	1.638(1.001, 2.682)
ANIPC(RMB Yuan)	–	–	− 8.039*	0.000(0.000, 0.558)
EP(%)	–	–	− 2.055	0.128(0.000, 35.929)
PCMLF(RMB Yuan)	–	–	−0.001	0.999(0.998, 1.000)
AFP	–	–	0.100	1.105(0.948, 1.288)
Individual Level:				
Gender				
1 = male	–	–	–	–
2 = female	− 0.205**	0.814(0.787, 0.842)	− 0.205**	0.814(0.787, 0.842)
Age				
1 = 15 to 24	–	–	–	–
2 = 25 to 44	0.128**	1.137(1.053, 1.227)	0.128**	1.137(1.054, 1.227)
3 = 45 to 59	−0.068	0.935(0.862, 1.013)	−0.068	0.935(0.863, 1.013)
4 = ≧60	−0.125**	0.882(0.812, 0.958)	−0.125**	0.882(0.812, 0.959)
Nationality				
1 = Han	–	–	–	–
2 = Minority	−0.176	0.839(0.685, 1.028)	−0.175	0.839(0.685, 1.028)
Family history of mental illness				
0 = no	–	–	–	–
1 = yes	0.227**	1.254(1.170, 1.344)	0.227**	1.254(1.170, 1.345)
Marital status				
1 = married	–	–	–	–
2 = unmarried	0.223**	1.250(1.206, 1.295)	0.223**	1.250(1.206, 1.295)
Economic status				
1 = poverty	–	–	–	–
2 = non-poverty	−0.494**	0.610(0.579, 0.642)	−0.494**	0.610(0.579, 0.643)
Education level				
1 = illiteracy/semiliterate	–	–	–	–
2 = elementary education and above	−0.123**	0.884(0.855, 0.914)	−0.123**	0.884(0.855, 0.914)
Diagnosis type				
1 = schizophrenia	–	–	–	–
2 = schizoaffective disorder	−0.044	0.957(0.845, 1.083)	−0.045	0.956(0.845, 1.082)
3 = paranoid psychosis	0.042	1.043(0.826, 1.316)	0.041	1.042(0.826, 1.315)
4 = bipolar affective disorder	−0.123*	0.885(0.802, 0.976)	−0.123*	0.884(0.802, 0.975)
5 = mental disorders due to epilepsy	−0.262**	0.769(0.712, 0.831)	−0.262**	0.769(0.712, 0.831)
6 = mental retardation with mental disorders	−1.096**	0.334(0.302, 0.370)	−1.096**	0.334(0.302, 0.370)
Duration of illness				
1 = < 10 years	–	–	–	–
2 = 10 to 19 years	0.118**	1.125(1.084, 1.168)	0.118**	1.125(1.084, 1.168)
3 = 20 to 29 years	0.142**	1.153(1.104, 1.204)	0.142**	1.153(1.104, 1.204)
4 = ≧30 years	0.152**	1.165(1.106, 1.226)	0.152**	1.165(1.107, 1.226)

Table 5 Two-level Poisson regression analyses for associates with high risk behavior of patients with severe mental illness in rural households of Sichuan Province *(Continued)*

Variables	Model1		Model2	
Fixed effect	Coefficient	IRR(95% CI)	Coefficient	IRR(95% CI)
Antipsychotic treatment				
0 = no	–	–	–	–
1 = yes	0.039*	1.040(1.002, 1.079)	0.039*	1.040(1.003, 1.079)
Participation in 686 project				
0 = no	–	–	–	–
1 = yes	−0.266**	0.767(0.734, 0.801)	– 0.266**	0.766(0.733, 0.801)
Random effect				
Level 2: Region ($\sigma^2_{u_0}$)	0.502(0.168)**		0.417(0.165)*	

*$P<0.05$, **$P<0.01$

Full description of regional variables as follows: annual net income of rural residents per capita (**ANIPC**), employment proportion of rural residents (**EP%**), and per capita minimal livelihood funds for rural residents under basic provision protection (**PCMLF**), number of psychiatric practitioners (including assistant psychiatric practitioners) per one hundred thousand people (**NPP/100,000**), the average number of follow-ups of patients in rural region (**AFP**)

The incidence rate of high risk behavior by municipality

This study demonstrated that from 2011 to 2013, when the NS system was solidly in place, there was a significant downward trend in the incidence rate among the studied patient population, from 23.92% per person year (2011) to 6.70% (2013). This downward trend reflected a positive effect of the health care management of SMD, particularly the development of community mental health services. More specifically, such declining trends were observed among all municipalities except for one PZ, where the incidence rate increased from 9.74 to 30.05% during the three year period. There are a number of possible reasons to explain the rise of such an outcome in this municipality. First, PZ is a typical region of migrants with a large floating population proportion who are more vulnerable to mental disorders than others [24]. Second, PZ is on the border with the LY Yi Minority Autonomy Prefecture, which has much better mental health care services. Many patients of Yi ethnic minority migrated from LY to work or live in PZ; hence, they were registered as crossing the border. Third, according to an internal report, many new patients came into the system since 2012 for the benefits of the NS, such as free treatment, free medical examination, and free training, etc. All these factors resulted in the unstable incidence rate in PZ. Another notable rise of the high risk behavior incidence was the BZ municipality, where the outcome was 56.46% (2011), 15.66% (2012), and up to 51.29% (2013). A common reason shared with the LY was a large proportion of floating population from BZ to other locations, due to its poor economic conditions, i.e. the lowest per capita net annual income of rural residents in Sichuan province. Many migrants returned to their hometowns after they were found to be mentally ill.

These findings suggest that both central and provincial health authorities should pay special attention, and perhaps invest more in the development of mental health care services to areas where economic development is low, transportation might be difficult, large populations of migrants and health system indicators are poorer than other regions.

Associates of high risk behavior at individual level

This study identified a number of factors at the individual level in different categories that were positively associated with an increase of high risk behavior. The demographic factors included being of male gender, between the ages of 25 and 44, an ethnic minority, and unmarried. The socioeconomic factors included illiteracy/semi-literacy and poverty. The disease related factors included having a family history of mental disorders, with schizophrenia diagnosis, and longer illness duration. Environmental factors were not part of the government "686 Project". Most of those factors were supported by previous national and international studies [25–28]. The mechanisms of their association with risk behaviors have been well examined in the fields of psychiatry and forensic psychiatry, and are mostly known. Patients who were involved in the "686 Project" showed lower risk outcomes. This might indicate that the "686 Project" created benefits for the patients, both from the management level and treatment effect. Future research could examine the predictive power of these factors in order to develop a screening tool for high risk groups for management and treatment purposes in the community.

Associates of high risk behavior of patients at municipal level

We found that a reduced regional socioeconomic advantage, measured by the annual net income of rural residents per capita, and an increased regional mental health human resource, measured by the number of psychiatric practitioners (including assistant psychiatric practitioners) per 100,000 population, were associated with an increased high risk behavior of patients in the study. Together, these two factors explained about 17% of the outcome variance among municipalities in Sichuan.

The association between socioeconomic disadvantage and worsening mental health outcomes might be explained by the supply and needs relationship [29]. However, an explanation for the association of larger mental health workforce with the increased risk behavior of patients is not intuitive. We speculated on the main cause: the recently increased number of mental health workforce improved the management activity in identifying preventive outcomes such as the risk behavior of patients. In China, psychiatrists and licensed psychiatric nurses are accredited by the NHFPC, psychological counsel or accredited by the Ministry of Human Resources and Social Security, and psychotherapists by both Ministries [4]. In 2004, China only had 16,103 licensed psychiatrists and psychiatric registrars (1.24/100,000 population) and 24,793 licensed psychiatric nurses (1.91/100,000 population) [30], in contrast to 4. 15 psychiatrists and 12.97 psychiatric nurses per 100,000 population, respectively, for the average global mental health workforce in the same year [31].

By 2013, in Sichuan province, there were 1621 registered psychiatrists, 1757 (assistant) psychiatrists and 3952 psychiatric nurses in psychiatric hospitals, in conjunction with 25,676 practicing physicians, 41,263 practicing (assistant) physicians, and 24,031 registered nurses in primary healthcare institutions for all primary health care services [32]. The management of mental disorders in communities was only one task of the services, and the professional workforce was small. However, for the NS system services, additional locally trained mental health workers could have been recruited to contribute to the national task of identifying and managing patients with SMD in the community. As a consequence, more risk behaviors of patients would be reported. Further investigations into the quality of services in patient treatment, and the prevention of risk behavior, at both individual and health care facility levels will be required on this account.

Limitations

A number of limitations in the study should be noted. Firstly, the NS was originally a response to the government's concern regarding social harmony and stability, as part of the "686 Program" [4]. It only focuses on SMD patients in terms of their violent or socially disruptive behaviors [18]. Meanwhile, information sharing between different surveillance systems was constrained by the incompatibility of their independent software and hardware [33]. As such, the variables employed in this study are limited and non-comprehensive. Secondly, the quality of the data is unoptimistic. The main problems include underreporting, missing values, and errors, which were due to the increasing gap between the demand and supply of mental health care, and the social stigma rooted in the moral and political context [5]. The problem could be higher in rural areas, with less training for rural staff, coupled with increased difficulties in accessing widely dispersed rural residents of regions with poor transportation systems [34, 35]. Quality issues may affect the accuracy of outcomes; however, they should have less impact on risk factor analysis, which is based on relative comparisons. Thirdly, as NS system was built from 2006, the patients enrolled in the first few years were very limited. The incidence rates in 2006-2009 could only represent the cohort, while not the local actual level. Fourthly, accessing data from the system is extremely difficult in China. No report on national psychosis surveillance has yet been released, except for a few papers published by local surveillance staff based on data from their regions [36]. Hence, a nationwide comparison of the study outcome could not be made.

Implications

The present study provides evidence to support the primary goal of the movement for Global Mental Health [37], and the WHO Mental Health Gap Action Program [38], to promote the scaling up of mental health services in low-income and middle-income countries [39]. Sichuan represents provinces in western China where development in economic and health care have lagged behind the rest of China. This puts mental health care issues in the rural areas of Sichuan on par with those of low income countries. As the researches on risk behavior in patients with SMD were mainly carried in the developed countries, our study findings may fill the knowledge gap regarding the quantity and quality of how the system operates, and to what degree patient risk behaviors were controlled for, and what possible associates might be linked with their risk behavior in developing countries. Changing trends in the registration and incidence rates suggested several positive impacts of the system over the last five years. A further in-depth study of the effects of the system might be a way to progress, based on epidemiological facts. Evidence regarding the significant variations in the incidence of the high risk rate between municipalities with known socioeconomic and human resource factors, and with identified municipal low and high patient outcomes, might advocate for the health authority to make decisions based on health resource distribution with clear localized targets. Risk factors at the individual level identified in this study may be used to develop a risk screening tool to earlier identify patients with the highest risk factors for targeted risk management by grass-level mental health workers. The above findings may be generalized to other developing countries in future.

Conclusions

The registration rate and incidence rate of risk behavior varied widely across municipalities in rural areas of west China. The factors in association of increased high risk behavior include males, aged 25 to 44, unmarried, in poverty, illiterate or semiliterate, having a family history of mental disorders and antipsychotic treatments, longer duration illnesses at the individual level; and higher psychiatric practitioner visits, the lower annual net income of rural residents per capita at the regional level.

Endnotes

[1]Based to the Household Registration System in China, residents are divided into urban and rural according to their registration in the system no matter where they live. In the aspect of geographical distribution, people natively live in level regions below township level are usually rural household registration [15].

Abbreviations

"686 Project": The National Continuing Management and Intervention Program for Psychoses (also known as Central Government Support for the Local Management and Treatment of Severe Mental Illnesses Project); ANIPC: Annual net income of rural residents per capita; CDCs: Centers for Disease Control and Prevention; CDPF: China Disabled Persons' Federation; EP%: Employment proportion of rural residents; IR: Incidence rate; IRRs: Incident rate ratios; MHCs: Mental Health Centers; NASMD: Number of agencies for severe mental disordered; NBPHS: National Basic Public Health Services; NBSMD: Number of inpatient beds for severe mental disordered; NHFPC: National Health and Family Planning Commission (previously been called the Ministry of Health); NPP/100,000: Number of psychiatric practitioners (including assistant psychiatric practitioners) per one hundred thousand people; NS: National System of Basic Information Collection and Analysis for Psychoses; PCMLF: Per capita minimal livelihood funds for rural residents under basic provision protection; SMD: Severe mental disorders

Funding

Supported by the Central Government Support for the Local Management and Treatment of Severe Mental Illnesses Project, China Medical Board (CMB 12-106), and Education Department of Sichuan Province Project.

Authors' contributions

YYL* and XL* participated in the study design, literature search, data analysis and interpreting, and drafting the manuscript. HW*, DW, XMY, WWT, YXL and TZ participated in the study design and provided access to the dataset and interpretation of data. MY designed the study, supervised data analysis, and provided critical revisions for the concepts and contents of the manuscript. All authors read and approved final version for the submission. *These authors contributed equally to this work.

Competing interests

The authors declare that they have no competing interests.

Author details

[1]Department of Epidemiology and Health Statistics, West China School of Public Health, Sichuan University, Chengdu, Sichuan, People's Republic of China. [2]Department of Health and Social Behavior, West China School of Public Health, Sichuan University, Chengdu, Sichuan, People's Republic of China. [3]Sichuan Provincial Mental Health Centre, Mianyang, Sichuan, People's Republic of China. [4]West China Research Center for Rural Health Development, Sichuan University, No.17 Section 3, South Renmin Road, Chengdu, Sichuan 610041, People's Republic of China.

References

1. Ministry of Health of the People's Republic of China. Chinese managerial and treatment regulations for severely mentally disordered patients, 104 C.F. R. 2012. (in Chinese).
2. Phillips MR, Zhang J, Shi Q, Song Z, Ding Z, Pang S, et al. Prevalence, treatment, and associated disability of mental disorders in four provinces of China during 2001-05: an epidemiological study. Lancet. 2009;373:2041-53.
3. Yang G, Wang Y, Zeng Y, Gao G, Liang X, Zhou M, et al. Rapid health transition in China, 1990–2010: findings from the global burden of disease study 2010. Lancet. 2013;381:1987–2015.
4. Liu J, Ma H, He Y, Xie B, Xu Y, Tang H, et al. Mental health system in China: history, recent service reform and future challenges. World Psychiatry. 2011;10:210–6.
5. Qian J. Mental health care in China: providing services for under-treated patients. J Ment Health Policy Econ. 2012;15:179–86.
6. Ministry of Health of the People's Republic of China. Notice to implement National Continuing Management and Intervention Program for Psychoses. 2012. Available at: http://www.nhfpc.gov.cn/zwgk/wtwj/201304/6ab6413a7e6741a1a6e2deab8a6c36b3.shtml. (in Chinese)
7. Ma H. Integration of hospital and community services—the '686 project'—is a crucial component in the reform of China's mental health services. Shanghai Arch Psychiatry. 2012;24:172–4.
8. Good BJ, Good MD. Significance of the 686 program for China and for global mental health. Shanghai Arch Psychiatry. 2012;24:175–7.
9. Ministry of Health of the People's Republic of China. National Basic Public Health Services. 2011. Available at: http://www.moh.gov.cn/jws/s3577/201105/51780.shtml (in Chinese).
10. Standing Committee of the National People's Congress. Mental health law of the People's republic of China. 2012. Available at: http://www.gov.cn/jrzg/2012-10/26/content_2252122.htm (in Chinese).
11. Chen H, Phillips MR, Cheng H, Chen Q, Chen X, Fralick D, et al. Mental health law of the People's republic of China (English translation with annotations). Shanghai Arch Psychiatry. 2012;24:305–21.
12. Law yearbook of China 2012: Peking: China Law Yearbook Press; 2012. (in Chinese)
13. The Bureau of Sichuan Province. Sichuan statistical yearbook. 2014. (in Chinese).
14. Chen H, Phillips MR, Cheng H, Chen Q, Chen X, Fralick D. The state of death and the cause of death in severe psychotic patients who were managed in Sichuan, 2011-2013. Sichuan Mental Health. 2014;27:337–40. (in Chinese)
15. Long J, Huang G, Liang W, Liang B, Chen Q, Xie J, et al. The prevalence of schizophrenia in mainland China: evidence from epidemiological surveys. Acta Psychiatr Scand. 2014;130:1–13.
16. Gu Y, Singh JP, Yun L, Hu Z. A review of violence risk assessment for mentally disordered patients in mainland of China. Crim Justice Behav. 2014;41:1398–405.
17. Chen X, Xiao S. The current development and future prospects of prevention for the mental illnesses in China's rural community. Prac Prevent Med. 2004;11:205–6. (in Chinese)
18. Zhou W, Xiao S. Existing public health surveillance systems for mental health in China. Int J Ment Health Syst. 2015;9:3.
19. Zhou W, Xiao S. Reporting on China's mental health surveillance. Am J Psychiatry. 2015;172:314–5.
20. Huang Y. Epidemiological study on mental disorder in China. Chin J Epidemiol. 2012;33:15–6. (in Chinese)
21. Yang M, Li X. Introduction to multilevel models in medical and public Health Research. Beijing: Beijing University Publish House; 2007. (in Chinese)
22. Chan KY, Zhao F, Meng S, Demaio AR, Reed C, Theodoratou E, et al. Global Health epidemiology reference group (GHERG), prevalence of schizophrenia in China between 1990 and 2010. J Glob Health. 2015;5:010410.
23. General Office of the Ministry of Health. Evaluation plan on the work of management and intervention for psychoses. 2012. Available at: http://www.nhfpc.gov.cn/jkj/s5888/201208/4517bc0f7a3b458cb65bd52da4eb3319.shtml (in Chinese).

24. Chen L, Ping H, Yang G. A study of forensic psychotic patients among the floating population. Shanghai Arch Psychiatry. 2005;17:80–2. (in Chinese)
25. James DV, Fineberg NA, Shan AK, Priest RG. An increase in violence on an acute psychiatric ward: a study of associated factors. Br J Psychiatry. 1990;156:846.
26. Fazel S, Yu R. Psychotic disorders and repeat offending: systematic review and Meta-analysis. Schizophr Bull. 2011;37:800–10.
27. China Law Society. Law yearbook of China 2012. Peking: China Law Yearbook Press. 2012. (in Chinese)
28. Gu Y, Hu Z. More attention should be paid to schizophrenic patients with risk of violent offences. Psychiatry Clin Neurosci. 2009;63:592–3.
29. Saxena S, Thornicroft G, Knapp M, Whiteford H. Resources for mental health: scarcity, inequity, and inefficiency. Lancet. 2007;370:878–89.
30. World Health Organization. Death and DALY estimates for 2004 by cause for WHO member states. Geneva: World Health Organization; 2004.
31. World Health Organization. Mental health atlas 2005. Geneva: World Health Organization; 2005.
32. The Bureau of Sichuan Province. Sichuan statistical yearbook of health and family planning. 2014. (in Chinese).
33. Yang C. The present situation of disease surveillance in China. Shanghai J Prevent Med. 2012;24:336–42. (in Chinese)
34. Luo B, Xiao S, Fu W, Li X. Quality evaluation on national system of basic information collection and analysis for psychoses. Chin J Public Health. 2014;30:958–9. (in Chinese)
35. Li J, Jing L, Pan Y, Lai Q, Yu W, Jing Y. An investigation of present situation in health management of patients with severe psychotic disorders in rural areas of the western region of China: problems and countermeasures analysis. Chinese Gen Pract. 2014;17:2684–7. (in Chinese)
36. Li Q, Huang X, Wen H, Liang X, Lei L, Wu J. Retrospective analysis of treatment effectiveness among patients in Mianyang municipality enrolled in the national community management program for schizophrenia. Shanghai Arch Psychiat. 2012;24:131–9.
37. The Lancet. A movement for global mental health is launched. Lancet. 2008;372:1274.
38. WHO. Mental health gap action program (mhGAP): scaling up care for mental, neurological, and substance use disorders. Geneva: World Health Organization; 2008.
39. Lancet Global Mental Health Group. Scale up services for mental disorders: a call for action. Lancet. 2007;370:1241–52.

2

Diagnosis of somatoform disorders in primary care: diagnostic agreement, predictors, and comaprisons with depression and anxiety

Katharina Piontek[1,2*], Meike C. Shedden-Mora[2], Maria Gladigau[2], Amina Kuby[2] and Bernd Löwe[2]

Abstract

Background: To investigate (a) the diagnostic agreement between diagnoses of somatoform disorders, depressive and anxiety disorders obtained from a structured clinical interview and diagnoses reported from primary care physicians (PCPs) and (b) to identify patient and PCP-related predictors for the diagnostic agreement regarding the presence of a somatoform disorder.

Methods: Data from a cross-sectional study comprising 112 primary care patients at high risk for somatoform disorders were analyzed. Diagnoses according to International Classification of Diseases, 10th revision (ICD-10) for somatoform, depressive and anxiety disorders were obtained from the Composite International Diagnostic Interview (CIDI) and compared with the diagnoses of the patients' PCPs documented in their medical records. Using multiple regression analyses, predictors for the PCPs' diagnosis of a somatoform disorder were analyzed.

Results: The agreement between PCP diagnoses and CIDI diagnoses was 32.3% for somatoform disorders, 48.0% for depressive disorders and 25.0% for anxiety disorders. Multiple regression analyses revealed the likelihood of being diagnosed with a somatoform disorder by PCP increased with somatic symptom severity (OR = 1.22, 95% CI 1.03–1.44). Regarding PCP-related characteristics, a specialization in internal medicine (OR = 5.95, 95% CI 1.70–20.80) and working in a solo practice (OR = 2.92, 95% CI 1.02–8.38) increased the likelihood that patients were diagnosed with a somatoform disorder.

Conclusions: The present results indicate that the process of diagnosing somatoform disorders in primary care needs to be improved. Findings further underline the necessity to implement appropriate strategies to improve early detection of patients.

Keywords: Somatoform disorders, Depressive disorder, Anxiety disorder, Primary care Diagnostic agreement, Detection rate, Structured clinical interview

* Correspondence: katharina.piontek@uni-greifswald.de
[1]Institute for Medical Psychology, University Medicine Greifswald, Greifswald, Germany
[2]Department of Psychosomatic Medicine and Psychotherapy, University Medical Center Hamburg-Eppendorf, Hamburg, Germany

Background

The burden of disease due to non-specific, functional and somatoform disorders is high and the presence of recurrent or persistent medically unexplained symptoms is associated with impaired physical and mental quality of life, increased utilization of healthcare services and the development of comorbidities like depressive and anxiety disorders [1, 2]. Available data regarding the prevalence of somatoform disorders are inconsistent and vary considerably in dependence on the underlying study population and the diagnostic criteria applied in the single studies (e.g. [3–6]). A recent meta-analysis of 32 studies investigated the prevalence of somatoform disorders and medically unexplained symptoms in primary care patients using both strict diagnostic criteria according to clinical assessments (*International Classification of Diseases; ICD* [7], *Diagnostic and Statistical Manual of Mental Disorders; DSM* [8]) and standardized questionnaires [9]. That study revealed a high heterogeneity of the primary studies and substantial differences in the prevalence rates in the diagnoses of somatoform disorders according to ICD or DSM criteria with prevalence rates of 34.8% and 26.2%, respectively. Further, in 40% to 49% of the primary care patients, at least one medically unexplained symptom was detected using questionnaires. These numbers underline that somatoform disorders pose a highly relevant public health problem, but existing literature suggests that the process of diagnosing somatoform disorders is challenging and that the different diagnostic criteria may have a substantial impact on the detection rate. The low detection rate in primary care is one key problem in the management of somatoform disorders [6]. It has been demonstrated that only 33% to 60% of the patients are correctly diagnosed by their primary care physician (PCP) and referred to a specialist for further treatment [4]. This is particularly alarming as the primary care practice serves as the patient's first point of entry into the health care system and access to mental health services. Furthermore, according to current guidelines for non-specific, functional, and somatoform bodily complaints [1], management of somatoform disorders is recommended within a stepped care model according to the course of disease, in collaboration with other physicians and therapists and coordinated by the PCP, thereby emphasizing the high responsibility of the PCP in the diagnostic and therapeutic procedure [10].

Several barriers have been identified with respect to the diagnosis of somatoform disorders in primary care settings [11]. Present data indicate that a lack of specific training, a lack of experience and a lack of reliable diagnostic tools may hinder the diagnosis of somatoform disorders [11]. It has been further demonstrated that the application of the diagnostic criteria seem to be problematic for many PCPs and existing classification systems have been described as being difficult to use, impractical, not distinct, overlapping or too restrictive [11]. Besides these conceptual barriers, both patient and PCP-related characteristics might contribute to a correct diagnosis, and it is of importance to identify relevant predictors of a correct PCP diagnosis of a somatoform disorder to improve early detection of the disease.

The aims of the present study are, first, to investigate the level of agreement between diagnoses of somatoform disorders and its comorbidities depression and anxiety disorder obtained from a structured clinical interview and diagnoses reported from PCPs and, second, to identify patient and PCP-related predictors of PCPs' diagnoses of a somatoform disorder.

Methods

Sample recruitment

Data were collected within the project "Network Somatoform and Functional disorders" (*Sofu-Net*), a sub-project of the Hamburg Network for Mental Health *psychenet* [12, 13]. The study is registered at ISRCTN (ISRCTN55870770). *Sofu-Net* aimed to improve early detection of patients with somatoform disorders in primary care and to refer patients more quickly into effective treatment [14].

Between September and December 2012, all patients at least 18 years old attending the participating primary care practices were asked to take part in a screening regarding bodily complaints and well-being. Patients with severe physical illness, cognitive impairment or insufficient German language skills were excluded from the study. Patients with a positive screening result were asked to participate in a telephone interview within 4 weeks after the screening. All patients gave informed written consent. The study protocol is consistent with the principles of the Declaration of Helsinki and was approved by the ethics committee Medical Chamber Hamburg, Germany.

Measures

The self-administered screening questionnaire included data on the patients' age, gender, marital status, and school education. The Patient-Health-Questionnaire (PHQ) [15] was used to screen for somatoform disorders (PHQ-15), depression (PHQ-9) and anxiety (Generalized Anxiety Disorder Assessment; GAD-7) [16]. The PHQ-15 comprises of 15 items assessing somatic symptoms and their severity within the last 4 weeks. The 3-point Likert scale ranges from *not bothered* (0) to *bothered a lot* (2). The PHQ-9 comprises nine items assessing depressive symptoms and their severity within the last 2 weeks. The 3-Point Likert Scale ranges from *not at all* (0) to *nearly every day* (2). The GAD-7 comprises of seven items assessing anxiety-related symptoms within the last 2 weeks. The 3-Point Likert Scale ranges from *not at all* (0) to *nearly every day* (2). On all three scales, cutoff-values of 5, 10 and 15 represent mild, moderate and severe symptom levels, respectively [15]. Patients were considered screening positive if one the following conditions was fulfilled: (a) PHQ-15 ≥ 15, (b) PHQ-15 ≥ 10 and GAD-7 or PHQ-9 ≥ 10. Further, patients were asked how often they talk about psychosocial complaints and private problems with their PCP using the following question: 'Do you talk about psychological complaints and private problems with your primary care physician?' Patients responded on a 6-point Likert Scale ranging from *never* (1) to *always* (6).

The telephone interview encompassed the sections for somatoform disorders, depressive and anxiety disorders of the Composite International Interview (CIDI) [17]. The CIDI assesses mental disorders according to the criteria of the *International Classification of Diseases, 10th revision* (ICD-10) [7] and the criteria of the *DSM-IV Diagnostic and Statistical Manual of Mental Disorders, 4th edition* (DSM-IV) [8]. For the present analyses, diagnostic codes according to ICD-10 were analyzed. ICD-10 diagnoses obtained from the CIDI were considered as reference standard. CIDI interviews were conducted by research assistants who were extensively trained and supervised. Patients fulfilling the diagnostic criteria within the last 6 months were classified as having a current somatoform disorder, depressive or anxiety disorder. The category of somatoform disorders included somatization disorder (F45.0), undifferentiated somatoform disorder (F45.1), and persistent pain disorder (F45.4). Within a decision tree, it was assessed for each reported complaint whether it was medically unexplained. Mild, moderate and severe depressive episodes as well as dysthymia were summarized in the category depressive disorders (F32-F34). Anxiety disorders included agoraphobia, social phobia, specific phobias (e.g. animal phobias), phobic anxiety disorder, panic disorder, and generalized anxiety disorder (F40-F41).

PCP data form

The PCPs completed a form assessing their patients' medical history based on the data in their medical records. This form consisted of 6 sections encompassing the following topics: (1) reason for the patients' consultation (using ICD-10 codes), (2) present somatic diseases (list of 26 diseases and an additional open question, e.g. cardiovascular, endocrine, neurological, lung and autoimmune diseases), (3) present mental disorders (list of 13 disorders and an additional open question, e.g. dementia, alcohol, drug and medication dependence, schizophrenia, depression, anxiety disorder, somatoform disorder), (4) somatic explanation of the patients' bodily symptoms from the PCPs' perspective, (5) recommendation of psychological treatment by PCP, and (6) intake of medication (antidepressants, analgesics, benzodiazepines, and antipsychotic drugs). The form was completed by PCPs for all screening-positive patients when the screening procedure had been finished.

Data from treating physicians

Using a questionnaire, the following characteristics of the participating PCPs were assessed: age, gender, specialization, training in psychosomatic basic care, years in general practice, and type of practice.

Data analyses

Data are reported as means (standard deviation) for continuous variables and as numbers (percentages) for categorical variables. Group comparisons were performed using t-tests (mean) for continuous variables and Pearson χ^2-tests for categorical variables. Tests were considered statistically significant at a two-sided p-value < 0.05. Kappa-statistics were calculated to determine the diagnostic agreement between diagnoses of somatoform disorders, depressive and anxiety disorders obtained from the CIDI and diagnoses obtained from PCPs. The following agreement levels were considered: discrete (0–0.20), regular (0.21–0.40), moderate (0.41–0.60), substantial (0.61–0.80), almost perfect (0.81–1.00) [18].

Two multiple logistic regression analyses were conducted to identify predictors for a PCP diagnosis of a somatoform disorder. The diagnoses obtained from CIDI were used as reference standard. The first model included the following patient-related predictors: age, gender, marital status, school education, comorbid depressive disorder, comorbid anxiety disorder, discussion of psychosocial problems with PCP, somatic symptom severity, and the number of PCP visits within the last 6 months. The second model included the following PCP-related predictors: age, gender, specialization, years in general practice, training in psychosomatic basic care, and type of practice.

Data analyses were conducted using STATA 13.0 (Stata Corporation, College Station, TX, USA).

Results

Characteristics of the study population

From 1826 screening participants, 283 (15.5%) were screened positive for somatoform disorders, depression and anxiety. From those screening positive, 137 (48.4%) patients participated in the telephone interview. After the exclusion of patients with incomplete interviews and missing data, 112 cases were available for the present analyses (Fig. 1).

Among the study population, the majority of patients was female. Data showed that patients with and without somatoform disorders did not differ in their sociodemographic and clinical characteristics (Table 1).

Within the study population, 65 (58.0%) patients were diagnosed with a current somatoform disorder according to CIDI and 29 (25.9%) patients were diagnosed with a current somatoform disorder according to their PCP.

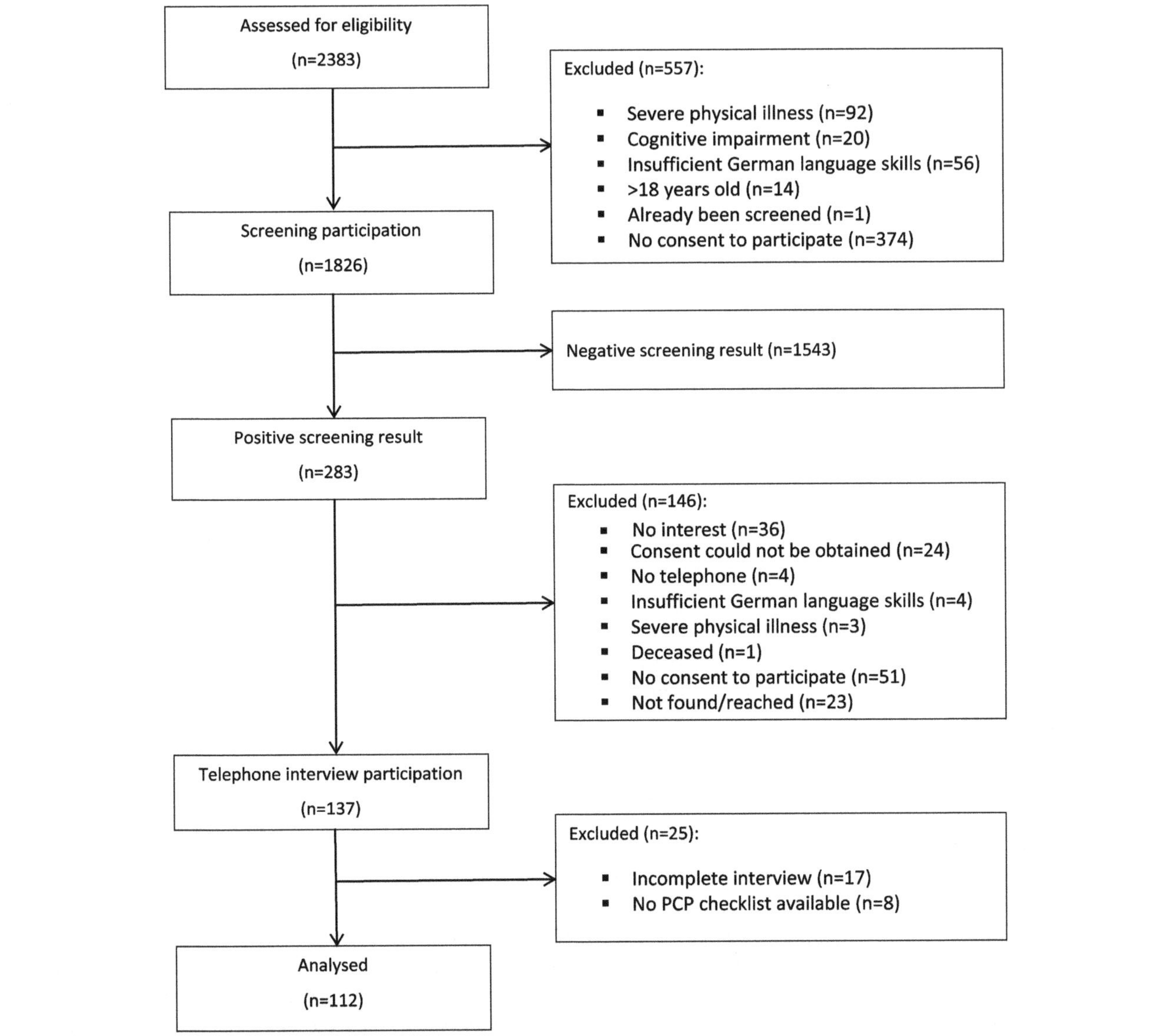

Fig. 1 Flow-chart according to sample recruitment

The rates of comorbidity with current depressive or anxiety disorders according to CIDI were 43.1 and 47.7%, respectively, while 26.6% of the patients presented both disorders (data not shown).

Characteristics of the participating PCPs

The characteristics of the participating PCPs are illustrated in Table 2. PCPs were on average 49.3 years old, and 53.7% were female. Most PCPs had a specialization in general medicine (58.5%) and 85.4% had completed training in psychosomatic basic care. Most frequently, PCPs worked in a group practice (75.6%) and had worked in general practice for on average 10.5 years.

Diagnostic agreement

The results of the analyses regarding the diagnostic agreement are displayed in Table 3. Using the CIDI diagnosis as gold standard, data analyses revealed that PCPs diagnosed 21 (32.3%) patients with a somatoform disorder, while they did not reach agreement with the CIDI diagnosis in 44 (67.7%) patients. PCPs classified 8 (17.0%) patients as having a somatoform disorder although a negative result was obtained using CIDI. Diagnostic agreement of not having a somatoform disorder according to CIDI or PCPs was found for 39 (83.0%) patients. Kappa value was 0.14 ($P < .05$), indicating a significant discrete diagnostic agreement.

Table 1 Characteristics of the study population according to the presence of a somatoform disorder as diagnosed using CIDI

	Total	With somatoform disorder	Without somatoform disorder
	$n = 112$	$n = 97$ (86.0%)	$n = 15$ (14.0%)
Female sex, n (%)	88 (78.6%)	79 (81.4%)	9 (60.0%)
Age (years), M (SD)	47.1 (15.9)	45.5 (15.2)	57.5 (17.1)
School education, n (%)			
< 10 years	28 (25.5)	25 (26.0)	3 (21.4)
10 years	35 (31.8)	29 (30.2)	6 (42.9)
> 10 years	47 (42.7)	42 (43.8)	5 (35.7)
Marital status, n (%)			
Married	42 (37.8)	35 (36.5)	7 (46.7)
Unmarried	38 (34.2)	35 (36.5)	3 (20.0)
Separated, divorced, widowed	31 (27.9)	26 (27.1)	5 (33.3)
PHQ-15 score, M (SD)	14.6 (3.3)	14.9 (3.4)	13.2 (2.6)
Age (years) at the onset of somatoform symptoms, M (SD)	19.3 (13.7)	19.3 (13.7)	n/a
Comorbid depressive disorder (CIDI) within the last 6 months, n (%)	50 (44.6)	43 (44.3)	7 (46.7)
Comorbid anxiety disorder (CIDI) within the last 6 months, n (%)	48 (42.9)	43 (44.3)	5 (33.3)
Currently in psychotherapy, n (%)	24 (22.0)	21 (22.3)	3 (20.0)
PCP visits within the past 6 months, M (SD)	6.1 (4.8)	6.0 (4.4)	6.6 (6.7)
Discussion of psychosocial distress with PCP, n (%)			
Never, seldom/rarely, sometimes	69 (61.6)	59 (60.8)	10 (66.7)
Often, very often, always	43 (38.4)	38 (39.2)	5 (33.3)

CIDI Composite International diagnostic interview
PHQ-15 Patient Health Questionnaire
PCP Primary care physician

Regarding depressive disorders, PCPs diagnosed 24 (48.0%) patients, while they did not reach agreement with the CIDI diagnosis in 26 (52.0%) patients. In contrast, PCPs classified 14 (22.6%) patients as having a depressive disorder although a negative result was obtained using CIDI. Diagnostic agreement of not having a depressive disorder according to CIDI or PCPs was found for 48 (77.4%) patients. Kappa value was 0.26 ($P < 0.01$), indicating a significant regular diagnostic agreement.

Regarding anxiety disorders, PCPs diagnosed 12 (25.0%) of patients, while they did not reach agreement with the CIDI diagnosis in 36 (75.0%) patients. In contrast, PCPs classified 5 (7.8%) patients as having an anxiety disorder

Table 2 Characteristics of PCPs ($n = 41$)

Age (years), M (SD)	49.3 (7.7)
Female sex, n (%)	22 (53.7)
Specialization, n (%)	
General medicine	24 (58.5)
Internal medicine	12 (29.3)
Other specialization	5 (12.2)
Training in psychosomatic basic care, n (%)	35 (85.4)
Type of practice, n (%)	
Solo practice	10 (24.4)
Group practice	31 (75.6)
Years in general practice, M (SD)	10.5 (5.6)

Table 3 Diagnostic agreement between PCP ratings and CIDI results ($n = 112$)

		CIDI	
		n (%) yes	n (%) no
Somatoform disorder			
PCP rating	n (%) yes	21 (32.3)	8 (17.0)
	n (%) no	44 (67.7)	39 (83.0)
Depressive disorder			
PCP rating	n (%) yes	24 (48.0)	14 (22.6)
	n (%) no	26 (52.0)	48 (77.4)
Anxiety disorder			
PCP rating	n (%) yes	12 (25.0)	5 (7.8)
	n (%) no	36 (75.0)	59 (92.2)

although a negative result was obtained using CIDI. Diagnostic agreement of not having an anxiety disorder according to CIDI or PCPs was found for 59 (92.2%) patients. Kappa value was 0.19 ($P < 0.01$), indicating a significant discrete diagnostic agreement.

Patient and PCP-related predictors for the diagnosis of a somatoform disorder by PCPs

Regarding patient-related characteristics, multiple regression analysis revealed that with every point increase in PHQ-15 mean score, the chance of being diagnosed with a somatoform disorder increased by 1.2 (OR = 1.22; 95% CI 1.03–1.44) (Table 4).

Regarding PCP-related characteristics, multiple regression analysis revealed that a specialization in internal medicine was associated with a 6-fold higher chance that patients were diagnosed with a somatoform disorder by their PCP (OR = 5.95; 95% CI 1.70–20.80) (Table 5). Further, working in a solo practice was associated with a 3-fold higher chance of patients being diagnosed with a somatoform disorder (OR = 2.92; 95% CI 1.02–8.38). With respect to the PCPs' age, younger age was associated with a higher chance of patients being correctly diagnosed with a somatoform disorder (OR = 0.90; 95% CI 0.81–1.00). This effect was borderline significant (p = 0.06). In the single models, all predictors explained 11.8 and 17.2% of the model variance, respectively.

Discussion

In the present population of primary care patients at high risk for somatoform disorders, the diagnostic agreement between PCPs' diagnoses and diagnoses obtained from a structured clinical interview was highest for depressive disorders, followed by somatoform disorders and anxiety disorders. Our analyses further revealed that somatic symptom severity was a relevant patient-related predictor for PCPs' diagnosis of a somatoform disorder, while a specialization in internal medicine and working in a solo practice were relevant physician-related predictors for PCPs' diagnosis of a somatoform disorder.

Table 4 Patient-related predictors for PCPs' diagnosis of a somatoform disorder (n = 85)

Patient-related characteristics	OR (95% CI)	P-value
Age	1.00 (0.97; 1.05)	0.75
Female gender	0.42 (0.10; 1.67)	0.22
Marital status, married	1.52 (0.75; 3.10)	0.25
At least 10 years of schooling	1.45 (0.71;2.96)	0.31
Comorbid depressive disorder	1.70 (0.52; 5.55)	0.38
Comorbid anxiety disorder	0.92 (0.20; 4.32)	0.92
Discussion of psychosocial distress	1.90 (0.60; 6.00)	0.27
Somatic symptom severity (PHQ-15)	1.22 (1.03; 1.44)	0.04
Number of PCP visits within the last 6 months	0.94 (0.80; 1.10)	0.44

Results of multiple logistic regression analysis
PHQ-15 Patient Health Questionnaire
PCP Primary care physician

Table 5 Physician-related predictors for PCPs' diagnosis of a somatoform disorder (n = 99)

Physician-related characteristics	OR (95% CI)	P-value
Age	0.90 (0.81; 1.00)	0.06
Female sex	2.26(0.74; 6.85)	0.15
Specialization internal medicine	5.95 (1.70; 20.80)	<.01
Years in general practice	1.06 (0.93; 1.21)	0.38
Training in psychosomatic basic care	0.58 (0.15; 2.96)	0.51
Solo practice	2.92 (1.02; 8.38)	<.05

Results of multiple logistic regression analysis

We showed that PCPs identified 32.3% of the patients with a somatoform disorder using the CIDI diagnosis as reference. This finding is in line with data from previous studies which revealed agreement rates ranging from 18% to 56%, depending on the investigated populations and the methods applied in the single studies [19–22]. This variety may reflect the difficulties in the terminology and conceptualization of somatoform type disorders which have often been discussed in previous research [11]. Regarding conceptual barriers in the process of diagnosing somatoform disorders, existing classification systems have been described by PCPs as being difficult to use, as providing little information about the illness, or as too restrictive [11].

In the present study, all PCPs participating in *Sofu-Net* had attended network meetings and quality circles which were an inherent part of the network providing information about diagnostic approaches and management of somatoform disorders. Moreover, participating PCPs were prompted to use the PHQ as screening tool for early detection and contemporary referral to psychotherapeutic co-treatment. We therefore suppose that participation in *Sofu-Net* has promoted the PCPs' awareness for patients with somatoform complaints and their diagnostic knowledge and skills. Further, among the participating PCPs, 85% had a training in psychosomatic basis care, suggesting that these PCPs may be particular interested in the field of psychosomatic care which might has enhanced the detection of patients with somatoform complaints. In addition, PCPs were aware of the patients' positive screening result, giving advice that somatoform complaints were present in their patients. Nevertheless, using CIDI as reference, a large part of the patients with somatoform as disorders remained unrecognized by their PCPs. However, it is of importance to note that among all patients who had been "overlooked" by their PCPs (67.7%), PCPs stated for 54.6% of these patients that they do not consider the patients' complaints as medically explained and therefore suspect the presence of a somatoform disorder. This finding suggests that PCPs were aware of somatization in their patients, although not having labelled their patients as having a somatoform disorder. A recent qualitative study by our group among PCPs investigated the process of coding somatoform disorders in primary care [23]. In that study, PCPs reported that coding is done for reimbursement purposes, that they use other information in their personal documentation, for example about the patients' psychosocial background or potential causes about the presented symptoms, and that they do not necessarily need to document a confirmed diagnosis for treatment. Moreover, PCPs reported that they restrain their coding to protect patients from stigma trough certain diagnoses or other negative consequences. Inaccurate coding was further described to arise from uncertainties regarding the diagnostic criteria and that finding the definite diagnosis is seen as the responsibilities of psychiatric specialists [23]. Although we have not investigated these processes in the present study, it might be assumed that the described factors were of relevance among the PCPs in the present study and have contributed to the relatively low detection rate.

In the present study, the diagnostic agreement was highest for depressive disorders (48%). It has been argued that PCPs are better acquainted with depression than with other mental disorders and may therefore have a greater ability to detect depressive disorders [24]. Regarding the presence of an anxiety disorder, the diagnostic agreement was only 25.0%. When interpreting this result, it needs to be considered that the diagnostic classification of anxiety disorders in the present study encompassed conditions of differential severity (i.e. panic disorder, animal phobia). It is possible that PCPs did not to diagnose light cases, given that symptoms might not have been apparent or might not have been associated with severe impairments. In turn, patients might have not disclosed their symptoms when feeling only slightly impaired.

We demonstrated that somatic symptom severity was a relevant predictor for a diagnosis of a somatoform disorder by PCPs, while the patient's sociodemographic characteristics had no impact on the detection rate. Possibly, an increasing symptom severity presumably has prompted patients to describe their bodily complaints more often and striking to their PCPs, thereby facilitating the detection of a somatoform disorder.

We further showed that a specialization in internal medicine and working in a solo practice were relevant physician-related predictors for a diagnosis of a somatoform disorder. This result is in line with findings from a study demonstrating that physicians who saw themselves as more effective in dealing with somatoform symptoms were more likely to be working in a solo practice [25]. Data from that study further showed that PCPs working in solo practices and those who were in the same practice for 5 years felt most comfortable in dealing with patients with somatoform disorders. It might be assumed that these PCPs had a better chance to establish a close relationship with their patients and had more time to explore their patients' complaints and psychosocial background facilitating the diagnostic process. With regard to the PCPs' education, we found that PCPs with training in internal medicine were more successful in diagnosing somatoform disorders compared to PCPs with training in general medicine, suggesting that training in internal medicine encompasses knowledge and skills facilitating the process of diagnosing somatoform disorders. It might be further possible that training in internal medicine makes PCPs more confident of declaring symptoms as medically explained, and thus diagnosing somatoform disorders. Taken together, the present findings underline that structural circumstances are essential for improving early detection and care for patients with somatoform disorders.

Strengths of the present study encompass the well characterized population of primary care patients at high risk for somatoform disorders as identified using established screening instruments and the structured diagnostic procedure using CIDI interviews. Our analyses are further based on different data sources including patient self-report, diagnoses obtained from CIDI interviews, and a PCP questionnaire, thereby integrating different perspectives on somatoform disorders diagnoses. Limitations may arise from the low response rate in the telephone interview, which potentially has introduced a selection bias. However, screening-positive patients who participated in the telephone interview did not differ from those who dropped out with regard to age, gender and PHQ-scores. Another weakness of the present study is the lack of data from screening-negative patients, which may has led to a misclassification bias underrepresenting the rate of patients with somatization. On the other hand, the PHQ has been demonstrated to be a well-validated measure for detecting and monitoring somatization, depression, and anxiety [15]. Nevertheless, as data on screening-negative patients are lacking, no data are available regarding PCPs diagnostic assessment of these patients.

Conclusions

Our data demonstrate that the process of diagnosing somatoform disorders in primary care remains challenging. We showed that the diagnostic agreement between diagnoses obtained from CIDI and diagnoses obtained from PCPs was low, but there is reason to assume that PCPs were aware of somatization in their patients without labelling them as having a somatoform disorder. Even with the release of the DSM-5, conceptual and practical problems of the previous classification remain unresolved. However, our data indicate that structural circumstances are crucial in the diagnostic process, as

PCPs training in internal medicine and working in a solo practice were associated with a higher chance of detecting a somatoform disorder. As structural circumstances are changeable, more research is necessary to assess and overcome situational barriers. Our data further suggest that there might be particular knowledge and skills taught during the education in internal medicine helping PCPs to detect patients with somatoform disorders. Likewise demonstrated in previous studies, the restricted time during consultations may hinder PCPs to build a strong doctor-patient relationship and to explore the psychosocial background of their patients, thereby impeding the correct diagnosis. Thus, continuity of care, as provided potentially stronger in solo practices, might facilitate the diagnosis of somatoform disorders in primary care. Furthermore, collaborative networks of PCPs and psychotherapists like *Sofu-Net* may contribute to the improvement of care in somatoform type disorders.

Abbreviations

CI: Confidence interval; CIDI: Composite International Interview; DSM: Diagnostic and Statistical Manual of Mental Disorders; GAD: Generalized Anxiety Disorder Assessment; ICD: International Classification of Diseases; OR: Odds Ratio; PCP: Primary care physician; PHQ: Patient-Health-Questionnaire

Acknowledgments

The authors would like to thank all patients for participating in the study and all network partners for their work.

Funding

The study was funded by the German Federal Ministry of Education and Research (BMBF) as part of *psychenet - Hamburg Network for Mental Health*, a large health services research study in the Hamburg Metropolitan Area (sub-project somatoform disorders; principal investigator: Bernd Löwe, grant number 01KQ1002B). The sponsor of the study was not involved in the design of the study, data collection, data analysis, data interpretation and writing the manuscript.

Authors' contributions

KP analyzed and interpreted the data and wrote the manuscript. MSM, MG, AK contributed to writing the manuscript. BL designed the study and was a major contributor in writing the manuscript. All authors read and approved the final manuscript.

Authors' information

Not applicable.

Consent for publication

Not applicable.

Competing interests

The authors declare that they have no competing interests.

References

1. Schaefert R, Hausteiner-Wiehle C, Hauser W, Ronel J, Herrmann M, Henningsen P. Non-specific, functional, and somatoform bodily complaints. Dtsch Arztebl Int. 2012;109(47):803–13.
2. Shedden-Mora M, Lau K, Kuby A, Gross B, Gladigau M, Fabisch A, Loewe B. Improving health Care for Patients with somatoform and functional disorders: a collaborative stepped care network (Sofu-net). Psychiatr Prax. 2015;42(Suppl 1):S60–4.
3. Loewe B, Spitzer RL, Williams JB, Mussell M, Schellberg D, Kroenke K. Depression, anxiety and somatization in primary care: syndrome overlap and functional impairment. Gen Hosp Psychiatry. 2008;30(3):191–9.
4. Steinbrecher N, Koerber S, Frieser D, Hiller W. The prevalence of medically unexplained symptoms in primary care. Psychosomatics. 2011;52(3):263–71.
5. de Waal MW, Arnold IA, Eekhof JA, van Hemert AM. Somatoform disorders in general practice: prevalence, functional impairment and comorbidity with anxiety and depressive disorders. Br J Psychiatry. 2004;184:470–6.
6. Fink P, Sorensen L, Engberg M, Holm M, Munk-Jorgensen P. Somatization in primary care. Prevalence, health care utilization, and general practitioner recognition. Psychosomatics. 1999;40(4):330–8.
7. World Health Organization. The ICD-10 classification of mental and behavioural disorders: clinical description and diagnostic guidelines. Geneva: World Health Organization; 1992.
8. American Psychiatric Association. Diagnostic and statistical manual of mental disorders (4th ed., text rev.). Washington, DC: American Psychiatric Publishing; 2000.
9. Haller H, Cramer H, Lauche R, Gobos G. Somatoform disorders and medically unexplained symptoms in primary care-a systematic review and meta-analysis of prevalence. Dtsch Arztebl Int. 2015;112:279–98.
10. Hanel G, Henningsen P, Herzog W, Sauer N, Schaefert R, Szecsenyi J, Löwe B. Depression, anxiety, and somatoform dirsorders: vague or distinct categories in primary care? Results from a large cross-sectional study. J Psychosom Res. 2009;67:189–97.
11. Murray AM, Toussaint A, Althaus A, Lowe B. The challenge of diagnosing non-specific, functional, and somatoform disorders: a systematic review of barriers to diagnosis in primary care. J Psychosom Res. 2016;80:1–10.
12. Haerter M, Brandes A, Hillebrandt B, Lambert M. psychenet - Das Hamburger Netz psychische Gesundheit [psychenet - The Hamburg Network for Mental Health]. Psychiatr Prax. 2015;42(Suppl 1):S4–8.
13. Shedden-Mora MC, Gross B, Lau K, Gumz A, Wegscheider K, Loewe B. Collaborative stepped care for somatoform disorders: a pre-post-intervention study in primary care. J Psychosom Res. 2016;80:23–30.
14. Loewe B, Piontek K, Daubmann A, Harter M, Wegscheider K, Koenig HH, Shedden-Mora M. Effectiveness of a stepped, collaborative, and coordinated health care network for somatoform disorders (Sofu-net): a controlled cluster cohort study. Psychosom Med. 2017;79(9):1016–24.
15. Kroenke K, Spitzer RL, Williams JB, Loewe B. The patient health questionnaire somatic, anxiety, and depressive symptom scales: a systematic review. Gen Hosp Psychiatry. 2010;32(4):345–59.
16. Spitzer RL, Kroenke K, Williams JB, Loewe B. A brief measure for assessing generalized anxiety disorder: the GAD-7. Arch Intern Med. 2006;166(10):1092–7.
17. Kessler RC, Ustun TB. The world mental health (WMH) survey initiative version of the World Health Organization (WHO) composite international diagnostic interview (CIDI). Int J Methods Psychiatr Res. 2004;13(2):93–121.
18. Landis JR, Koch GG. The measurement of observer agreement for categorical data. Biometrics. 1977;33(1):159–74.
19. Pols RG, Battersby MW. Coordinated care in the management of patients with unexplained physical symptoms: depression is a key issue. Med J Aust. 2008;188(12 Suppl):S133–7.
20. Norton J, de Roquefeuil G, David M, Boulenger JP, Ritchie K, Mann A. Prevalence of psychiatric disorders in French general practice using the patient health questionnaire: comparison with GP case-recognition and psychotropic medication prescription. Encéphale. 2009;35(6):560–9.
21. Pilowsky I. Dimensions of hypochondriasis. Br J Psychiatry. 1967;113(494):89–93.
22. H G, Henningsen P, Herzog W, Sauer N, Schaefert R, Szecsenyi J, Lowe B. Depression, anxiety, and somatoform disorders: vague or distinct categories in primary care? Results from a large cross-sectional study. J Psychosom Res. 2009;67(3):189–97.
23. Pohontsch NJ, Zimmermann T, Jonas C, Lehmann M, Lowe B, Scherer M. Coding of medically unexplained symptoms and somatoform disorders by general practitioners - an exploratory focus group study. BMC Fam Pract. 2018;19(1):129.

3

Barriers to effective diabetes management – a survey of people with severe mental illness

Kathleen Mulligan[1,2*], Hayley McBain[1], Frederique Lamontagne-Godwin[3], Jacqui Chapman[4], Chris Flood[1], Mark Haddad[1], Julia Jones[5] and Alan Simpson[1,2]

Abstract

Background: People with severe mental illnesses (SMI) such as schizophrenia and bipolar disorder have an increased risk of developing type 2 diabetes and have poorer health outcomes than those with diabetes alone. To maintain good diabetes control, people with diabetes are advised to engage in several self-management behaviours. The aim of this study was to identify barriers or enablers of diabetes self-management experienced by people with SMI.

Methods: Adults with type 2 diabetes and SMI were recruited through UK National Health Service organisations and mental health and diabetes charities. Participants completed an anonymous survey consisting of: Summary of Diabetes Self-Care Activities (SDSCA); CORE-10 measure of psychological distress; a measure of barriers and enablers of diabetes self-management based on the Theoretical Domains Framework; Diabetes UK care survey on receipt of 14 essential aspects of diabetes healthcare. To identify the strongest explanatory variables of SDSCA outcomes, significant variables ($p < .05$) identified from univariate analyses were entered into multiple regressions.

Results: Most of the 77 participants had bipolar disorder (42%) or schizophrenia (36%). They received a mean of 7.6 (SD 3.0) diabetes healthcare essentials. Only 28.6% had developed a diabetes care plan with their health professional and only 40% reported receiving specialist psychological support. Engagement in self-management activities was variable. Participants reported taking medication on 6.1 (SD 2.0) days in the previous week but other behaviours were less frequent: general diet 4.1 (2.3) days; specific diet 3.6 (1.8) days, taking exercise 2.4 (2.1) days and checking feet on 1.7 (1.8) days. Smoking prevalence was 44%. Participants reported finding regular exercise and following a healthy diet particularly difficult. Factors associated with diabetes self-management included: the level of diabetes healthcare and support received; emotional wellbeing; priority given to diabetes; perceived ability to manage diabetes or establish a routine to do so; and perceived consequences of diabetes self-management.

Conclusions: Several aspects of diabetes healthcare and self-management are suboptimal in people with SMI. There is a need to improve diabetes self-management support for this population by integrating diabetes action plans into care planning and providing adequate psychological support to help people with SMI manage their diabetes.

Keywords: Diabetes, Severe mental illness, Service users, Self-management, Theoretical domains framework

* Correspondence: Kathleen.Mulligan.1@city.ac.uk
[1]School of Health Sciences, City, University of London, Myddelton Street, London EC1V 0HB, UK
[2]East London NHS Foundation Trust, London, UK
Full list of author information is available at the end of the article

Background

People with severe mental illnesses (SMI), such as schizophrenia and bipolar disorder, have poorer physical health than the general population [1, 2]. Among the health disparities experienced is a two-fold risk of developing diabetes [3, 4], which has a prevalence of approximately 13% in people with SMI [5]. Diabetes outcomes are also poorer in this group as they experience a higher risk of acute [6] and macrovascular complications [7] and higher mortality [8] than those with diabetes alone.

To maintain good diabetes control and thus reduce the risk of complications, people with diabetes are advised to engage in several self-management behaviours. These may include taking medication, eating a healthy diet, taking regular physical activity, giving up smoking, monitoring blood glucose levels, examining their feet and attending regular health checks, including retinopathy screening. The DAWN2 cross-national survey of diabetes concluded that performance of these behaviours in the general diabetes population is sub-optimal in most countries, particularly for glucose monitoring, physical activity and foot care [9]. A study in Taiwan that used the same measure of self-management behaviour as DAWN2 found that performance was poorer in people with diabetes and schizophrenia than in those with diabetes alone [10].

Very little research has explored factors that may influence diabetes self-management in people with SMI. In a recent qualitative interview study that informed the current research [11], we found that sub-optimal diabetes self-management in people with SMI did not appear to be explained by a lack of knowledge of the recommended self-management behaviours or of the potential consequences of poor diabetes control; people with SMI reported awareness of both but found it difficult to adopt and/or maintain the recommended behaviours. Barriers to effective diabetes self-management that have been found among people with SMI include psychological factors such as stress and isolation [12] or periods of deteriorating mental health [11]; low self-efficacy [10], lack of social support [12] and poor relationships with health providers or fragmented care [12]. Conversely, receipt of support from family and health professionals has been reported as an enabler of diabetes self-management [11].

The aim of the current study was to enhance our understanding of factors that may influence diabetes self-management among people with SMI by using a theoretical framework to explore a comprehensive range of potential barriers and enablers. The findings will inform the development of an intervention to help support diabetes self-management among people with SMI.

Methods

Design

An anonymous cross-sectional survey was conducted between November 2015 and October 2016.

Participants

People were eligible to participate if they:

- were aged 18 years or over,
- had a SMI (defined as schizophrenia, schizoaffective disorder, bipolar disorder or depression with psychotic features)
- had type 2 diabetes
- were able to read English

In the case of participants who were recruited through the UK National Health Service (NHS) (see below), a member of the clinical team checked eligibility criteria, including diagnoses, before sending out the survey, however, this check was not possible in the case of participants recruited through other routes.

Procedures

Following advice received from patient and public involvement (PPI) representatives, recruitment was undertaken through both NHS organisations, relevant charities and service user networks. These included a national diabetes charity, a community database of people with diabetes in South West England, five national and five local mental health charities (four in London and one in South West England), one national service user network and a local service user group in London. The NHS organisations were five NHS Trusts (three in North and East London, one in South West England and one in East England) and 16 general practice (GP) surgeries (15 in North and East London and one in a city in the Midlands) .

The charities and service user groups advertised the survey through their websites and/or newsletters and provided a link to the online version of the survey. NHS organisations identified eligible service users from their databases and posted a paper version of the survey questionnaire to them with a freepost envelope for return of the questionnaire to the research team. The correspondence also contained details of the link to the online version of the survey, which participants could complete instead of the paper version, if preferred. Participants were advised that a contribution of £2 would be made to a diabetes or mental health charity for each completed questionnaire.

Measures

The survey was developed in collaboration with established research advisory groups of mental health service users and carers [13] and people with diabetes [14]. The survey comprised questions on the following:

- Performance of diabetes self-management behaviour was the primary study outcome and was assessed using the Summary of Diabetes Self-Care Activities (SDSCA) scale [15]. This is a validated and widely used measure of performance of diabetes self-management. The measure has 11 core items - self-monitoring of blood glucose (2 items), foot care (2 items), general diet (2 items), specific diet items about eating fruit and vegetables and high fat foods (2 items), physical activity (2 items) and smoking status (1 item); we also included two of the optional items about medication (2 items). Participants are asked on how many of the last 7 days they performed each behaviour. Summary scores are calculated for each behaviour using the mean number of days. For smoking, participants are asked whether or not they smoked in the last 7 days, producing a categorical outcome variable. We added a question asking participants to indicate which one of these aspects of their diabetes they find most difficult to manage.
- Psychological distress over the previous week was assessed using the CORE-10 [16]. This validated measure comprises 10 items scored on a 5-point scale ranging from 0 ('not at all') to 4 ('most or all the time'). A total score is calculated by adding the values of all 10 items to give a score from 0 to 40, with a higher score representing greater psychological distress. A score of ≤10 is in the non-clinical range, a score of 11–14 is considered 'mild' distress, 15–19 'moderate', 20–24 'moderate-to-severe' and 25+ 'severe' psychological distress.
- Barriers and enablers of diabetes self-management were examined using a 27-item questionnaire. Questionnaire items were generated from a previous interview study with service users about the barriers and enablers to diabetes self-management they experience [11]. The interview schedule and subsequent questionnaire were based on the Theoretical Domains Framework (TDF) [17], a synthesis of 33 theories of behaviour change, which comprises 14 theoretical domains found to influence behaviour. The 14 domains are 1) knowledge, 2) skills, 3) social/professional role and identity, 4) beliefs about capabilities, 5) optimism, 6) beliefs about consequences, 7) reinforcement, 8) intentions, 9) goals, 10) memory, attention and decision processes, 11) environmental context and resources, 12) social influences, 13) emotion and 14) behavioural regulation. The questionnaire included items which were deemed relevant from the interview study, and covered each of these 14 domains (see Additional file 1). Items were scored on a 7-point Likert scale ranging from 'strongly disagree' to 'strongly agree', with higher sores representing stronger agreement. Subscales representing the 14 domains of the barriers and enablers questionnaire were created by calculating means of the items in each domain. Items 6 and 18 (see Additional file 1) were reverse-scored.
- The Diabetes UK care survey was used to measure participants' experience of receiving recommended diabetes care [18]. The survey explores whether respondents have received diabetes 'healthcare essentials' [19] to which the response options are 'Yes', 'No' or 'Don't Know'. We excluded three questions that ask about care for children with diabetes, giving a 15-item measure, 14 of which ask about receipt of healthcare essentials plus one that asks if the quality of diabetes care received over the past 12 months had improved, stayed the same or worsened. The total number of healthcare essentials received was calculated. In addition, we asked participants to indicate if they would be interested in receiving diabetes education (if they had not already received any) or more education (if they had already attended diabetes education).
- Demographic characteristics (age, education, employment status, ethnicity, gender, relationship status).
- Clinical characteristics: participants were given a list of mental health diagnoses and asked to tick all that applied to them. They were also asked how long ago, in years, they were diagnosed with a) diabetes and b) their mental health problem. Participants were asked how they managed their diabetes (response options: tablets; insulin; lifestyle; don't know) and which medication they take for their mental health (free text response box).

Statistical analysis

Data were analysed using IBM SPSS Statistics v.23.

Composite variables representing the 14 domains of the barriers and enablers questionnaire were created. To test the internal consistency, inter-item correlations were calculated for each domain. In the case of scales with fewer than 10 items it is more appropriate to report the mean inter-item correlation, rather than Cronbach alpha. It is recommended that average inter-item correlations should fall between 0.15 and 0.50 [20]. Inter-item correlations were found to range from 0.31 to 0.73, with two domains (*Memory, Attention and Decision Processes*; *Environmental Context and Resources*) exceeding the recommended higher limit of 0.50. The composite variables were used in the remainder of the analyses.

To examine which factors were associated with performance of self-management behaviours, univariate analyses were initially performed. The independent variables (IVs) were demographic and clinical variables, psychological distress, diabetes care received and the 14 domains from the barriers and enablers questionnaire. The relationship between SDSCA variables and continuous IVs was examined by Pearson r correlations. In the case of categorical IVs (e.g. gender), differences in SDSCA between categories were examined by t-test or analysis of variance (ANOVA), as applicable.

To examine which were the strongest explanatory variables of SDSCA outcomes, significant IVs ($p < .05$) identified from the univariate analyses were included in stepwise multiple linear regressions. Separate regression analyses were performed for each of the behaviours assessed in the SDSCA. As smoking was a categorical variable, logistic regression analysis was performed for this outcome. Before entering categorical IVs into the regressions, dummy variables were created for those with more than two categories.

To enter all of the 26 IVs outlined above in the multiple regression analysis, based on a medium effect size of 0.15, with 80% power and alpha 0.05, would require a sample size of 175. However, only variables that were significantly associated with the outcome of interest in the univariate analysis ($p < 0.05$) were entered into the multiple regression analyses.

Results

A total of 486 questionnaires were mailed out to service users. Ninety-seven people opened the online survey, of whom 70 consented into the study, and 52 people completed the paper survey, giving a total sample of 122 participants. Eleven participants were excluded as they reported mental health and/or diabetes diagnoses that did not meet the study inclusion criteria. We excluded cases who had missing data for more than 50% of variables, a threshold above which imputation is not recommended [21, 22]. This gave a final sample of 77 (63.1%). Little's Missing Completely at Random (MCAR) test was non-significant (Chi-squared = 443.641, df = 444, $p = 0.496$), indicating that data were MCAR. Missing data were managed using multiple imputation methods in IBM SPSS version 23. Full Conditional Specification (FCS), an interactive Markov chain Monte Carlo (MCMC) procedure, was used as the missing data pattern was arbitrary. Constraints and rounding were used to ensure that the imputed scale level data was meaningful and corresponded to possible values. The model used to generate the imputed values corresponded with the model used for the analysis. Ten scale level imputation iterations were used to eliminate bias; it has been suggested that between 3 and 10 imputations are sufficient [23]. All analysis was performed on each of these 10 datasets and then pooled to give a final result.

Participant demographic and clinical characteristics are shown in Table 1. A majority of participants were male, of white British ethnicity, with an average age of 52.3 years (SD 11.5). Just over half of the sample were educated to A-Level standard (a national exam taken at 18 years of age) or above but this varied from 70.3% of those with bipolar disorder, 58.8% of those with depression with psychotic features, 50% with schizoaffective disorder and 44.4% of participants with schizophrenia. Few participants were in employment. Approximately half of the sample was living alone. Participants had been diagnosed with SMI for an average of 19.5 years and with diabetes for an average of 5 years. Most participants were taking tablets to manage their diabetes, but 10 (13%) were taking insulin. The most commonly occurring SMI in our sample was bipolar disorder, followed by schizophrenia. Over half of the sample reported experiencing at least moderate psychological distress over the previous week (Table 2).

Diabetes self-management behaviour

The average number of days on which participants reported engaging in recommended self-management behaviours is shown in Table 3. Following recommended behaviour was most common for medication and least common for exercise and foot care. Participants reported eating a healthy diet roughly half of the time. The aspects of diabetes self-management that participants reported finding most difficult were taking regular exercise and eating a healthy diet. Over 40% of participants had smoked in the past 7 days and of these, only 21% considered not smoking to be the most difficult aspect of diabetes management.

Diabetes care received

Table 4 shows the number of participants who reported receiving each of the diabetes healthcare essentials. The responses of participants in the Diabetes UK survey [18] are also shown for comparison. Participants in the current study reported receiving a mean of 7.6 (SD 3.0) of the 14 healthcare essentials. Almost a quarter of the sample reported that their diabetes care had improved over the past 12 months, but for 14% it had worsened. The most commonly received aspects of care were blood pressure and eye checks, received by 85.7 and 83.1% of participants respectively. The least common were: being seen by a diabetes specialist if in hospital (20.3%); developing a care plan with their healthcare professional (28.6%); and being offered specialist psychological support (40.3%). Other aspects of care were each received by approximately two-thirds of participants.

Table 1 Demographic and clinical characteristics

Age in years, mean (SD)	52.3 (11.5)
Gender, n (%) Male	41 (53.2)
Ethnicity, n (%)	
White, British	47 (61.0)
White, other	7 (9.1)
South Asian	8 (10.4)
Black African Caribbean	6 (7.8)
Other	8 (10.4)
Missing data	1 (1.3)
Relationship status, n (%)	
Married/Living with Partner	20 (26.0)
Living alone	39 (50.6)
Living with relatives/friends/supported accommodation	16 (20.8)
Missing data	2 (2.6)
Education – highest qualification, n (%)[a]	
Higher education/professional or vocational equivalent	27 (35.1)
A Levels / vocational level 3 or equivalent	13 (16.9)
GCSE A*- C/O Level/vocational level 2 or equivalent	13 (16.9)
None or Qualifications at level 1 and below	13 (16.9)
Other qualifications: level unknown	8 (10.4)
Missing data	3 (3.9)
Employment	
Full time work	4 (5.2)
Part time work	3 (3.9)
Full time homemaker	3 (3.9)
Unemployed	33 (42.9)
Other	8 (10.4)
Retired	7 (9.1)
Missing	19 (24.7)
Diabetes duration (years), median (IQR)	5.0 (2.0–9.0)
Diabetes medication, n, %	
Tablets only	52 (67.5)
Insulin only	4 (5.2)
Tablets and insulin	6 (7.8)
Lifestyle only	15 (19.5)
SMI duration (years), median (IQR)	19.5 (10.75–30.25)
SMI diagnosis, n, % (may have more than one diagnosis)	
Schizophrenia	28 (36.4)
Schizoaffective disorder	13 (16.9)
Depression with psychotic features	17 (22.1)
Bipolar disorder	32 (41.6)

[a]A levels – national exams taken at age 18 years; GCSE – national exams taken at age 16 years

Of the 50 participants who had been offered diabetes education, 40 (80.0%) reported that they would be interested in receiving more education. Of 27 participants who had not been offered education, 19 (70.4%) reported that they would be interested in receiving education.

Barriers and enablers to performing diabetes self-management behaviours

Responses concerning the individual barriers and enablers are shown in Fig. 1. A majority of respondents (> 75%) agreed that they know about diabetes and how to manage it. They were also aware that poor diabetes control would have adverse health consequences, with almost all participants reporting that if they did not manage their diabetes properly they would have poor health. However, a smaller percentage (57.2%) felt that poor diabetes management would have an impact on their mental health.

Most people saw diabetes management as their responsibility and intended to take steps to manage their diabetes in the future. Diabetes management was considered important, with over 80% wanting to control their diabetes to protect their health and do the things they want to in life; however managing mental health was considered more important than managing diabetes by approximately half the sample.

Just over 60% felt confident in their ability to manage their diabetes and felt optimistic that they would be able to do so in future. However, difficulty in establishing a routine to manage diabetes was reported by approximately half of the respondents and about a third reported that they found managing diabetes confusing or struggled to remember all the things they needed to do to manage their diabetes. Controlling sugar intake was reported as difficult by over 40% of participants. Managing diabetes was a worry for over 60% of participants and 75% reported that they find it difficult to manage their diabetes if their mental health is poor.

The extent to which other people were perceived as helping with diabetes management varied, with over two-thirds (69%) agreeing that primary care staff helped them to manage their diabetes, but this was lower for diabetes specialists (49%) and their mental health team (35%) and only 30% felt friends and family helped them to manage their diabetes.

Factors associated with diabetes self-management

Univariate associations between diabetes self-management behaviours (SDSCA variables) and continuous and categorical IVs are shown in Tables 5 and 6 respectively. Several factors were significantly correlated ($p < 0.05$) with one or more self-management behaviour, but none were significant across all behaviours.

Table 2 Mental Health

CORE-10 measure of global distress, mean (SD)	16.65 (7.81)
CORE-10 classifications, n, %	
Non-clinical range 0–10	18 (23.4)
Mild 11–14	16 (20.8)
Moderate 15–19	16 (20.8)
Moderate to severe 20–24	14 (18.2)
Severe 25+	13 (16.9)

Scale 0–40, higher score = more distress. A score of ≤10 = non-clinical range, score 11+ = clinical range - 11-14 = mild, 15–19 = moderate, 20–24 = moderate-to-severe, 25+ = severe

Variables that were statistically significant in the multiple regression analyses and logistic regression analysis are shown in Tables 7 and 8 respectively. Findings for each of the self-management behaviours are summarised below.

Medication taking

Frequency of medication taking was higher in participants who received more of the diabetes healthcare essentials. Associations between medication taking and all other IVs were not statistically significant in univariate analyses therefore multiple regression analysis was not performed.

Blood glucose testing

More frequent blood glucose testing was associated with psychological distress and *Behavioural Regulation* in the

Table 3 Diabetes self-management behaviour

Summary of Diabetes Self-Care Activities (SDSCA)	Mean	SD
Number of days in last 7 that participant has engaged in		
Taking medication	6.1	2.0
Blood sugar testing[a]	3.8	2.7
General diet	4.1	2.3
Specific diet	3.6	1.8
Exercise	2.4	2.1
Foot Care	1.7	1.8
	n	%
Smoked	34	44.2
Which aspect of your diabetes do you find most difficult to manage?		
Exercising for at least 30 min, 5 days a week	29	37.7
Following a healthy eating plan	27	35.1
Not smoking	7	20.6[b]
Testing blood sugar	5	6.5
Taking diabetes medication	5	6.5
Checking feet	4	5.2

[a]not all participants had been supplied with a blood glucose monitor – these data relate to 40 participants who had received a monitor
[b]of those who reported being smokers

Table 4 Diabetes healthcare essentials received

	Current study		Diabetes UK survey	
	n	%	n	%
Over the past 12 months, in general has the overall quality of diabetes care that you receive:				
Improved	18	23.4	709	10.6
Stayed the same	41	53.2	4776	71.3
Worsened	11	14.3	851	12.7
I don't know	7	9.1	366	5.5
In the last year, or as part of your most recent annual review, have you had an HbA_{1c} blood test carried out, to measure your overall blood glucose control?				
Yes	56	72.7	6319	94.2
No	7	9.1	389	5.8
Don't know	14	18.2		
In the last year, or as part of your most recent annual review, have you had your blood pressure measured?				
Yes	66	85.7	6225	92.8
No	5	6.5	480	7.2
Don't know	6	7.8		
In the last year, or as part of your most recent annual review, have you had your blood fats (cholesterol) measured?				
Yes	53	68.8	5730	85.8
No	12	15.6	945	14.2
Don't know	12	15.6		
Your eyes should be screened for retinopathy each year, using a specialised digital camera. In the last year, or as part of your most recent annual review, have you had your eyes looked at?				
Yes	64	83.1	6271	93.4
No	13	16.9	446	6.6
In the last year or as part of your most recent annual review, have you had your legs and feet checked?				
Yes	50	64.9	5131	76.4
No	25	32.5	1587	23.6
Don't know	2	2.6		
In the past year, or as part of your most recent annual review, have you had a urine or blood test to monitor your kidney function?				
Yes	50	64.9	5163	78.6
No	19	24.7	791	12.0
Don't know	8	10.4	616	9.4
In the last year, or as part of your most recent annual review, have you had your weight checked and your waist measured?				
Yes	52	67.5	4549	69.5
No	22	28.6	2000	30.5
Don't know	3	3.9		
If you are a smoker, in the last year, or as part of your most recent annual review, have you had support and advice on how to quit?				
Yes	23	62.2	366	56.5
No	11	29.7	282	43.5

Table 4 Diabetes healthcare essentials received *(Continued)*

	Current study		Diabetes UK survey	
	n	%	n	%
Don't know	3	8.1		
Don't smoke	40		5904	
Have you developed a care plan with your healthcare professional, which has been decided by discussing your individual needs with them to set targets?				
Yes	22	28.6	2339	35.9
No	55	71.4	4184	64.1
Have you ever been offered an education course about diabetes, either when you were first diagnosed or later on?				
Yes	50	64.9	3676	56.2
No	27	35.1	2867	43.8
Don't know			65	13.7
If you have had to go into hospital, for whatever reason, has somebody from a diabetes specialist team come to see you about your diabetes while you were there?				
Yes	14	20.3	803	30.4
No	55	79.7	1835	69.6
Not applicable	8		3667	
If you are planning a pregnancy, or you are pregnant, have you been offered specialist healthcare advice before and during your pregnancy?				
Yes	4	40.0	158	60.1
No	6	60.0	105	39.9
Not applicable	67		3667	
Do you think that, when the need arises, you are referred to the care of specialists who can help you with different aspects of your diabetes?				
Yes	53	68.8	4294	69.4
No	24	31.2	1894	30.6
If you have needed it, have you been offered emotional or psychological support from a specialist healthcare professional or service?				
Yes	31	40.3	723	24.1
No	46	59.7	2277	75.9
Not applicable			3293	

univariate analysis. Both variables remained significant in the multiple regression analysis and explained 37% of the variance in blood glucose testing. More frequent testing was reported by those who scored higher on psychological distress and those who found it less difficult to establish a routine to manage their diabetes.

General diet

In univariate analysis, following a healthy diet was more frequent in participants who received a higher number of the diabetes healthcare essentials and who reported less psychological distress. All of the TDF domains, with the exception of *Skills* and *Social/Professional Role and Identity*, were also associated with general diet. In the multiple regression analysis, 42% of the variance in general diet was explained by the domains *Beliefs about Consequences, Goals* and *Beliefs about Capabilities.* Eating a healthy diet was more frequent among those who expressed a stronger belief that failure to manage their diabetes would damage their health, gave diabetes a higher goal priority and had greater confidence in their ability to manage their diabetes.

Specific diet

Seven of the TDF domains - *Behavioural Regulation, Beliefs about Capabilities, Environmental Context and Resources, Goals, Optimism, Reinforcement* and *Social influences* - were associated with frequency of specific healthy diet in the univariate analysis. In multiple regression, 19% of the variance in specific diet was explained by the domains *Goals* and *Behavioural Regulation.* Eating a healthy diet was more frequent among those who gave diabetes a higher goal priority and who reported less difficulty in establishing a routine to manage their diabetes.

Exercise

In univariate analysis, exercise was more frequent among participants who received a higher number of the diabetes healthcare essentials and who reported less psychological distress. Six of the TDF domains - *Beliefs about Capabilities, Environmental Context and Resources, Goals, Intentions, Reinforcement* and *Social Influences* - were also associated with frequency of exercise. In multiple regression, *Goals* and *Environmental Context and Resources* remained significant, explaining 15% of the variance. Exercise was more frequent among those who gave diabetes a higher goal priority and who reported greater access to relevant services for their diabetes.

Foot care

In univariate analysis, more frequent foot care was reported by those who scored lower on diabetes-related *Emotion* and those whose diabetes was managed with tablets rather than lifestyle only. Both variables remained significant in the multiple regression analysis, explaining 15% of the variance.

Smoking

Smoking was more prevalent in men than women and in those who scored lower on diabetes-related *Emotion.* Only the domain *Emotion* remained statistically significant in the logistic regression analysis, with smokers scoring lower on diabetes-related emotion.

Discussion

To the authors' knowledge, this is the first survey that has asked people with SMI about the factors that affect

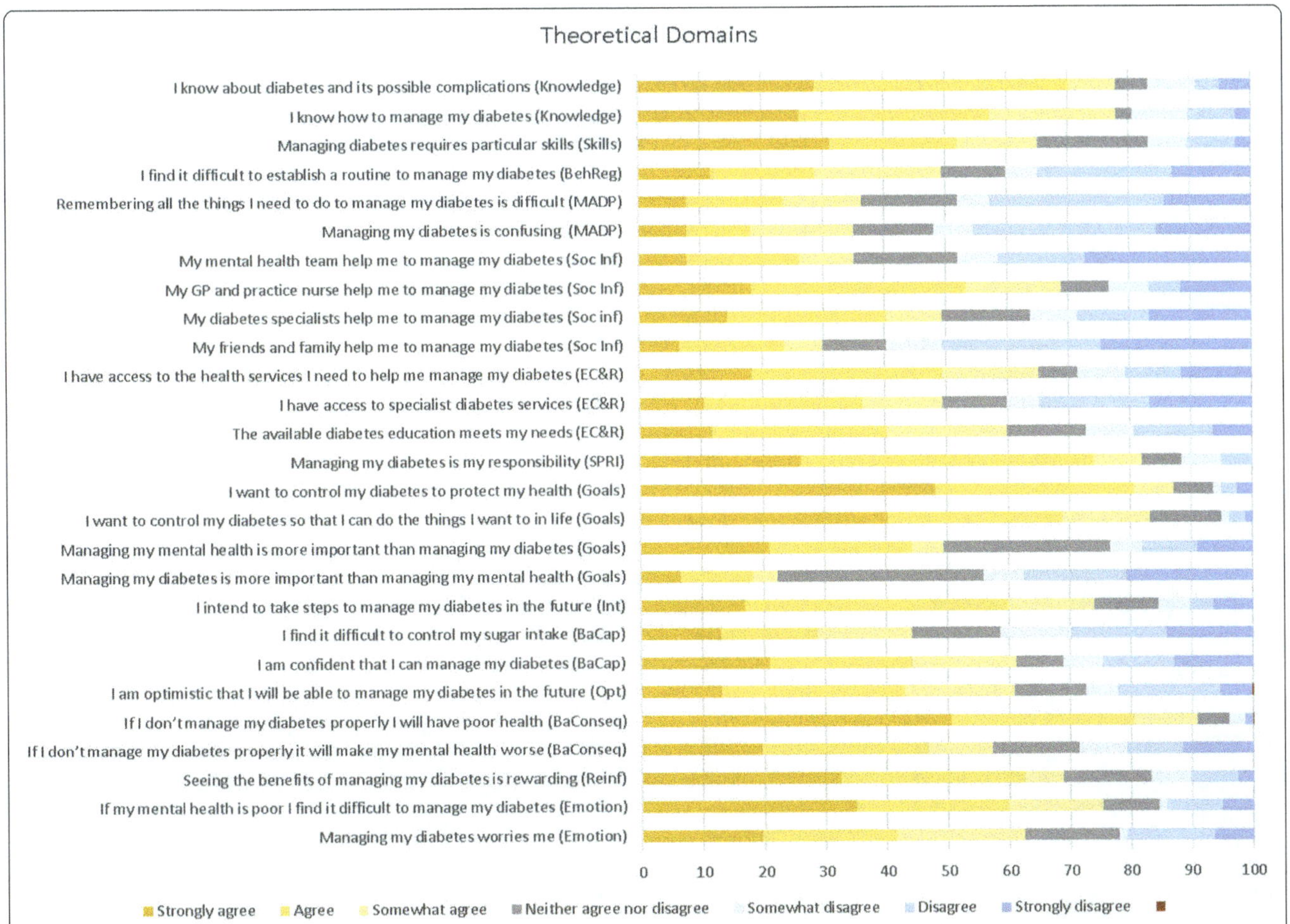

Fig. 1 Responses to questions in the Theoretical Domains Framework questionnaire

their ability to manage their diabetes. We found that several aspects of diabetes healthcare and self-management are suboptimal in people with diabetes and SMI and some, though not all, are poorer than in the general diabetes population. Several factors emerged as important for diabetes self-management, including the degree to which participants were receiving recommended diabetes healthcare, the support they received, their emotional wellbeing, the priority they give to diabetes, their perceived ability to manage diabetes or establish a routine to do so and the perceived consequences of not managing their diabetes.

There was variability in the average number of days on which the different diabetes self-management behaviours were performed. The most commonly reported behaviour was taking medication, with most participants reporting taking their diabetes medication every day. However, foot care was infrequent and exercise was taken on average 2 days per week. Participants reported following a healthy diet for approximately half of the week. When compared to both UK and international data from the DAWN2 study in the general diabetes population [9], participants in the current study took their medication and checked their blood sugar at about the same frequency as those in the DAWN2 study, but eating a healthy diet, taking exercise and checking feet were less frequent in the current sample. The rate of smoking in our sample was almost three times the rate in the general population [24], but is similar to smoking prevalence among people with SMI in the UK [25]. Researchers in the DAWN2 study concluded that diabetes self-management is sub-optimal in the general population with diabetes [9] and our findings indicate that people with SMI experience even greater difficulty in self-managing some aspects of their diabetes.

Participants reported that they found taking regular exercise and following a healthy diet particularly difficult. A recent systematic review [26] identified only one small trial ($n = 64$) of a lifestyle intervention for people with diabetes and SMI [27, 28]. The trial reported a small improvement in physical activity immediately following the intervention, which was not maintained at 6-month follow-up. Self-reported calorie intake did not change as a result of the intervention however,

Table 5 Univariate relationships between continuous independent variables and self-management behaviours

	Summary of Diabetes Self Care Activities variables						
	Pearson correlations (*p* value in brackets)						t-test (*p* value)
	Blood Glucose Testing	Medication	General Diet	Specific Diet	Exercise	Foot Care	Smoking
Age	.045	.047	.243	.120	.172	.139	1.154
	(.818)	(.766)	(.071)	(.381)	(.206)	(.310)	(.249)
Diabetes duration in years	–.140	–.204	–.138	–.023	.066	–.203	1.471
	(.439)	(.141)	(.265)	(.854)	(.598)	(.100)	(.141)
SMI duration in years	–.180	–.076	.169	.196	.177	.059	–.389
	(.295)	(.588)	(.162)	(.105)	(.144)	(.627)	(.697)
Diabetes healthcare essentials_total	–.144	.277	.371	.139	.264	.173	.129
	(.386)	(.030)	(.001)	(.231)	(.021)	(.136)	(.897)
CORE Total Score	.334	–.065	–.250	–.082	–.304	–.078	–.265
	(.037)	(.625)	(.028)	(.478)	(.007)	(.500)	(.791)
TDF Behavioural Regulation	–.344	–.236	–.348	–.344	–.216	–.159	1.188
	(.031)	(.067)	(.002)	(.002)	(.059)	(.168)	(.235)
TDF Beliefs about Capabilities	.091	.146	.466	.350	.313	.117	–1.228
	(.585)	(.259)	(.000)	(.002)	(.005)	(.315)	(.220)
TDF Beliefs about Consequences	.250	–.045	.297	.090	.175	–.088	1.507
	(.125)	(.734)	(.008)	(.437)	(.128)	(.446)	(.132)
TDF ECR	.088	.023	.382	.269	.333	.220	.602
	(.597)	(.860)	(.001)	(.018)	(.003)	(.055)	(.547)
TDF Emotion	–.115	–.136	–.371	–.180	–.210	–.263	2.631[a]
	(.486)	(.294)	(.001)	(.120)	(.067)	(.021)	(.009)
TDF Goals	–.076	.172	.547	.377	.328	.065	.628
	(.646)	(.184)	(.000)	(.001)	(.003)	(.574)	(.530)
TDF Intention	–.036	–.107	.301	.202	.236	.151	–.480
	(.830)	(.412)	(.008)	(.080)	(.042)	(.191)	(.631)
TDF Knowledge	.173	.040	.261	–.005	.129	.058	1.799
	(.296)	(.763)	(.022)	(.966)	(.263)	(.619)	(.072)
TDF MADP	–.100	.098	–.272	–.158	–.156	–.161	.217
	(.547)	(.459)	(.016)	(.174)	(.178)	(.165)	(.828)
TDF Optimism	–.142	.240	.414	.229	.092	.188	.534
	(.391)	(.062)	(.000)	(.045)	(.432)	(.103)	(.593)
TDF Reinforcement	–.059	.062	.475	.233	.232	.100	1.157
	(.723)	(.638)	(.000)	(.042)	(.042)	(.391)	(.247)
TDF Skills	.059	.138	.135	.138	.105	.148	–.502
	(.722)	(.294)	(.243)	(.233)	(.367)	(.200)	(.616)
TDF Social Influence	–.176	.157	.392	.315	.291	.256	0.330
	(.283)	(.226)	(.000)	(.005)	(.010)	(.025)	(.741)
TDF SPRI	–.108	–.240	–.136	–.128	–.074	.052	1.008
	(.524)	(.063)	(.240)	(.272)	(.523)	(.659)	(.313)

[a]Non-smokers more likely to agree with emotion items

ECR – Environmental Context and Resources; MADP – Memory, Attention and Decision Processes; SPRI – Social/Professional Role and Identity

Table 6 Univariate relationships between categorical independent variables and self-management behaviours

	Summary of Diabetes Self Care Activities variables												
	Blood glucose testing		Medication		General diet		Specific diet		Exercise		Foot care		Smoker/ non-smoker
	Mean	Statistic *P* value	Mean	Statistic *P* value	Mean	Statistic *P* value	Mean	Statistic *P* value	Mean	Statistic *P* value	Mean	Statistic *P* value	Statistic *P* value
Gender													
Male	4.2085	$t = 0.757$	6.42	$t = 1.426$	4.4878	$t = 1.683$	3.4504	$t = -0.865$	2.5976	0.949	1.6724	$t = -0.024$	**$\chi^2 = 4.467$**
Female	3.6591	$p = 0.454$	5.66	$p = 0.159$	3.5893	$p = 0.097$	3.8154	$p = 0.390$	2.1324	0.346	1.7453	$p = 0.981$	**$p = 0.039$**
Ethnicity													
Asian	4.4000	F = 1.965	5.92	F = 0.561	3.9537	F = 1.062	3.4231	F = 1.596	1.9722	F = 2.235	1.5981	F = 0.828	$\chi^2 = 2.930$
Black	0.9667	$p = 0.137$	5.67	$p = 0.643$	5.4214	$p = 0.371$	4.8571	$p = 0.198$	3.2857	$p = 0.091$	2.7286	$p = 0.483$	$p = 0.403$
White	3.0000		6.33		3.6500		3.2050		3.1000		1.7000		
Mixed	3.0000		7.00		4.7000		4.2000		3.7000		1.4000		
Relationship status													
Married/Living with partner	4.5000	F = 1.639	6.15	F = 0.399	4.2000	F = 0.393	3.2775	F = 0.587	2.0750	F = 0.315	1.4250	F = 0.304	$\chi^2 = 3.362$
Living alone	4.2159	$p = 0.208$	5.81	$p = 0.673$	3.8962	$p = 0.677$	3.5769	$p = 0.599$	2.4231	$p = 0.731$	1.8231	$p = 0.739$	$p = 0.186$
Living with friends /relatives/supported accommodation	2.4563		6.34		4.5000		3.9594		2.6250		1.6750		
Employment													
Not employed	3.8069	$t = -1.458$	6.06	$t = 0.290$	4.1265	$t = -1.056$	3.6931	$t = -0.804$	2.2157	$t = -1.945$	1.6843	F = 0.370	$\chi^2 = 0.044$
Employed	6.5000	$p = 0.156$	5.75	$p = 0.773$	5.1429	$p = 0.296$	4.2929	$p = 0.425$	3.9286	$p = 0.057$	1.4286	$p = 0.713$	$p = 1.000$
Education level													
Below A level	4.0750	$t = 0.260$	5.97	$t = -0.502$	4.2794	$t = 0.358$	3.7941	$t = 0.848$	2.3676	$t = 0.135$	1.3824	$t = -1.206$	$\chi^2 = 2.410$
A level or above	3.8447	$p = 0.796$	6.23	$p = 0.617$	4.0863	$p = 0.722$	3.4225	$p = 0.399$	2.3000	$p = 0.893$	1.8975	$p = 0.232$	p = 0.159
SMI diagnosis													
Schizophrenia	3.5909	F = 0.767	6.07	F = 0.378	4.3182	F = 0.391	3.9348	F = 1.264	2.8261	F = 1.260	2.2273	F = 1.748	$\chi^2 = 6.777$
Schizoaffective disorder	3.6429	$p = 0.520$	6.10	$p = 0.823$	3.9500	$p = 0.815$	3.9500	$p = 0.292$	2.9000	$p = 0.294$	1.4500	$p = 0.149$	$p = 0.148$
Bipolar disorder	5.3333		6.86		4.7778		4.0556		2.5000		2.4444		
Depression + psychotic feature	3.7000		5.88		3.7308		2.9231		1.6346		1.1731		
More than one diagnosis	–		5.92		4.0556		4.0000		2.5000		1.3889		
Diabetes management													
Tablets	3.3111	F = 2.128	6.07	F = 0.212	4.2779	F = 1.836	3.8433	F = 2.547	2.6442	F = 1.450	**2.0846**	**F = 3.120**	$\chi^2 = 4.679$
Insulin	5.8750	$p = 0.114$	6.50	$p = 0.810$	4.8750	p = 0.148	4.5000	$p = 0.062$	2.1250	$p = 0.235$	**0.8750**	**$p = 0.031$**	$p = 0.197$
Tablets and lifestyle	5.8750		5.67		2.0833		2.2500		0.9167		**1.4167**		
Lifestyle only	3.3000		–		4.0000		2.9033		2.0000		**0.6000**		

Table 7 Multiple linear regressions

SDSCA Outcome variable	Independent variables	Variable Coefficients B	Std. Error	p	Model Summary Cumulative adjusted R^2
Blood glucose testing	CORE-10 Total	.189	.049	<.001	0.37
	Behavioural regulation	−.740	.188	<.001	
Diet General	Beliefs about Capabilities	.494	.126	<.001	0.42
	Beliefs about Consequences	.363	.156	.020	
	Goals	.745	.198	<.001	
Diet Specific	Behavioural Regulation	−.245	.098	.012	0.19
	Goals	.500	.171	.003	
Exercise	Environmental Context & Resources	.328	.132	.013	0.15
	Goals	.481	.199	.016	
Foot Care	Diabetes mgt – tablets	1.360	.445	.002	0.15
	Emotion	−.307	.120	.011	

improvement was reported in body mass index. The reviewers concluded [26] that there is insufficient evidence to show whether diabetes self-management interventions are effective for people with SMI and further trials of theoretical and evidence-based interventions are needed.

Although the smoking rate was very high in the current study, only 20% of smokers considered that not smoking was the most difficult aspect of managing their diabetes. It may be that people with SMI do not associate smoking with diabetes self-management even though it increases the risk of complications [29]. Over 60% of smokers in our sample reported that they had been given support and advice on how to quit but unfortunately this was clearly ineffective. A recent systematic review of smoking cessation in severe mental illness concluded that specialised smoking cessation programmes did not show evidence of benefit, but effective pharmacological interventions are available [30]. It is crucial that diabetes self-management interventions for people with SMI include appropriate support to give up smoking to help reduce the risk of diabetes complications.

We examined whether people with SMI received recommended diabetes healthcare and whether their diabetes self-management was related to the level of care received. In a replication of the survey conducted by Diabetes UK [18], we found that the percentages reporting receipt of diabetes healthcare essentials were lower in the current sample for some, but not all, aspects of care. Percentages were lower for checks of HbA1c, BP, cholesterol, eyes, feet and kidney function and for developing a care plan with their healthcare professional. Percentages were similar for weight checks and referral to diabetes specialists. The percentage of participants in the current study being offered diabetes education, given advice to quit smoking and offered specialist psychological support was higher than in the Diabetes UK survey. Participants who reported receiving fewer of the healthcare essentials also reported less frequent performance of three diabetes self-management behaviours: taking medication, eating a healthy diet and exercise. Several participants were unaware of whether or not they had received some of the health checks, perhaps suggesting that they are not fully engaged in their diabetes care. In previous research in the UK, two comparisons between diabetes care for those with and without SMI have been conducted in primary care [31, 32]. Whyte et al. [32] examined 17 quality indicators and reported that having SMI did not result in poorer diabetes care. The only significant difference was on target HbA_{1c} level which was better in those with SMI, however the proportions achieving target HbA_{1c} levels were relatively low in both populations (54% in those with SMI v 47% in those without SMI). Mathur et al. [31] found no significant differences in statin prescribing or cholesterol control between people with or without SMI. They found that people with SMI had better HbA_{1c} and blood pressure control than those without SMI but less than half in both populations were within the target range for HbA_{1c}. However, those with SMI were more likely than people without SMI to be smokers and to be obese and were less likely to have had retinopathy screening [31]. Our findings on smoking, diet and exercise are consistent with Mathur et al's [31] finding of higher rates of

Table 8 Logistic regression

SDSCA Outcome	Independent variables	B	Std. Error	Wald χ2	p	Nagelkerke R^2
Smoking	Emotion	−.367	.157	5.431	.020	0.10

smoking and obesity. Whyte et al. [32] and Mather et al. [31] did not ask about several aspects of diabetes care, including foot checks, referral to structured education, care plans, psychological support or being seen by a diabetes specialist if admitted to hospital. The percentages of participants in the current study who reported receipt of these aspects of care ranged from 20% being seen by a diabetes specialist in hospital to 65% being offered an education course. It is encouraging that 23% of participants reported that their diabetes care had improved over the previous 12 months, perhaps reflecting the greater emphasis now being placed on the physical health of people with SMI [33]. However, these findings indicate that several aspects of diabetes care remain suboptimal for people with SMI. The finding that survey participants who received more complete diabetes care were significantly more likely to be engaging in self-management activities, such as exercise and healthy eating, indicates the potentially motivating aspects of service contact. It has been suggested that factors such as the high number of contacts people with SMI have with health professionals may confer a benefit for their diabetes medication adherence [34], however the cross-sectional nature of this research means that we cannot infer causation.

The current study identified a number of other important factors that were related to performance of diabetes self-management behaviours. When these factors were examined in multiple regression analyses, the domains of *Goals*, *Behavioural regulation* and *Emotion* or psychological distress were statistically significant across more than one behaviour. The findings suggest that setting diabetes-related goals and action plans, including how to manage diabetes in the face of fluctuations in mental health, may be important for optimising diabetes self-management, supporting our previous qualitative work [11]. Few participants (28.6%), however, had developed a diabetes care plan with their healthcare professional. Emotional factors were also important, but only 40% of participants reported that they had received emotional or psychological support from a specialist healthcare professional or service, which is of particular concern given that all participants had a SMI and over half reported at least moderate psychological distress. A recent study of community mental health care planning found that few service users felt they were adequately involved in developing meaningful care plans [35]. The current study indicates that this is the case for their physical as well as their mental health and only a minority of service users feel that their mental health teams support their diabetes care. Community mental healthcare pathways will therefore need to be radically revised in order to improve physical health outcomes in those with SMI.

Identification of the theoretical domains that appear to be important for diabetes self-management in people with SMI is a step towards the development of an intervention to support this population. Recent expert consensus work [29, 30] has produced a method for mapping theoretical domains onto appropriate behaviour change techniques (BCTs) [31]. For example, *Goal-setting*, *Review of [outcome and behaviour] goals* and *Action planning* are BCTs suggested to bring about a change in behaviour by altering a person's *Goals* related to that behaviour [36]. One example of the successful use of action planning in mental health is the Wellness Recovery Action Plan (WRAP) [37] which has been widely-used to help people develop plans for maintaining their health when well and action plans to help manage if they become unwell. Use of WRAPs was found to improve psychiatric symptoms and quality of life [37] and reduce the need for and use of mental health services [38]. WRAPs can be seen to incorporate several of the BCTs listed and could potentially be adapted to include diabetes self-management as well as offering a format for developing more meaningful care plans for people with SMI.

Self-management education has been shown to improve outcomes for the general diabetes population [39–41] and it is encouraging that participants in this study were as likely as the general population with diabetes (perhaps somewhat more likely) to be offered an education course. However this still equated to less than two-thirds being offered an education course and only 60% of participants felt that the available diabetes education met their needs. The recent Cochrane review [26] identified only one education course that had been developed specifically for people with diabetes and SMI [27, 28], and evaluations of other diabetes education programmes often exclude people with SMI [42–44]. Given the challenges that people with SMI face when attempting to manage their diabetes, it is important that appropriate education and support is developed and provided on an ongoing basis. Opportunities for provision of diabetes education and skills development should not be limited to diabetes specialist services but also optimised in primary care and mental health services. The current study has identified several factors associated with diabetes self-management behaviour in people with SMI and suggested some strategies that may help to address these. Development and testing of interventions that target these factors may generate more effective diabetes self-management education programmes for this population.

The study had a number of limitations. The use of online recruitment methods meant that we are unable to estimate response rate, which is a limitation of all surveys that recruit in this way. As the study is cross-sectional, we are also unable to infer causation. Although we tried several routes to recruit participants, the sample size achieved was small, which resulted in some of the analyses being underpowered. Similar difficulties in recruitment have been found in other studies in SMI. For example, a telephone survey of mental health service users conducted across NHS sites between 2008 and 2014 obtained response rates ranging from 6 to 11% [45] and the 2016 Community Mental Health Survey achieved a response rate of 28% [46]. We used an anonymous postal and online survey in the hope that providing anonymity would encourage response and we also offered a small donation to relevant charities. However, providing anonymity meant that we could not send reminders to non-responders, a strategy that has been found to increase response rates in survey research [47], and which was used in the Community Mental Health Survey [46]. Anonymity also precluded us from making payments direct to participants, which may also have improved recruitment.

Given the small sample size, univariate screening was used to identify potentially relevant predictors for the regression models. Although this method has limitations [48], we chose a widely adopted approach that should be seen as hypothesis generating, suggesting avenues for future research. Although this study measured several self-management behaviours, we did not adjust the *p*-value to account for multiple outcomes as it would have increased the likelihood of type II error which is no less important than a type I error. We took this approach as the study is exploratory, but we acknowledge that we may have identified some chance findings.

To avoid the questionnaire being onerously long, we included only one measure of mental health - a short measure of psychological distress [16]. This meant that other potentially important barriers to effective diabetes self-management, such as positive and negative symptoms of psychosis, were not assessed.

Although the education level of participants is similar to that of the general UK population [49], this may not be representative of people with SMI, in whom lower levels of educational attainment have been reported [50]. It is possible that we recruited a sample of participants who are particularly interested in managing their diabetes and that this is an area of relatively low priority for many people with diabetes and SMI. Furthermore, those least likely to be able to manage their diabetes are probably also unlikely to complete a survey. Giving greater priority to physical health, including diabetes, is an important area to be promoted among people with SMI and those involved in their care.

Conclusions

This study demonstrates that people with SMI find it difficult to manage aspects of their diabetes and many do not receive all of the recommended diabetes healthcare essentials. The ability of respondents to manage their diabetes was influenced by the level of diabetes healthcare and support they received, their emotional wellbeing, the priority they give to diabetes, their perceived ability to manage diabetes or establish a routine to do so and the perceived consequences of their diabetes management. The development and evaluation of tailored interventions that address these areas are needed to help improve diabetes self-management support for people with SMI.

Abbreviations

ANOVA: Analysis of variance; BCT: Behaviour change techniques; BP: Blood pressure; EC&R: Environmental Context and Resources; GP: General Practice; HbA_{1c}: Glycated haemoglobin (A1c); IV: Independent variables; MADP: Memory, Attention and Decision Processes; MCAR: Missing Completely at Random; NHS: National Health Service; PPI: Patient and public involvement; SDSCA: Summary of Diabetes Self-Care Activities; SMI: Severe mental illness; SPRI: Social/Professional Role and Identity; TDF: Theoretical Domains Framework; WRAP: Wellness Recovery Action Plan

Acknowledgements

The authors wish to thank all participants for volunteering to take part in the study. We also wish to thank the charities and NHS organisations through which we recruited study participants.

Funding

This study was funded by a grant from Barts Charity, reference number: 477/2314. The funding body did not have any role in the design of the study or collection, analysis, or interpretation of data or in writing the manuscript.

Authors' contributions

All authors were involved in the conception and design of the study. FLG collected the data and HM and KM analysed the data. All authors were involved in data interpretation and either drafting or revising the manuscript and approving the final version for publication.

Competing interests

The authors declare that they have no competing interests.

Author details

[1]School of Health Sciences, City, University of London, Myddelton Street, London EC1V 0HB, UK. [2]East London NHS Foundation Trust, London, UK. [3]School of Human and Social Sciences, University of West London, London,

UK. [4]Diabetes Specialist Nursing Service, East London NHS Foundation Trust, London, UK. [5]Centre for Research in Primary & Community Care (CRIPACC), University of Hertfordshire, Hatfield, Hertfordshire, UK.

References

1. De Hert M, Correll CU, Bobes J, Cetkovich-Bakmas M, Cohen D, Asai I, et al. Physical illness in patients with severe mental disorders. I. Prevalence, impact of medications and disparities in health care. World Psychiatry. 2011;10:52–77.
2. Walker ER, McGee RE, Druss BG. Mortality in mental disorders and global disease burden implications: a systematic review and meta-analysis. JAMA Psychiatry. 2015;72:334–41.
3. Osborn DP, Wright CA, Levy G, King MB, Deo R, Nazareth I. Relative risk of diabetes, dyslipidaemia, hypertension and the metabolic syndrome in people with severe mental illnesses: systematic review and metaanalysis. BMC Psychiatry. 2008;8:84.
4. Stubbs B, Vancampfort D, De HM, Mitchell AJ. The prevalence and predictors of type two diabetes mellitus in people with schizophrenia: a systematic review and comparative meta-analysis. Acta Psychiatr Scand. 2015;132:144–57.
5. Ward M, Druss B. The epidemiology of diabetes in psychotic disorders. Lancet Psychiatry. 2015;2:431–51.
6. Becker T, Hux J. Risk of acute complications of diabetes among people with schizophrenia in Ontario, Canada. Diabetes Care. 2011;34:398–402.
7. Wu CS, Lai MS, Gau SS. Complications and mortality in patients with schizophrenia and diabetes: population-based cohort study. Br J Psychiatry. 2015;207:450–7.
8. Vinogradova Y, Coupland C, Hippisley-Cox J, Whyte S, Penny C. Effects of severe mental illness on survival of people with diabetes. Br J Psychiatry. 2010;197:272–7.
9. Nicolucci A, Kovacs BK, Holt RI, Comaschi M, Hermanns N, Ishii H, et al. Diabetes attitudes, wishes and needs second study (DAWN2): cross-national benchmarking of diabetes-related psychosocial outcomes for people with diabetes. Diabet Med. 2013;30:767–77.
10. Chen SR, Chien YP, Kang CM, Jeng C, Chang WY. Comparing self-efficacy and self-care behaviours between outpatients with comorbid schizophrenia and type 2 diabetes and outpatients with only type 2 diabetes. J Psychiatr Ment Health Nurs. 2014;21:414–22.
11. Mulligan K, McBain H, Lamontagne-Godwin F, Chapman J, Haddad M, Jones J, et al. Barriers and enablers of type 2 diabetes self-management in people with severe mental illness. Health Expect. 2017;20:1020–30.
12. Blixen CE, Kanuch S, Perzynski AT, Thomas C, Dawson NV, Sajatovic M. Barriers to self-management of serious mental illness and diabetes. Am J Health Behav. 2016;40:194–204.
13. Simpson A, Jones J, Barlow S, Cox L. Adding SUGAR: service user and carer collaboration in mental health nursing research. J Psychosoc Nurs Ment Health Serv. 2014;52:22–30.
14. Queen Mary Univeristy of London. Diabetes Research Lay Panel Group. Engagement and Enterprise Awards 2017. Public Engagement Category. https://www.qmul.ac.uk/publicengagement/prizes/engagement-and-enterprise-awards-2017/public-engagement-2017/. 2017. 7-11-2017.
15. Toobert DJ, Hampson SE, Glasgow RE. The summary of diabetes self-care activities measure: results from 7 studies and a revised scale. Diabetes Care. 2000;23:943–50.
16. Barkham M, Bewick B, Mullin T, Gilbody S, Connell J, Cahill J, et al. The CORE-10: a short measure of psychological distress for routine use in the psychological therapies. Couns Psychother Res. 2012;13:3–13.
17. Cane J, O'Connor D, Michie S. Validation of the theoretical domains framework for use in behaviour change and implementation research. Implement Sci. 2012;7:37.
18. Diabetes UK. Care survey results 2013. https://www.diabetes.org.uk/Guide-to-diabetes/Monitoring/15-healthcare-essentials/Care-survey-results-2013. 2014.
19. Diabetes UK. Diabetes 15 healthcare essentials. https://www.diabetes.org.uk/Guide-to-diabetes/Managing-your-diabetes/15-healthcare-essentials. 2014.
20. Clark LA, Watson D. Constructing validity: basic issues in objective scale development. Psychol Assess. 1995;7:309–19.
21. Graham JW. Missing data analysis: making it work in the real world. Annu Rev Psychol. 2009;60:549–76.
22. Garson GD. Missing Values Analysis and Data Imputation. Asheboro: Statistical Associates Publishing; 2015. http://www.statisticalassociates.com/missingvaluesanalysis.
23. Rubin DB. Multiple imputation for nonresponse in surveys. USA: Wiley; 2009.
24. Office for National Statistics. Adult smoking habits in the UK; 2016. p. 2017.
25. Health and Social Care Information Centre. Smoking rates in people with serious mental illness (SMI) https://indicators.hscic.gov.uk/webview/. 2016.
26. McBain H, Mulligan K, Haddad M, Flood C, Jones J, Simpson A. Self management interventions for type 2 diabetes in adult people with severe mental illness. Cochrane Database Syst Rev. 2016;4:CD011361.
27. McKibbin CL, Patterson TL, Norman G, Patrick K, Jin H, Roesch S, et al. A lifestyle intervention for older schizophrenia patients with diabetes mellitus: a randomized controlled trial. Schizophr Res. 2006;86:36–44.
28. McKibbin CL, Golshan S, Griver K, Kitchen K, Wykes TL. A healthy lifestyle intervention for middle-aged and older schizophrenia patients with diabetes mellitus: a 6-month follow-up analysis. Schizophr Res. 2010;121:203–6.
29. Fagard RH, Nilsson PM. Smoking and diabetes - the double health hazard! Primary Care Diabetes. 2009;3:205–9.
30. Peckham E, Brabyn S, Cook L, Tew G, Gilbody S. Smoking cessation in severe mental ill health: what works? An updated systematic review and meta-analysis. BMC Psychiatry. 2017;17:252.
31. Mathur R, Hull SA, Boomla K, Robson J. Ethnic differences in primary care management of diabetes and cardiovascular disease in people with serious mental illness. Br J Gen Pract. 2012;62:e582–8.
32. Whyte S, Penny C, Phelan M, Hippisley-Cox J, Majeed A. Quality of diabetes care in patients with schizophrenia and bipolar disorder: cross-sectional study. Diabet Med. 2007;24:1442–8.
33. Working Group for Improving the Physical Health of People with SMI. Improving the physical health of adults with severe mental illness: essential actions (OP100): Royal College of Psychiatrists; 2016.
34. Kreyenbuhl J, Dixon LB, McCarthy JF, Soliman S, Ignacio RV, Valenstein M. Does adherence to medications for type 2 diabetes differ between individuals with vs without schizophrenia? Schizophr Bull. 2010;36:428–35.
35. Simpson A, Hannigan B, Coffey M, Barlow S, Cohen R, Jones A, et al. Recovery-focused care planning and coordination in England and Wales: a cross-national mixed methods comparative case study. BMC Psychiatry. 2016;16:1–18.
36. Michie S, Johnston M, Francis J, Hardeman W, Eccles M. From theory to intervention: mapping theoretically derived behavioural determinants to behaviour change techniques. Appl Psychol. 2008;57:660–80.
37. Cook JA, Copeland ME, Jonikas JA, Hamilton MM, Razzano LA, Grey DD, et al. Results of a randomized controlled trial of mental illness self-management using wellness recovery action planning. Schizophr Bull. 2012;38:881–91.
38. Cook JA, Jonikas JA, Hamilton MM, Goldrick V, Steigman PJ, Grey DD, et al. Impact of wellness recovery action planning on service utilization and need in a randomized controlled trial. Psychiatr Rehabil J. 2013;36:250–7.
39. Chrvala CA, Sherr D, Lipman RD. Diabetes self-management education for adults with type 2 diabetes mellitus: a systematic review of the effect on glycemic control. Patient Educ Couns. 2016;99:926–43.
40. Taylor SJC, Pinnock H, Epiphaniou E, Pearce G, Parke HL, Schwappach A, et al. A rapid synthesis of the evidence on interventions supporting self-management for people with long-term conditions: PRISMS – practical systematic Review of self-management support for long-term conditions. Health Serv Delivery Res. 2014;2(53).
41. Steinsbekk A, Rygg L+, Lisulo M, Rise MB, Fretheim A: Group based diabetes self-management education compared to routine treatment for people with type 2 diabetes mellitus. A systematic review with meta-analysis. BMC Health Serv Res 2012, 12: 213.
42. Davies MJ, Heller S, Skinner TC, Campbell MJ, Carey ME, Cradock S, et al. Effectiveness of the diabetes education and self management for ongoing and newly diagnosed (DESMOND) programme for people with newly diagnosed type 2 diabetes: cluster randomised controlled trial. BMJ. 2008;336:491–5.
43. The Look AHEAD Research Group. Long term effects of a lifestyle intervention on weight and cardiovascular risk factors in individuals with type 2 diabetes: four year results of the look AHEAD trial. Arch Intern Med. 2010;170:1566–75.
44. Krakow D, Feulner-Krakow G. LINDA: the diabetes self-management training programme for people with type 1 or type 2 diabetes. Eur Diabetes Nurs. 2007;4:106–12.

45. Corker E, Hamilton S, Robinson E, Cotney J, Pinfold V, Rose D, et al. Viewpoint survey of mental health service users' experiences of discrimination in England 2008 - 2014. Acta Psychiatr Scand. 2016;134:6–13.
46. Care Quality Commission. 2016 Community mental health survey. Statistical release 2016.
47. Edwards PJ, Roberts I, Clarke MJ, DiGuiseppi C, Wentz R, Kwan I, et al. Methods to increase response to postal and electronic questionnaires. Cochrane Database Syst Rev. 2009; Issue 3. Art. No.: MR000008
48. Babyak MA. What you see may not be what you get: a brief, nontechnical introduction to overfitting in regression-type models. Psychosom Med. 2004;66:411–21.
49. Office for National Statistics. Graduates in the UK Labour Market: 2013. 2013.
50. Tempelaar WM, Termorshuizen F, MacCabe JH, Boks MPM, Kahn RS. Educational achievement in psychiatric patients and their siblings: a register-based study in 30 000 individuals in the Netherlands. Psychol Med. 2017;47:776–84.

4

Treatment results for severe psychiatric illness: which method is best suited to denote the outcome of mental health care?

Edwin de Beurs[1,2*], Matthijs Blankers[3,4], Philippe Delespaul[5], Erik van Duijn[6], Niels Mulder[7,8], Annet Nugter[9], Wilma Swildens[10], Bea G. Tiemens[11,12], Jan Theunissen[13^], Arno F. A. van Voorst[14] and Jaap van Weeghel[7,15,16]

Abstract

Background: The present study investigates the suitability of various treatment outcome indicators to evaluate performance of mental health institutions that provide care to patients with severe mental illness. Several categorical approaches are compared to a reference indicator (continuous outcome) using pretest-posttest data of the Health of Nation Outcome Scales (HoNOS).

Methods: Data from 10 institutions and 3189 patients were used, comprising outcomes of the first year of treatment by teams providing long-term care.

Results: Findings revealed differences between continuous indicators (standardized pre-post difference score ES and ΔT) and categorical indicators (SEM, JT_{RCI}, JT_{CS}, $JT_{RCI\&CS}$, $JT_{revised}$) on their ranking of institutions, as well as substantial differences among categorical indicators; the outcome according to the traditional JT approach was most concordant with the continuous outcome indicators.

Conclusions: For research comparing group averages, a continuous outcome indicator such as ES or ΔT is preferred, as this best preserves information from the original variable. Categorical outcomes can be used to illustrate what is accomplished in clinical terms. For categorical outcome, the classical Jacobson-Truax approach is preferred over the more complex method of Parabiaghi et al. with eight outcome categories. The latter may be valuable in clinical practice as it allows for a more detailed characterization of individual patients.

Keywords: Clinical significance, HoNOS, Routine outcome monitoring, Severe mental illness, Treatment outcome

Background

Routine Outcome Monitoring (ROM) is gathering momentum as an adjunct to treatment [1, 2] and as a basis for outcome management [3]. In the Netherlands, ROM has been stimulated by health insurers, resulting in a nationwide implementation of ROM in clinical practice to serve both goals: providing feedback on individual treatment progress and on outcomes attained with groups of patients (aggregated outcomes). The present paper focuses on the latter. Currently about 45% of all remunerated treatments can be evaluated, and results are aggregated and used to give feedback to institutions on their performance in terms of outcome [4]. For ROM assessments of patients with severe mental illness (SMI), the Health of Nation Outcome Scales (HoNOS) [5] is used, a well-known rating scale generally completed by the professional who delivers care. The HoNOS comprises 12 items, each with five response options (scoring range is 0–48), and has good psychometric properties [6]. Outcome on clinical problems and psychosocial functioning is assessed by comparing pretest and posttest total scores on the HoNOS for each patient. The simplest, most straightforward and most commonly used outcome indicator in treatment outcome research is the average change from pretest to posttest score, converted into a standardized change score or within- group effect size (ES) indicator [7, 8]. For benchmarking in the Netherlands, we have adapted this approach to a change

* Correspondence: edwin.debeurs@sbggz.nl
^Deceased
[1]Stichting Benchmark GGZ, Rembrandtlaan 46, 3723 BK Bilthoven, Netherlands
[2]Leiden University, Wassenaarseweg 52, 2333 Leiden, AK, Netherlands
Full list of author information is available at the end of the article

score based on transformed T-scores (ΔT) [9]. However, average change offers rather abstract information on the performance of treatment institutions. It would be informative to know what proportion of patients have benefitted from treatment or can be considered as recovered, yielding a performance indicator with direct appeal.

Jacobson et al. [10–12] have proposed a method to delineate the treatment results of individual patients, comprising criteria for clinically significant and statistically reliable change. The outcome is deemed significant if a patient's posttest score is within the functional range; a patient has reliably changed if the pretest-posttest change is larger than a chance fluctuation due to instrument measurement error. Various revisions of the Jacobson-Truax (JT) approach have been proposed [13–15], finding extensive application in comparing outcomes of groups of patients [16–18] as well as in ROM for individual patients [19]. Recently we evaluated the practicality of this approach as an indicator of institutional performance, using pretest and posttest scores on self-report measures. The JT approach was deemed a worthy addition to traditional performance indicators such as pretest-posttest ES or change in T-score (ΔT), as it illustrates these numerical values in a clinically meaningful manner with children and adolescents [20], and with adults with common mental disorders such as depression and anxiety disorders [9].

Application of JT to rating scales, such as the HoNOS, is less common than its application to self-report measures. The results appear of limited use when the JT approach is applied to HoNOS for the SMI population, as usually a very large proportion of patients is deemed unchanged. This may reflect the chronicity of SMI, where change – let alone(clinical) recovery or remission – is relatively uncommon within the time frame of one or two years. It may be caused by lack of responsiveness to change of the HoNOS, especially for patients with low pretest scores to begin with [21], but it may also be due to the stringency of JT criteria, particularly for reliable change [22]. In a paper published in 2005, Parabiaghi et al. [23] proposed for the HoNOS total score that a change of at least 8 points is required to deem a patient as statistically reliably changed. Such a change in score is substantial and infrequent in care provided to the majority of patients with SMI, but is also a stringent criterion when the HoNOS is applied to evaluate outpatient care for common mental disorders [21]. Other values for reliable change and alternative statistical approaches to arrive at performance indicators for use with the HoNOS have been proposed by Burgess et al. [24]. They discuss the merits of effect size (ES), reliable change index (RCI), and standard error of measurement (SEM), proposing various threshold values for these indicators to distinguish unchanged from changed patients (improved or deteriorated), varying in statistical uncertainty. Utilization of each threshold score yields three possible outcomes: no significant change, significant improvement, and significant deterioration.

In order to obtain an improved categorization for use with HoNOS data, in a more recent paper from 2014 Parabiaghi et al. [22] describe a revised approach to JT. This approach ($JT_{revised}$) focuses more on outcome than on change, underlining the significance of slightly changed and unchanged subjects. Where JT distinguishes two classes of patients (dysfunctional and functional), Parabiaghi et al. propose three classes of severity for the HoNOS total score: mild (< 10), moderate (10–13), and severe (> 13). They also propose two levels of meaningful change: reliably changed (RCI 90%; at least 8 points) and minimally changed (at least 4 points change). Potentially, the method proposed by Parabiaghi et al. [22] is an improvement over the traditional JT approach: as it allows for a more comprehensive categorization of treatment results, it seems better suited to meet the demands of clinical reality.

In the present study, we compared several categorical approaches as clinical illustrations of ES and ΔT: classifications into three categories (improved, unchanged, and deteriorated) based on ES and RCI threshold values, dichotomous classifications (JT_{RCI} and JT_{CS}), the more complex classification of JT into four categories (recovered, improved, unchanged, deteriorated, or $JT_{RCI\&CS}$), and the proposed revised JT of Parabiaghi et al. [22] into eight categories ($JT_{revised}$). We evaluated which categorical method is most suitable to denote outcome for patients with SMI by comparing the ranking of institutions according to ES and/or ΔT with their ranking based on categorical outcomes. ES/ΔT was chosen as the reference method, as this outcome indicator is appropriate given the continuous nature of the data, and it is the most commonly used effect indicator to denote within-group effect size in treatment outcome research [8]. We therefore examined which of the categorical methods revealed the largest differences in outcome between mental health institutions, whether rankings based on continuous and categorical methods were concordant and evaluated the informative value of each method.

It is important to note that the aim of the present study was to compare performance indicators for their ability to assess differences in outcome of care among institutions. Variation in outcome between providers enables us to compare performance indicators. The aim was *not* to compare the performance of the participating institutions per se. Case mix differences and differences in completeness of the data among institutions preclude firm conclusions regarding their comparative performance. We consequently choose to anonymize institutions. The reader should take note of the fact that ranking of institutes does not necessarily reflect an order in the quality of care provided; it is merely a reflection of differences in outcome, which may well be due to case mix differences or other factors affecting outcome, such as timing of assessments, proficiency in use of the HoNOS, etc.

Methods

Design and participants

This is an observational study, using data from real-life patients in everyday clinical practice. Data were collected from 10 integrated mental health institutions in the Netherlands and pertain to first-year-of-care episodes completed in 2013 and 2014. Participating institutions offer a mix of inpatient and intensive outpatient treatments, day-clinic treatment, and what is known as (Flexible) Assertive Community Treatment ((F)ACT). Patients receiving short-term crisis intervention were excluded. Data were collected as part of the treatment and anonymized before analysis. Patients were informed about use of the data for routine outcome monitoring [2], and Dutch law allows use of these anonymized ROM data for research [25]. The Central Committee on Medical Research (CCMO) approved the use of anonymized data. The study included data from N = 3189 patients. Institutions contributed between 199 and 505 cases (M = 318,9; SD = 106.7; see Table 1). Institutions are given a number that represents their position in the rank order from worst to best outcome according to ES and ΔT (both rankings are almost identical; where ties occur in one indicator, ranking of tied institutions is based on the other indicator).

Instrument

Health of nation outcome scales (HoNOS)

The Health of Nation Outcome Scales (HoNOS) was developed in 1993 by the Research Unit of the Royal College of Psychiatrists to evaluate clinical treatment outcome [5]. The HoNOS is a rating scale, to be administered by a trained practitioner or research assistant. The instrument is short and easy to complete, and it was designed for routine clinical work. Its use is widespread, as it is the prime outcome measure for mental health care in the UK [6], Australia [26], and New Zealand [27]. In the Netherlands, use of the HoNOS is limited to patients with SMI, who receive "integrated care , i.e. support living, work, and social relations in addition to psychiatric treatment" [25]. It consists of 12 items that cover clinical problems and social functioning. Each item is evaluated on a 5-point (0–4) Likert scale, resulting in a total score ranging from 0 to 48. Response options vary for each item and are anchored with a comprehensive description. Several studies have evaluated the HoNOS and found support for its reliability, validity, and sensitivity to change [25, 27, 28].

Methods for rendering treatment outcome

Continuous indicators (ES and ΔT)

A popular estimate of treatment outcome is the within-group effect size estimator ES, denoting the size of the pretest-posttest change in standardized units [8]. It provides a clear indication of what has been achieved in treatment [29], and is calculated as the difference of pretest and posttest scores divided by the pretest standard deviation of the instrument for patients.

ΔT is an outcome indicator similar to ES, but based on the difference between pretest and posttest scores transformed to standardized T-scores [30] with a normal distribution of scores. Raw HoNOS scores are asymmetrical and skewed to the right, which implies that intervals in the lower scale range are not equal to intervals in the higher range. Normalization turns the HoNOS into a true interval scale, a measurement level required for subtraction [31]. T-scores have a standard deviation of 10, therefore ΔT is similar to ES but 10 times larger. For the present study, categorical indicators based on raw scores were compared to ES, and categorical indicators based on T-scores were compared to ΔT.

Table 1 Number of patients, gender, age, pretest-posttest response rate, and length of treatment (days) per institution

Institution		1	2	3	4	5	6	7	8	9	10	Total
Included	N	1056	771	968	4754	2061	9221	2177	2076	1304	589	16,771
Assessed	N	265	192	215	290	336	342	505	438[a]	407	199	3189
	%	8.3	6.0	6.7	9.1	10.5	10.7	15.8	13.7	12.8	6.2	100.0
Response	%	25.1	24.9	22.2	6.1	16.3	33.7	23.2	21.1	31.2	33.8	19.1
Length of	M	337.7	328.9	326.8	284.1	312.4	314.0	288.6	294.8	225.6	329.9	297.9
treatment	SD	51.8	57.4	54.6	99.2	73.2	80.5	91.8	85.8	138.9	41.8	93.5
Males	N	164	121	130	238	170	227	282	155	248	123	1858
	%	61.9	63.0	60.5	82.1	50.6	66.4	55.8	35.4	60.9	61.8	58.3
Age	M	40.0	40.2	42.7	38.8	42.5	37.8	42.7	40.6	39.0	42.6	40.7
	SD	12.4	12.8	11.5	10.6	11.6	13.0	12.3	11.9	12.4	13.8	12.3
HoNOS	M	9.7	14.0	13.6	14.9	13.3	11.2	11.5	12.3	13.3	10.3	12.4
pretest	SD	5.4	3.0	2.0	7.5	6.0	5.8	6.1	6.4	7.2	6.1	6.5
HoNOS	M	9.4	12.1	12,8	13.8	11.5	9.5	9.6	9.8	10.5	7.9	10.5
posttest	SD	6.4	6.8	7.0	6.9	5.9	5.8	6.0	6.2	6.8	5.8	6.5

[a]For 112 (12.1%) of 438 patients of institution 8 no information on gender was provided

Categorical indicators based on ES, RCI and RCI threshold values

Burgess, Pirkis and Coombs [24] propose various threshold values for ES, RCI, and SEM when using raw HoNOS scores to classify patients as unchanged, improved or deteriorated. Significantly changed are patients with a change of at least $ES_{medium} = 4$ or $ES_{large} = 6$, four RCI thresholds with different confidence levels ($RCI_{95} = 10$, $RCI_{90} = 9$; $RCI_{80} = 7$ and $RCI_{67} = 5$), and a single threshold value based on SEM proposed by McHorney and Tarlov [32]. SEM is calculated by multiplying the standard deviation by the square root of 1 minus the reliability coefficient. For the HoNOS when used with inpatients Burgess et al. [24] propose SEM = 5.

Categorical indicators based on the JT approach

Traditional Jacobson-Truax (JT_{CS}, JT_{RCI} and $JT_{RCI\&CS}$) JT is a widely accepted approach to denote clinically significant change in patients and to identify meaningful individual improvement [16]. Based on the criteria described in the Introduction, JT yields three indicators: (a) clinical significance composed of a cut-off point where "the patient moves outside the dysfunctional population or within functional population" (JT_{CS}); (b) reliable change index, which indicates whether the change that occurred was statistically significant (JT_{RCI}); and (c) the combination of these two ($JT_{RCI\&CS}$), which categorizes outcome of treatment into "deteriorated", "unchanged", "improved" or "recovered" [11]. We applied the traditional JT approach to raw scores (RCI = 8, CS = 5) [23] and to transformed T-scores (RCI = 5 and CS = 42.5) [9, 20].

Revised JT model

Parabiaghi et al. [22] proposed a revised model of JT to denote meaningful clinical outcome for patients with SMI, using two change and two endstate threshold values. First, they proposed three levels of change: reliable change (RCI: change ≥8), minimal change (based on the SEM: change ≥4), or no change or stability (change < 4). They also proposed distinguishing three levels of severity: mild (HoNOS score < 10), moderate (score = 10–13), and severe (score > 13). All in all, this combination of two change criteria and two severity cut-offs leads to a complex "research model" comprising 23 outcome categories (see Parabiaghi et al. [22]; Fig. 1, p. 299). For clinical use they propose a simplified version using a single change criterion (at least 4 points change, the more lenient criterion for a minimally detectable change based on SEM; the chosen value of 4 is based on data of Italian and Dutch patients) and the two CS values (10 and 13). Combination of three possible outcomes according to SEM-based minimally detectable change (improved, unchanged, or worsened) and three severity levels (mild, moderate, and severe) results in a categorization into nine groups (see Parabiaghi et al. [22]; Fig. 2, p. 300). Stable patients are categorized into three levels: "stability in mild illness", "stability in moderate illness", and "stability within severe illness", utilizing the cut-off values of 10 and 13 on the means of their pretest and posttest HoNOS scores. Based on the posttest HoNOS score, three improved groups are distinguished: "improved to mild illness", "improved to moderate illness", and "improved within severe illness". As worsening to a mild level is a relatively rare event, those who showed significant worsening from pretest to posttest were allocated to only two categories: "worsening to mild or moderate illness" and "worsening to severe illness", using the cut-off value of 13 to distinguish between the two groups [22]. Hence the simplified $JT_{revised}$ model results in eight outcome categories (see Table 5).

Statistical analysis

Outcomes between institutions were compared and the ability of the various indicators to distinguish between them was investigated. A repeated-measures ANOVA for a 2 (time) × 10 (institution) design was conducted on transformed T-scores to test for main effects of time and institution as well as for their interaction to compare outcome slopes of institutions over time. Post hoc pairwise comparisons were conducted to assess which institutions differed from each other. For the categorical outcomes we assessed the differences in proportions with chi-squared tests. Ranking of institutes according to each outcome indicator is presented and compared to ranking according to ES or ΔT (the reference indicator for raw scores or T-scores, respectively). Concordance between rankings is assessed with the Spearman Rank correlation coefficient.

Results

The initial dataset comprised 16,771 patients who received treatment; 8402 (50.1%) were assessed at pretest and for 38.0% of these posttest data were available, yielding a final sample of 3189 patients with complete pretest and posttest data and an overall response rate of 19.1%. Table 1 presents background information on the participating patients. The duration of care episodes ranged from 30 to 446 days (M = 297.8; SD = 93.4), with no significant differences between institutions. Pretest selection, posttest attrition and overall response rates (the proportion of care episodes with complete pretest and posttest data) varied considerably between institutions (range: 6.1–33.8%).

There were statistically significant, albeit small, differences between institutions in mean age and gender; overall 58.3% of patients were males and gender was unevenly distributed among the 10 institutions ($\chi^2(9) = 103.44$; $p < .001$), with Institution 4 treating more males (82.1% vs. 58.3% for the total population). Participants' age ranged from 17 to 84 years (M = 40.7; SD = 12.3) and varied among institutions ($F(9) = 7.34$; $p < .001$; $\eta^2 = .02$), with

Institutions 4, 6, and 9 treating somewhat younger patients. The mean pretest score on the HoNOS differed significantly between institutions ($F(9) = 18.04$; $p < .001$; $\eta^2 = .05$), with Institutions 1, 6, and 10 having lower scores (i.e. less impairment in function) than the others according to Bonferroni corrected pairwise comparisons.

There were large differences in diagnostic composition of the case mix among institutions. Table 2 presents this diagnostic information. The largest group among the diagnoses is psychotic disorders (47.3%), followed by mood/anxiety/somatoform disorders (17.9%) and personality disorders (11.4%). The smallest groups are pervasive developmental disorders (10.5%), substance abuse (5.0%), and bipolar disorder (4.9%). Patient composition differs significantly among institutions ($\chi^2(54) = 1583.09$; $p < .001$), with Institution 4 treating more patients with substance-related disorders (36.9%) and fewer psychotic disorders (13.4%), Institution 5 treating more patients with mood/anxiety/somatoform disorders (36.0%) and fewer personality disorders (18.8%), Institution 6 treating more patients with pervasive developmental disorders (44.7%), and Institutions 8, 5, and 1 treating more personality disorders (19.4, 18.8 and 17.7%, respectively).

Difference between pretest-posttest change on HoNOS T-scores among institutions was analyzed in a 2 (time) × 10 (institution) repeated-measures ANOVA. This revealed statistically significant main effects of time ($F(1) = 233.4$; $p < .001$; $\eta^2 = .068$) and institution ($F(9) = 23.6$; $p < .001$; $\eta^2 = .063$), which reflects a difference over time as well as between institutions regardless of time. More importantly, there was a significant interaction effect (time x institution) revealing a difference in outcome slope between health institutions over time ($F(9,3179) = 3.33$; $p < .001$; $\eta^2 = .009$). Pairwise comparisons of institutions (with Bonferroni correction) revealed that Institutions 5 to 10 reported larger pretest-posttest differences than Institutions 1 to 4.

Ranking of institutions was based on ES and ΔT. Hence, institutions with a higher rank number have a larger ES than those with a low rank number, as Table 3 shows. This table also presents results using threshold values for ES, SEM, and JT_{RCI90}. All categorizations reveal significant differences among institutions (all $p < .001$). The proportions of reliably changed patients from Table 3 using the RCI threshold of at least 8 points as proposed by Parabiaghi et al. [23] varied among institutions ($\chi^2(9) = 58.1$; $p < .001$), as did the proportions of patients with a posttest score < 5, denoting a clinically significant change ($\chi^2(9) = 42.8$; $p < .001$). Finally, combining both indices in four outcome categories also reveals differences among institutions ($\chi^2(27) = 111.4$; $p < .001$). Institutions with a higher rank number had more recovered (= Institution 9: 17.4% vs. = Institution 1: 4.9%) and fewer deteriorated patients (= Institution 9: 10.6% vs. Institution 6: = 3.8%). The results indicate that 11.2% (n = 356) of patients had recovered, 6.1% (n = 196) had improved, 75.9% (n = 2421) remained unchanged, and 6.7% (n = 215) had deteriorated. The large proportion of unchanged patients results from the stringent RCI criterion of at least 8 points change. The ranking of institutes diverges considerably among indicators, and most indicators have no statistically significant association with ES, except for the improved and reliable change (JT_{RCI}) indicators, which correspond best with ES. All in all, most of the indicators proposed by Burgess et al. [24] and $JT_{RCI\&CS}$ based on raw scores are insufficiently concordant with ES.

Table 2 Overview of the case mix composition regarding main psychiatric diagnosis per institution

Institution		1	2	3	4	5	6	7	8	9	10	Total
Psych. Dis.	N	132	128	127	39	108	108	282	195	264	125	1508
	%	49.8	66.7	59.1	13.4	32.1	31.6	55.8	44.5	64.9	62.8	47.3
MAS	N	27	23	25	61	121	29	110	80	64	31	571
	%	10.2	12.0	11.6	21.0	36.0	8.5	21.8	18.3	15.7	15.6	17.9
Pers. Dis.	N	47	11	21	38	63	28	37	85	21	12	363
	%	17.7	5.7	9.8	13.1	18.8	8.2	7.3	19.4	5.2	6.0	11.4
Perv. DD	N	32	20	14	36	17	153	29	15	11	9	336
	%	12.1	10.4	6.5	12.4	5.1	44.7	5.7	3.4	2.7	4.5	10.5
Bipolar Dis.	N	18	5	7	4	14	17	12	23	38	18	156
	%	6.8	2.6	3.3	1.4	4.2	5.0	2.4	5.3	9.3	9.0	4.9
Substance	N	4	2	17	107	6	4	5	12	0	1	158
	%	1.5	1.0	7.9	36.9	1.8	1.2	1.0	2.7	0.0	0.5	5.0
Other	N	5	3	4	5	7	3	30	28	9	3	97
	%	1.9	1.6	1.9	1.7	2.1	0.9	5.9	6.4	2.2	1.5	3.0

Psych. Dis. Psychotic Disorders, *MAS* Mood, anxiety, and somatoform disorders, *Pers. Dis.* Personality Disorders, *Perv. DD* Pervasive Developmental Disorders, *Bipolar Dis.* Bipolar Disorders, *Substance* Substance Abuse

Table 3 Effect Size (ES) and percentage of patients in outcome categories based on raw HoNOS scores and classification according to various ES_{medium}, SEM, and $JT_{RCI\text{-}90}$ threshold values, and according to JT_{RCI95}, JT_{CS}, and $JT_{RCI\&CS}$

Institution		1	2	3	4	5	6	7	8	9	10	Total	Rank order[a]	Rho
Continuous:	ES	0.06	0.18	0.19	0.24	0.29	0.29	0.32	0.38	0.38	0.39	0.29	1 2 3 4 5/6 7 8/9 10	
Categorical:														
$ES_{medium} \leq -4$	deteriorated	20.0	19.3	20.5	20.7	15.2	11.4	17.8	14.8	20.9	14.1	17.3	9 4 3 1 2 7 5 8 10 6	.35
$-4 < ES_{medium} < 4$	unchanged	56.2	48.4	43.7	40.0	49.7	57.6	45.0	42.7	34.4	46.7	45.9	6 1 5 2 10 7 3 8 4 9	.38
$ES_{medium} \geq 4$	improved	23.8	32.3	35.8	39.3	35.1	31.0	37.2	42.5	44.7	39.2	36.8	1 5 2 8 4 3 6 9 10 7	.71*
$SEM \leq -5$	deteriorated	15.5	13.0	15.3	17.6	12.5	9.1	14.5	11.0	16.2	11.1	13.5	4 9 1 3 7 2 5 10 8 6	.35
$-5 < SEM < 5$	unchanged	63.4	60.4	56.3	49.3	57.1	68.1	53.7	52.7	45.9	54.8	55.5	6 1 2 5 3 10 7 8 4 9	.55
$SEM \geq 5$	improved	21.1	26.6	28.4	33.1	30.4	22.8	31.9	36.3	37.8	34.2	30.9	1 6 2 3 5 7 4 10 8 9	.79**
$JT_{RCI90} \leq -9$	deteriorated	8.3	4.2	7.0	9.3	3.6	2.3	5.1	3.9	7.6	2.5	5.4	4 1 9 3 7 2 8 5 10 6	.43
$9 < JT_{RCI90} < 9$	unchanged	85.3	82.8	80.0	71.4	87.5	88.0	82.2	79.2	69.0	83.9	80.6	6 5 1 10 2 7 3 8 4 9	.24
$JT_{RCI90} \geq 9$	improved	6.4	13.0	13.0	19.3	8.9	9.6	12.7	16.9	23.3	13.6	14.1	1 5 6 7 2/3 10 8 4 9	.51
JT_{RCI} (change ≥8)	reliable change	9.4	14.6	14.9	19.7	11.3	14.3	17.4	21.7	27.0	15.6	17.3	1 5 6 2 3 10 7 4 8 9	.64*
JT_{CS} (post < 5)	clinical change	13.6	9.9	7.0	7.2	8.6	14.9	16.0	15.5	15.2	21.1	13.3	3 4 5 2 10 1 6 8 7 9	.56
$JT_{RCI\&CS}$	deteriorated	9.1	5.2	8.4	10.3	3.9	3.8	5.9	5.7	10.6	4.5	6.7	9 4 1 3 7 8 2 10 5 6	.14
	unchanged	81.5	80.2	76.7	70.0	84.8	81.9	76.6	72.6	62.4	79.9	75.9	5 6 1 2 10 3 7 8 4 9	.39
	improved	4.5	4.7	3.3	4.1	3.0	6.1	6.3	8.7	9.6	8.0	6.1	5 3 4 1 2 6 7 10 8 9	.75*
	recovered	4.9	9.9	11.6	15.5	8.3	8.2	11.1	13.0	17.4	7.5	11.2	1 10 6 5 2 7 3 8 4 9	.24

$ES = \frac{M_{pretest} - M_{posttest}}{SD_{pretest}}$; $SEM = SD \times \sqrt{1 - r_{ii}}$; $JT_{RCI} = \frac{M_{pretest} - M_{posttest}}{SEM}$; $JT_{CS} = \frac{SD_{pre} * M_{post} + SD_{post} * M_{pre}}{SD_{pre} + SD_{post}}$

ES_{medium} implies a change of at least 4 points; SEM implies 5 points change or more; JT_{RCI90} implies 9 points change; JT_{RCI90}, JT_{CS}, and $JT_{RCI\&CS}$ imply 8 points change and transgression of a score of 5 from pretest to posttest. Rho is Spearman rank correlation coefficient between the ranking based on an indicator and ranking based on ES (*$p < .05$; **$p < .01$)

[a]Ranked from the worst (1) to the best (10) outcome according to the indicator; categories "unchanged" and "deteriorated" have a reversed rank order: the fewer the patients the better the outcome

Table 4 presents the results when we convert the HoNOS scores to T-scores. Again, institutions with a high rank number performed better (ΔT = range 3.3–4.3) than those with a lower rank number (ΔT range 0.9–3.0). Using the threshold of a change ΔT > 5 [9, 20], the proportions of reliably changed patients differed significantly among institutions ($\chi^2(9) = 29.8$; $p < .001$), as did the proportions of patients transgressing the threshold of CS = 42.5 (pretest ≥42.5; posttest < 42.5), denoting clinically significant change ($\chi^2(9) = 30.4$; $p < .001$). Combining the two indices into $JT_{RCI\&CS}$ with four categories also reveals significant differences among institutions ($\chi^2(27) = 76.1$; $p < .001$). Furthermore, with the traditional $JT_{RCI\&CS}$ method applied to T-scores, patients got more evenly distributed over the outcome categories: in total 18.8% (n = 598) of patients were considered recovered, 22.2% (n = 709) had improved, 40.0% (n = 1277) remained unchanged, and 19.0% (n = 605) had deteriorated. Institutions with a higher rank have more recovered patients (Institution 10: 24.6% vs. = Institution 1: 12.5%) and fewer deteriorated

Table 4 Mean ΔT and percentage of patients in outcome categories based on T-scores according to the JT approach

Institution		1	2	3	4	5	6	7	8	9	10	Total	Rank order[a]	Rho
Continuous:	Mean ΔT	0.9	2.0	2.0	2.6	2.8	3.0	3.3	4.1	4.3	4.3	3.1	1 2/3 4 5 6 7 8 9/10	
Categorical:														
$JT_{RCI\text{-}95}$ (> 5)	improved	33.6	34.4	37.7	40.0	37.5	36.5	43.0	46.8	46.9	45.7	41.0	1 2 6 5 3 4 7 10 8 9	.86**
JT_{CS} (42.5)	changed	14.0	14.1	19.1	14.8	17.6	20.5	23.6	23.1	23.8	25.6	20.2	1 2 4 5 3 6 8 7 9 10	.95**
$JT_{RCI\&CS}$	deteriorated	23.4	18.2	21.4	22.1	16.1	14.3	20.2	16.0	21.9	17.1	19.0	1 4 9 3 7 2 10 5 8 6	.38
	unchanged	43.0	47.4	40.9	37.9	46.4	49.1	36.8	37.2	31.2	37.2	40.0	6 2 5 1 3 4 8/10 7 9	.65*
	improved	21.1	21.4	19.1	26.9	22.0	18.7	21.4	24.9	23.6	21.1	22.2	6 3 1 10 2/7 5 9 8 4	.26
	recovered	12.5	13.0	18.6	13.1	15.5	17.8	21.6	21.9	23.3	24.6	18.8	1 2 4 5 6 3 7 8 9 10	.93**

[a]Institutions are rank ordered according to increased performance (the higher the rank number the more improved or recovered patients); categories "unchanged" and "deteriorated" have a reversed rank order (fewer patients means a higher rank and a better outcome)
*$p < .05$; **$p < .01$

patients (Institution 10: 17.1% vs. = Institution 1: 23.4%). The Rho correlation coefficients indicate that the rankings based on ΔT scores (in Table 4) are more concordant than rankings based on raw HoNOS difference scores (ES in Table 3), with $JT_{RCI\&CS}$ recovery having the highest concordance with ΔT, followed by the category of unchanged patients. However, lack of concordance is also noteworthy. Institution 9, for instance, has the second-highest ranking based on ΔT, but also the third-largest proportion of deteriorated patients (based on $JT_{RCI\&CS}$; see Table 4).

The results of Table 5 show the categorization according to the revised JT proposed by Parabiaghi et al. (2014). A significant difference among institutions in these categories is found, with higher rates of patients in the "mild illness" and "improvement to mild illness" categories and lower rates of "stability in severe illness" or "worsening in/to severe illness" among institutions with a high ranking ($\chi^2(63) = 230.9$; $p < .001$). Correspondence between ranking of institutes according to ES and the $JT_{revised}$ categorization is low, except for the category "improvement to mild illness".

Discussion

In the present study, we compared various categorical indicators on their usefulness to illustrate differences between institutions regarding treatment outcome. The primary aim of the study was to test the suitability of various categorical methods to denote treatment outcome in mental health care for patients with SMI using the HoNOS as assessment instrument. We were fortunate to find differences in outcomes between institutions and could use their data to evaluate various methods to delineate outcome. We also assessed the suitability of a number of methods to compare institutions. The results revealed differences in ranking institutions between the two continuous indicators (ES and ΔT) and the categorical indicators (SEM, JT_{RCI}, JT_{CS}, $JT_{RCI\&CS}$, $JT_{revised}$). Indicators based on categorical outcomes yielded quite divergent rankings; the categories of the traditional JT approach were most concordant with the continuous outcome indicators ES and ΔT, particularly JT_{RCI} and JT_{CS} based on T-scores.

The traditional JT approach ($JT_{RCI\&CS}$) with four categories is applied frequently in practice and provides useful information on patients' condition after treatment [9, 11, 16]. However, as an outcome indicator for aggregated data it has some serious drawbacks. As the indicator classifies patients into four categories, it is impossible to rank health institutions consistently: ranking according to proportion of recovered patients yields a different order than ranking according to proportion of reliably changed patients, and so forth. A possible solution would be to collapse the four categories into two, in order to get a ranking based on less complex information, but this reduces information value and statistical power. Fedorov, Mannino and Zhang [33] calculated that dichotomizing information leads to a substantial loss of statistical power (at least 36% reduction when data are made binary and 19% when data are converted to three categories). These percentages are based on optimal cut-off points. In practice, the loss of statistical power may be greater. Indeed, Markon, Chmielewski and Miller [34] showed that a sample needed to be twice as large when moving from a continuous to a dichotomous outcome. Statistical power can be increased by adding more categories, but this reintroduces the complexity of interpreting the outcome data.

Another drawback of the $JT_{RCI\&CS}$ method is that it will result in a large proportion of "unchanged" patients if a stringent criterion for $RCI \geq 8$ is applied to raw HoNOS scores. Such a large category provides little information and is hard to interpret, as we are unsure whether to regard this outcome as disappointing or as successful stabilization (this of course also depends on the goal of treatment or care). Using various alternative cut-off values for deterioration or improvement, as proposed by Burgess

Table 5 Percentage of subjects classified into 8 outcome categories based on raw scores according to the revised JT approach of Parabiaghi et al. [22]

institution	1	2	3	4	5	6	7	8	9	10	Total	Rank order[a]	Rho
Mild illness	40.4	17.7	21.4	15.2	22.9	36.3	29.3	24.9	21.1	34.2	26.4	4 2 9 3 5 8 7 10 6 1	.13
Improvement to mild illness	18.5	17.7	22.3	18.3	20.5	22.8	26.9	28.3	31.2	32.7	24.6	2 4 1 5 3 6 7 8 9 10	.92**
Improvement to moderate illness	3.8	6.8	7.0	11.4	7.7	4.4	6.9	8.2	7.1	4.5	6.9	1 6 10 2 7 3 9 5 8 4	.23
Improvement within severe illness	1.5	7.8	6.5	9.7	6.8	3.8	3.4	5.9	6.4	2.0	5.3	1 10 7 6 8 9 3 5 2 4	−.29
Stability in moderate illness	12.1	12.0	8.4	9.3	10.4	11.4	9.1	7.8	5.9	8.0	9.2		
Worsening to moderate illness	4.9	5.2	3.3	2.8	2.7	2.0	4.0	3.9	4.4	3.0	3.6	2 1 9 7 8 3 10 4 5 6	.26
Stability in severe illness	7.2	20.3	15.8	17.9	18.8	11.7	8.9	11.4	10.3	8.0	12.5		
Worsening in/to severe illness	11.7	12.5	15.3	15.5	10.1	7.6	11.5	9.6	13.5	7.5	11.4	4 3 9 2 1 7 5 8 6 10	.52

Improvement based on SEM: pre-to-posttest change ≤4
Mild illness: post < 10; moderate illness: post = 10–13; severe illness post > 13
[a]Rank order is not provided for stability categories; rank order of worsening is reversed
$^{**}p < .01$

et al. [24], does not lead to a categorization highly concordant with ES. The present results show that applying the JT categorization after raw scores have been converted into transformed T-scores yields a more even distribution of patients over the outcome categories. Moreover, ranking of institutes according to proportion of recovered patients based on transformed T-scores is more concordant with outcome according to ΔT than the ranking using raw scores. We therefore recommend using transformed T-scores with the proposed cut-off values RCI > 5 and CS = 42.5 – corresponding to RCI > 2 to RCI > 4 (depending on the position on the scale) and CS = 8 in raw score on the HoNOS – as the most suitable approach to convey differences in performance between institutions, given that this indicator is methodologically sound as it uses data that have been transformed into a normal distribution.

Parabiaghi et al. [22] evaluated a more refined approach for meaningful change and outcome. We examined this approach and compared it with the traditional JT approach, to investigate how these categorical methods compare in their convergence with the continuous method and how they compare in denoting outcome in a meaningful way. The results indicate that the proposed revision may have advantages over the traditional JT approach, as it provides a quite meticulous and clinically meaningful way to denote clinical status and outcome of care for individual patients with SMI. $JT_{revised}$ may thus be more informative for clinicians when monitoring progress and choosing the most appropriate course of treatment as compared to the traditional JT approach. Further validation of $JT_{revised}$ is needed to justify use of its more refined outcome categories. It should also be noted that the threshold value for change based on SEM (change ≥4 is deemed meaningful) needs validation, as it is far more lenient than the RCI90 ≥ 9 based on the formulas proposed by Jacobson and Truax and the reliability of the HoNOS may not justify the chosen low-threshold value. Future research, for instance directly comparing the predictive validity of the categorization according to the traditional JT approach and the $JT_{revised}$ in terms of further course of treatment, will reveal which approach best predicts need for care after the first year. However, the Parabiaghi approach is deemed too complex for research on groups of patients or for use as a performance indicator comparing aggregated outcomes of institutions: with eight categories it is not considered a practical or more appropriate alternative to the simpler traditional $JT_{RCI\&CS}$ with four categories.

A strength of the present study is its use of real-life data, collected in everyday clinical practice. The study also uses a considerably large data set, in number of both institutions and patients per institution, boosting confidence in the generalizability of the findings for clinical practice in the Netherlands and bringing about ample statistical power to find differences among methods to denote outcome. Indeed, substantial variation in outcome was found among institutions, offering a realistic test of the usefulness of various approaches to denote outcome of patients in care for SMI.

A limitation of the study is that only data from the first year of care were analyzed. Patients with SMI typically stay in care for a longer period. Their change in subsequent years of care is likely to be substantially smaller, as may also be the case for outcome variation between institutions. It should be noted that the substantial differences between institutions in case mix composition for demographics and clinical features of patients, as well as differences in completeness of provided data, imply that outcomes of institutions are potentially confounded by these pretest differences. For example, institutions' patient populations vary in pretest severity, a variable strongly associated with posttest scores and gain scores; this implies that the level of pretest severity is also associated with categorical outcomes. Higher average pretest levels leave more room for reliable improvement, lower pretest levels leave less room but make achieving recovery status more likely. In addition, case mix composition between institutions also differed in ratio of inpatients to community patients. This underscores the need for case mix correction when comparing institutional performance. We reanalyzed the data after case mix correction for several variables that appeared associated with outcome (pretest severity, age, and bipolar disorder). This case mix model explained 23% of outcome variation (predominantly by pretest HoNOS scores). Correction did influence average outcome of institutions, but overall the ranking of institutes remained the same. However, differences between institutions diminished somewhat, and with this smaller contrast between institutions the rankings of the various approaches were more diverse. Consequently, the concordance between approaches was also more varied. As a further limitation of the study, response rates for institutions ranged from 6.1 to 33.8%, compromising the representativeness of the data for the institutions. Hence, the present results do not necessarily reflect differences in quality of care between institutions and should be examined cautiously, also bearing in mind that comparing institutions was not our aim. Moreover, the overall response rate limits the generalizability of the study findings, as we do not know whether outcome data are missing systematically.

The HoNOS total score may be considered too small a basis to evaluate the outcome of an individual patient or appraise the overall performance of mental health institutions. Use of the HoNOS is widespread, not only for outcome monitoring but also to assign patients to clusters based on their treatment needs. Large datasets have thus become available to evaluate the psychometric quality of the instrument, and some negative findings have emerged. For instance, the HoNOS appears not to be associated with need-for-care as operationalized by costs of treatment in a large British cohort of 1343 patients with common mental health problems [35]. For this patient group, the sensitivity to change in severity of psychopathology of the HoNOS appears to be limited as only three items (7, 8, and 9) seem relevant and appropriate [21]. The utility of the HoNOS for clustering patients into groups of various need levels has been questioned as well [36]. Finally, the factorial structure of the HoNOS has been criticized: the HoNOS does not appear to be unidimensional, which casts doubt on the validity of calculating a total score. Various multidimensional factorial models have been proposed, but none appears to have sufficient fit to be deemed good over the full range of psychiatric disorders [37]. Further development of measurement instruments for appropriate outcome domains (assessing severity of symptomatology, functioning, and personal recovery) is therefore needed, and several such projects are currently underway, internationally as well as in the Netherlands. Finally, the present study lacks an external criterion to validate the various methods to denote outcome. Additional information on patients' posttreatment functioning is needed, such as continued use of mental health care after the first year of treatment or long-term follow-up data (e.g. several years after treatment has ended).

Conclusions

Methods based on continuous variables – ES on raw scores or ΔT based on transformed T-scores – are the most convenient choice for research or for comparing institutions, subdivisions or teams: they have the best statistical power and allow for a straightforward ranking of institutions. Based on this study, we conclude that the use of categorical approaches is complicated as it matters importantly which outcome category is considered for ranking institutions on their performance. However, information from categorical approaches is of *supplemental* value, as this illustrates what differences in rank order mean in clinically relevant terms and reveals what has been accomplished in clinically meaningful terms. We recommend the traditional JT approach as a good choice among the categorical indicators. The revision by Parabiaghi et al. [22] provides more detailed information, but eight outcome categories may be too complex for a practical comparison of institutions.

Abbreviations

CS: Clinical Significant change; ES: Effect Size; HoNOS: Health of Nation Outcome Scale; JT: Jacobson-Truax; RCI: Reliable Change Index; SEM: Standard Error of Measurement; ΔT: Difference T-score from pretest to posttest

Acknowledgements

The authors would like to thank the participating institutions for providing data for the study.

Authors' contributions

EdeB was the chief investigator. He aggregated, analyzed, and interpreted the data and wrote the first draft of the paper. MB, PD, EvD, NM, AN, WS, BT, JT, AvV, and JvW contributed to the formulation of the research question, analysis, and writing of this study. All authors read, revised, commented and approved intermediate versions of the paper. Sadly, JT passed away on October 16th, 2017. MB, PD, EvD, NM, AN, WS, BT, AvV, and JvW approved the final version of the paper.

Consent for publication

Not applicable.

Competing interest

The authors declare that they have no competing interest.

Author details

[1]Stichting Benchmark GGZ, Rembrandtlaan 46, 3723 BK Bilthoven, Netherlands. [2]Leiden University, Wassenaarseweg 52, 2333 Leiden, AK, Netherlands. [3]Arkin, Klaprozenweg 111, 1033 Amsterdam, NN, Netherlands. [4]Trimbos Institute, Da Costakade 45, 3521 Utrecht, VS, Netherlands. [5]Maastricht University, Minderbroedersberg 4-6, 6211 Maastricht, LK, Netherlands. [6]GGZ Delfland, Sint Jorisweg 2, 2612 Delft, GA, Netherlands. [7]Parnassia Bavo GGZ Zorgholding BV, Monsterseweg 93, 2553 Den Haag, RJ, Netherlands. [8]Erasmus University, Burgemeester Oudlaan 50, 3062 Rotterdam, PA, Netherlands. [9]GGZ Noord-Holland Noord, Postbus 18, 1850 Heilo, BA, Netherlands. [10]Altrecht Mental Health Care, Lange Nieuwstraat 119, 3512 Utrecht, PG, Netherlands. [11]Pro Persona Mental health Services ProCES, Indigo, Wolfheze 2, 6874 Wolfheze, BE, Netherlands. [12]Radboud University, Comeniuslaan 4, 6525 Nijmegen, HP, Netherlands. [13]GGZ Ingeest, VU University Medical Center Amsterdam, De Boelelaan 1117, 1081 Amsterdam, HV, Netherlands. [14]GGZ Centraal, Utrechtseweg 266, 3818 Amersfoort, EW, Netherlands. [15]Phrenos, Trimbos Institute, Da Costakade 45, 3521 Utrecht, VS, Netherlands. [16]Tilburg University, Warandelaan 2, 5037 Tilburg, AB, Netherlands.

References

1. Lambert MJ. Presidential address: what we have learned from a decade of research aimed at improving psychotherapy outcome in routine care. Psychother Res. 2007;17(1):1–14.
2. de Beurs E, den Hollander-Gijsman ME, van rood YR, van der wee NJ, Giltay EJ, van Noorden MS, van der Lem R, E vF, Zitman FG. Routine outcome monitoring in the Netherlands: practical experiences with a web-based strategy for the assessment of treatment outcome in clinical practice. Clin Psychol Psychother. 2011;18(1):1–12.
3. Ellwood PM. Shattuck lecture–Outcomes management. A technology of patient experience N Engl J Med. 1988;318(23):1549–56.
4. de Beurs E, Barendregt M, Warmerdam L, editors. Behandeluitkomsten: bron voor kwaliteitsbeleid in de GGZ [Treatment outcome: source of quality management in mental Health Care]. Amsterdam: Boom; 2017.
5. Wing JK, Beevor AS, Curtis RH, Park SB, Hadden S, Burns A. Health of the nation outcome scales (HoNOS). Research and development Br J Psychiatry. 1998; 172(1):11–8.
6. Pirkis JE, Burgess PM, Kirk PK, Dodson S, Coombs TJ, Williamson MK. A review of the psychometric properties of the health of the nation outcome scales (HoNOS) family of measures. Health Qual Life Outcomes. 2005;3(1):1–12.
7. Cohen J. Statistical power analysis for the behavioral sciences. 2nd ed. Hillsdale, NJ: Lawrence Erlbaum Associates; 1988.
8. Seidel JA, Miller SD, Chow DL. Effect size calculations for the clinician: methods and comparability. Psychother Res. 2014;24(4):470–84.
9. de Beurs E, Barendregt M, de Heer A, van Duijn E, Goeree B, Kloos M, Kooiman K, Lionarons H, Merks A. Comparing methods to denote treatment outcome in clinical research and benchmarking mental health care. Clin Psychol Psychother. 2016;23:308–18.
10. Jacobson NS, Roberts LJ, Berns SB, McGlinchey JB. Methods for defining and determining the clinical significance of treatment effects: description, application, and alternatives. J Consult Clin Psychol. 1999;67(3):300–7.
11. Jacobson NS, Truax P. Clinical significance: a statistical approach to defining meaningful change in psychotherapy research. J Consult Clin Psychol. 1991; 59(1):12–9.

12. Jacobson NS, Follette WC, Revenstorf D. Toward a standard definition of clinically significant change. Behav Ther. 1986;17:308–11.
13. Hageman WJJM, Arrindell WA. Establishing clinically significant change: increment of precision and the distinction between individual and group level of analysis. Behav Res Ther. 1999;37(12):1169–93.
14. Maassen GH. The unreliable change of reliable change indices. Behav Res Ther. 2001;39(4):495–8.
15. Tingey R, Lambert M, Burlingame G, Hansen N. Assessing clinical significance: proposed extensions to method. Psychother Res. 1996;6(2): 109–23.
16. Wise EA. Methods for analyzing psychotherapy outcomes: a review of clinical significance, reliable change, and recommendations for future directions. J Pers Assess. 2004;82(1):50–9.
17. Atkins DC, Bedics JD, McGlinchey JB, Beauchaine TP. Assessing clinical significance: does it matter which method we use? J Consult Clin Psychol. 2005;73(5):982–9.
18. Ogles BM, Lunnen KM, Bonesteel K. Clinical significance: history, application, and current practice. Clin Psychol Rev. 2001;21(3):421–46.
19. Lutz W, Stulz N, Martinovich Z, Leon S, Saunders SM. Methodological background of decision rules and feedback tools for outcomes management in psychotherapy. Psychother Res. 2009;19(4–5):502–10.
20. de Beurs E, Barendregt M, Rogmans B, Robbers S, van Geffen M, Van Aggelen-Gerrits M, Houben H. Denoting treatment outcome in child and adolescent psychiatry: a comparison of continuous and categorical outcomes. Eur Child Adolesc Psychiatry. 2015;23:553–63.
21. Audin K, Margison FR, Clark JM, Barkham M. Value of HoNOS in assessing patient change in NHS psychotherapy and psychological treatment services. Br J Psychiatry. 2001;178(6):561–6.
22. Parabiaghi A, Kortrijk HE, Mulder CL. Defining multiple criteria for meaningful outcome in routine outcome measurement using the health of the nation outcome scales. Soc Psychiatry Psychiatr Epidemiol. 2014;49(2): 291–305.
23. Parabiaghi A, Barbato A, D'Avanzo B, Erlicher A, Lora A. Assessing reliable and clinically significant change on health of the nation outcome scales: method for displaying longitudinal data. Aust N Z J Psychiatry. 2005;39(8): 719–24.
24. Burgess P, Pirkis J, Coombs T. Modelling candidate effectiveness indicators for mental health services. Aust N Z J Psychiatry. 2009;43(6):531–8.
25. Mulder CL, van der Gaag M, Bruggeman R, Cahn W, Delespaul PA, Dries P, Faber G, de Haan L, van der Heijden FM, Kempen RW, et al. Routine Outcpme monitoring voor patiënten met ernstige psychiatrische aandoeningen: een consensus document [routine outcome monitoring for patients with severe mental illness: a consensus document]. Tijdschr Psychiatr. 2010;52(3):169–79.
26. Trauer T, editor. Outcome measurement in mental health. Cambridge: Cambridge University Press; 2010.
27. Brooks R. The reliability and validity of the health of the nation outcome scales: validation in relation to patient derived measures. Aust N Z J Psychiatry. 2000;34(3):504–11.
28. Slade M, Beck A, Bindman J, Thornicroft G, Wright S. Routine clinical outcome measures for patients with severe mental illness: CANSAS and HoNOS. Br J Psychiatry. 1999;174(5):404–8.
29. Kazis LE, Anderson JJ, Meenan RF. Effect sizes for interpreting changes in health status. Med Care. 1989;27(3, S):S178–89.
30. McCall WA. How to measure in education. New York: MacMillan; 1922.
31. Stevens SS. On the theory of scales of measurement. Science. 1946; 103(2684):677–80.
32. McHorney CA, Tarlov AR. Individual-patient monitoring in clinical practice: are available health status surveys adequate? Qual Life Res. 1995;4(4):293–307.
33. Fedorov V, Mannino F, Zhang R. Consequences of dichotomization. Pharm Stat. 2009;8(1):50–61.
34. Markon KE, Chmielewski M, Miller CJ. The reliability and validity of discrete and continuous measures of psychopathology: a quantitative review. Psychol Bull. 2011;137(5):856–79.
35. Twomey C, Prina AM, Baldwin DS, Das-Munshi J, Kingdon D, Koeser L, Prince MJ, Stewart R, Tulloch AD, Cieza A. Utility of the health of the nation outcome scales (HoNOS) in predicting mental health service costs for patients with common mental health problems: historical cohort study. PLoS One. 2016;11(11):e0167103.
36. Speak BL, Hay P, Muncer SJ. HoNOS–their utility for payment by results in mental health. Int J Health Care Qual Assur. 2015;28(2):115–28.

5

Trajectories of antidepressant medication use in individuals before and after being granted disability pension due to common mental disorders

Syed Rahman[1*], Michael Wiberg[1,5], Kristina Alexanderson[1], Jussi Jokinen[2,3], Antti Tanskanen[2,4] and Ellenor Mittendorfer-Rutz[1]

Abstract

Background: Early retirement caused by disability pension (DP) due to common mental disorders (CMDs) is frequent in European countries. Inadequate treatment, e.g., suboptimal antidepressant (AD) medication before DP can be crucial in such DP. This explorative study aimed to disentangle trajectories of AD based on defined daily dose (DDD) before and after granted DP, and to characterize the trajectories by socio-demographics and medical factors.

Methods: All 4642 individuals in Sweden aged 19–64 with incident DP due to CMD in 2009–2010 were included. Trajectories of annual DDDs of AD were analysed over a 6-year period by a group-based trajectory method. Associations between socio-demographic or medical factors and different trajectories were estimated by chi^2-test and multinomial logistic regression.

Results: Five trajectories of ADs were identified. Three groups, comprising 34%, 34%, and 21% of the cohort, had constant AD levels before and after DP with mean annual DDDs of 29, 234, and 580, respectively. Two groups, each including 6% of the cohort, had increasing levels of DDDs, levelling off at around 1150 and 785 DDDs after DP. Particularly age, outpatient care due to mental diagnoses and DP diagnoses were significantly associated with different trajectories ($p < 0.05$). All the groups had a larger proportion of older individuals (> 50%, 45–64 years), except for the 'increasing low' group, where younger individuals were in majority (> 60%, 18–44 years), who more frequently exited labour market due to 'anxiety disorders', with lower education and more specialised healthcare before DP than the other groups.

Conclusion: The heterogeneity among the five trajectory groups was partly explained by age, the severity of the mental disorder and the DP diagnoses. DDDs of ADs, though on different levels, varied marginally before and after granted DP in the majority. Moreover, AD levels were very low in one third of the individuals. Early identification and focus on the 'increasing low' group might be important in order to identify individuals at risk for further increase in annual DDDs of ADs even after granted DP, and might also contribute in prevention of DP. Further detailed research regarding different groups is warranted.

Keywords: Common mental disorders, Antidepressant, Epidemiology, Psychiatry in Europe, Disability pension, Sick-leave, Group-based trajectories

* Correspondence: Syed.Rahman@ki.se
[1]Department of Clinical Neuroscience, Division of Insurance Medicine, Karolinska Institutet, SE-171 77 Stockholm, Sweden
Full list of author information is available at the end of the article

Background

Common mental disorders (CMDs) constitute one of the most frequent reasons for disability pension (DP) claims and rank among the main medical causes of labour market marginalisation in OECD (Organisation for Economic Co-operation and Development) countries [1–6]. CMDs have a strong impact on individuals' lives, e.g., adverse effect on social and occupational functioning [7], potentially leading to long-term sickness absence [8] and consequently even to disability pension [9].

CMDs are known to be positively affected by treatment and rehabilitation efforts and are likely to worsen with inactivity [10–12]. Adequate healthcare before DP, particularly adequate prescription of antidepressants (ADs) can reduce the burden of disease and hereby have an effect on improving work capacity and reducing premature exit from the labour market in terms of DP [13–15]. However, previous studies, which considered cognitive behavioural therapy (CBT), pharmacological treatment, and healthcare visits, have indicated inadequate treatment before being granted DP [16, 17].

Recent studies have reported an increase in psychotropic medications before DP due to mental disorders and an immediate decrease after DP [18–20]. It is likely that patterns of such medication may differ for different mental disorders and that such changes might be influenced by different socio-demographic and medical factors. To the best of our knowledge, no study has been conducted yet aiming at identifying potential variability of such trajectories before and after being granted DP and at focussing on one of the most frequent diagnostic DP groups, namely CMDs.

Aim

The aims of this explorative study were to, among individuals granted DP due to CMD, 1) identify and describe different trajectories of AD over a 6-year period (3 years prior, and 3 years after being granted DP), and 2) analyse the heterogeneity, if any, between the trajectories by characterizing them with regard to socio-demographics and medical factors.

Methods

Study population

All individuals aged 19–64 and living in Sweden who were granted DP due to CMD for the first time during 2009–2010 ($N = 4642$) comprised the study base. CMD was defined as 'depressive episode' (F32), 'recurrent depressive disorder' (F33), 'phobic anxiety disorder' (F40), 'other anxiety disorder' (F41), 'obsessive-compulsive disorder' (F42), and 'reaction to severe stress and adjustment disorder' (F43) [21–24], based on the corresponding codes of the International Classification of Diseases (ICD) version 10 [25].

The study population was identified through register linkage at individual level using the unique ten-digit personal number of all residents in Sweden. Information was obtained from the following nationwide registers:

1) Longitudinal integration database for health insurance and labour market studies (LISA) (with information on: sex, age, education, country of birth, type of living area, family situation, and emigration) from Statistics Sweden.

2) (i) National patient register (date and main diagnosis of in- and specialized outpatient care); (ii) Drug register (information on prescribed dispensed drugs, including dates, dosages, amount, Anatomical Therapeutic Chemical (ATC) Classification System code [26], defined daily dose per dispensed pack; and (iii) Cause of death register (date of death) – all three from the National Board of Health and Welfare.

3) Micro-data for analyses of social insurance (MiDAS) (date and main disability pension diagnosis) from the National Social Insurance Agency.

Antidepressants

Antidepressants were identified based on the respective ATC code (N06A) [26]. Levels of defined daily dose (DDD) of ADs per year during the 3 years before and 3 years after the date of being granted DP were assessed. The DDD, as defined by 'the WHO collaborating centre for Drug Statistics Methodology', is the tentative average maintenance daily dose for a drug, used as main indication in adults [27]. A time scale on an annual basis was introduced where t0 represented the first date of being on DP, t-1 to t-3 referred to the three respective years prior to DP, and t + 1 to t + 3 indicated the 3 years after. The total amount of DDDs for a given year was calculated by summing up the DDDs of any AD medication during that year. If more than one AD was purchased during a year, then annual DDDs of all AD were summed up together for that particular year.

Drug purchase subsidies in Sweden

There is an upper limit of how much an individual has to pay out of pocket for medication during a 12-months period. The limit was between 100 and 126 Euros during the study period [28, 29]. Individuals can buy for up to a maximum of 3 months of prescribed medication at a time.

Covariates

Socio-demographics (sex, age, education, country of birth, type of living area, and family situation) were measured on 31-Dec of the year preceding DP granting and categorised as shown in Table 1. Among the medical factors, previous healthcare was measured during the 3 years before starting DP (from t-3 to t0) and categorized as 'yes' and 'no'. Regarding underlying diagnoses of previous healthcare, F00-F99 (ICD-10) codes were categorized as mental and all other as somatic diagnoses. The main DP diagnosis was the main one given when granting the DP (t0). We did not consider alteration in the main DP diagnosis, if any, during the study period. Diagnoses were categorized as indicated in Table 1. Annual in- and specialized outpatient healthcare use was considered as a proxy of the severity of the underlying disorder.

Disability pension in Sweden

All residents in Sweden aged 19–64 years, with a reduced work capacity due to disease or injury, can be granted DP from the Social Insurance Agency, for full- (100%) or part-time (75, 50, or 25% of ordinary working hours) [3]. People aged 19–29 years can be granted temporary DP if their work capacity is reduced due to disease or injury, not only for paid work but also to complete upper-secondary education, and individuals between 30 and 64 years of age can be granted permanent DP [3].

Statistical analyses

We calculated the individual annual DDDs for each specific AD for the six studied years, considering the date of granted DP; t0. Then we summed up DDDs of all specific ADs the individual bought during a one-year interval. Annual cumulative DDDs exceeding 1500 (around 4 DDDs) were deemed unusual (might be due to special cases, large purchases before traveling abroad, or error in data). So any such annual DDDs were truncated at a level of 1500 (equals 194 yearly purchases).

Thereafter, we used group-based trajectory modelling to estimate trajectories of AD among individuals with incident DP due to CMD during 2009–2010, for six time points (i.e. within a six-year window, starting from 3 years before and ending at 3 years after the date being granted DP). These models estimate changes in AD patterns over time in multiple subgroups within the cohort and estimate a regression model for each discrete group, and assess proportions of individuals in each group.

Additionally, this flexible model allows for different polynomials of the outcome [30]. We used the Bayesian information criterion (BIC) to test the best-fitted model related to the number of groups between 2 to 8, and in parallel, we also considered the proportions of the individuals in each group. While six and seven group models had better BIC values compared to the five-group model, there were very few individuals in some of the groups. Therefore, the model with five groups was considered most appropriate.

Probabilities for an individual to be assigned to a specific trajectory group were calculated. The highest estimated probability was used to decide each individual's group belonging. Côté et al. recommend that the average probability for individuals of a trajectory group should be ≥0.70 [31]. Such average probability for individuals of our cohort was 0.89, indicating a very good fit. It should be noted that all the time points represented an interval of 1 year calculated on the basis of DP granting date (t0), but for the sake of graphical presentation, t0 was calculated as the average of t-1 and t + 1, though t0 represented a date and not an interval (Fig. 1).

We calculated descriptive statistics of the socio-demographics and medical factors prior to DP, after assessing potential sex differences in these factors by chi^2-test. We then estimated their associations in each AD trajectory group by chi^2-test and multinomial logistic regression. The likelihood ratio tests were used to evaluate whether socio-demographic and medical factors were associated with type of trajectory group in the full model. Moreover, Nagelkerke pseudo R^2 values were estimated to evaluate the strength of these associations. By consecutively excluding and re-including each factor from the full model, we calculated differences in R^2 for each factor in order to examine the contribution of a given factor to the full model.

Analyses were carried out for the entire study population with DP due to CMD regardless of grade (part-time/full-time) as sensitivity analyses revealed no differences in the trajectories between individuals with full-time and part-time DP.

In case of death or emigration during the study period, due to differences in the exposure time, the data on DDDs for an individual was considered as missing for the whole year of the event and onward.

Data processing was performed using statistical software SAS for Windows version 9.4 (SAS-based procedure "Traj" [32]) and SPSS for Windows version 22.0 (chi^2-test and multinomial logistic regression).

Results

In Table 1, descriptive statistics, including socio-demographics and medical factors for the cohort (individuals with incident DP due to CMD in 2009–2010) are presented. Two thirds of the cohort were women (62.4%) and 77.3% were born in Sweden. When granted DP, most of them were aged 45–64 years (57.8%), had proceeded to high school education (46.0%), lived in big cities (39.9%), and were single without any child at home (45.3%). A higher proportion of the women (14.5%) than of the men (3.3%) were single with children living at home. Depressive disorders were the most common (46.3%) DP diagnosis. A history of specialised outpatient care was more common than inpatient care due to mental or somatic diagnoses (57.6%, 74.0% compared to 16.7%, 29.1%, respectively).

Figure 1 shows the estimated five groups of different trajectories of AD. The groups were labelled as, 'low

Table 1 Descriptive statistics for all women ($n = 2897$) and men ($n = 1745$) granted disability pension (DP) due to common mental disorders in 2009–2010 in Sweden ($N = 4642$)

Characteristics, measured at the end of the year preceding granted DP	All		Women		Men	
	n 4642	% 100	*n* 2897	% 62.4	*n* 1745	% 37.6
Socio-demographic characteristics[b]						
Age[a]						
18–24	837	18.0	520	17.9	317	18.2
25–34	490	10.6	294	10.1	196	11.2
35–44	635	13.7	407	14.0	228	13.1
45–54	1112	24.0	730	25.2	382	21.9
55–64	1568	33.8	946	32.7	622	35.6
Education (years)[a]						
Compulsory (≤9)	1301	28.0	710	24.5	591	33.9
High school (10–12)	2134	46.0	1353	46.7	781	44.8
University (> 12)	1207	26.0	834	28.8	373	21.4
Country of birth[a]						
Sweden	3589	77.3	2314	79.9	1275	73.1
Other EU countries	278	6.0	180	6.2	98	5.6
Rest of the world	775	16.7	403	13.9	372	21.3
Type of living area[ac]						
Big cities	1852	39.9	1120	38.7	732	41.9
Medium sized cities	1576	34.0	988	34.1	588	33.7
Small towns/villages	1214	26.2	789	27.2	425	24.4
Family situation[a]						
Married[d] living without children	743	16.0	496	17.1	247	14.2
Married[d] living with children	967	20.8	598	20.6	369	21.1
Single[e] living without children	2103	45.3	1188	41.0	915	52.4
Single[e] living with children	478	10.3	420	14.5	58	3.3
Adolescents living with parents, < 20 years	351	7.6	195	6.7	156	8.9
Medical characteristics						
Main DP diagnosis[a]						
Depressive disorders	2150	46.3	1305	45.0	845	48.4
Anxiety disorders	1441	31.0	867	29.9	574	32.9
Stress-related mental disorders	1051	22.6	725	25.0	326	18.7
Previous healthcare[f]						
Mental inpatient care[a]	777	16.7	460	15.9	317	18.2
Specialized mental outpatient care[a]	2674	57.6	1588	54.8	1086	62.2
Somatic inpatient care	1349	29.1	864	29.8	485	27.8
Specialized somatic outpatient care[a]	3436	74.0	2225	76.8	1211	69.4

[a]Significant sex differences
[b]All socio-demographic variables are measured at t0
[c]Type of living area: big cities (Stockholm, Gothenburg and Malmö); medium sized cities (cities with more than 90,000 inhabitants within 30 km distance from the centre of the city); small cities/villages/rural
[d]Married includes all living with partner; cohabitant
[e]Single includes divorced, separated, or widowed
[f]Measured during t-3 to t0

constant', 'low increasing', 'middle constant', 'high constant', and 'high increasing'. Many of the individuals ('low constant' 33.5% of the cohort) had none or very low (less than 50) annual DDDs of AD. Nearly 6% percent ('low increasing') had very low annual DDDs 3 years before DP granting, and showed a steep increase

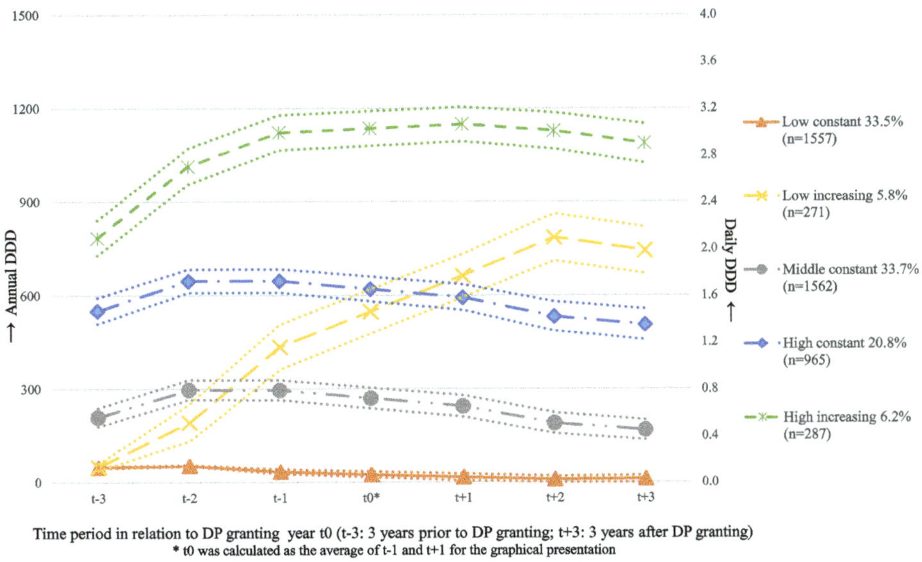

Fig. 1 Trajectory groups of antidepressants according to annual defined daily doses (DDDs) and percentages of individuals with granted disability pension (DP) due to common mental disorders granted in 2009–2010 ($N = 4642$) within each trajectory group in Sweden. (The dotted lines represent 95% confidence intervals)

in annual DDDs of AD up to 785 up until 2 years following DP. The group 'middle constant' (33.7%) had annual DDDs in between 200 and 300 during the study period. The group 'high constant' included 20.8% of the cohort, and had 500–600 DDDs per year throughout the study period. In the groups 'middle constant' and 'high constant', there was a slight decline in DDDs of AD following the DP. Six percent of the cohort had over 1000 DDDs per year since 2 years before DP granting until the end of follow-up (high increasing).

Table 2 describes the distribution of the socio-demographics and medical factors across the five identified trajectory groups. All socio-demographic and medical factors, but sex and previous healthcare due to somatic diagnoses, were significantly associated with different trajectory groups ($p < 0.05$) in the unadjusted analyses. In the full model, along with other variables, sex was significantly associated with the trajectory groups. The full model explained 17.2% of the variance between the groups (using Nagelkerke pseudo R^2). The highest estimated difference of 5% was observed for 'Previous mental outpatient care' (diff. in $R^2 = 0.05$), otherwise the individual factors, other than age and main DP diagnosis (diff. in $R^2 = 0.02$), merely effected the full model independently.

All the groups had a larger proportion of older individuals (> 50%, 45–64 years), except for the 'low increasing', where younger individuals constituted the absolute majority (>60%, 18-44 years), and notably 41.3% of those in this group were in the 18-24 age range. This group also had fewer individuals (17.3%) who have been to university compared to the other groups, whereas the 'high increasing' group had the highest proportions of individuals having attended high school or university (53.0% and 29.6%, respectively). In the 'low increasing' group, 80% of the individuals were single and did not have any children. Other socio-demographic factors were fairly equally distributed among all five groups.

Regarding the main DP diagnosis, the 'low increasing' group had equal proportions of depressive and anxiety disorders (43.2% each), whereas in all other trajectory groups, depressive disorders dominated. The percentage of the individuals with 'stress-related mental disorders' as main DP diagnosis was largest in the 'low constant' (31.5%) and followed by the 'middle constant' (21.0%) groups. The proportions of the individuals from the 'high increasing' group who had had previous in- or specialized outpatient care due to mental diagnoses were approximately twice as high compared to the proportions of the 'low constant' group (24.0%, 79.4% and 9.1%, 40.5%, respectively).

Approximately 41% ($n = 1906$) of the study population did not receive in- or specialized psychiatric care during the 3 years prior to DP grant. Further analyses showed that this group consisted individuals somewhat older (mean age 49 vs 44 years), with better educational level (university education: 32% vs 26%) than the whole study population (data not shown). Regarding the main DP diagnosis, more individuals without previous psychiatric specialised health care were granted DP due to stress-related mental disorders than in the whole study population (31.8% vs 22.6%), and fewer received DP due to anxiety disorders (22.5% vs 31%) (data not shown). Trajectory analyses revealed this group had similar patterns of trajectory groups, but larger proportions of 'low constant' and 'high constant' group (38.5% vs 33.5%,

Table 2 Distributions and associations of socio-demographic and medical characteristics in each trajectory group of antidepressants according to annual defined daily doses (DDDs), in individuals with disability pension (DP) due to common mental disorders granted in 2009–2010 ($N = 4642$) in Sweden

Characteristics	Low constant *n* (%) 1557(33.54)	Low increasing *n* (%) 271(5.84)	Middle constant *n* (%) 1562(33.65)	High constant *n* (%) 965(20.79)	High increasing *n* (%) 287(6.18)	Pearson's Chi-Square (*p*-value)[f]	Log-likelihood test Chi-Square (*p*-value)[g]	Diff. in R^2 *
Socio-demographic characteristics								
Sex[a]								
Men	604 (38.8)	102 (37.6)	598 (38.3)	347 (36.0)	94 (32.8)	5.2 (0.26)	10.7 (0.03)	0.002
Women	953 (61.2)	169 (62.4)	964 (61.7)	618 (64.0)	193 (67.2)			
Age[a]								
18–24	286 (18.4)	112 (41.3)	305 (19.5)	101 (10.5)	33 (11.5)	207.4 (< 0.001)	109.1 (< 0.001)	0.021
25–34	135 (8.7)	44 (16.2)	172 (11.0)	104 (10.8)	35 (12.2)			
35–44	202 (13.0)	23 (8.5)	207 (13.3)	144 (14.9)	59 (20.6)			
45–54	348 (22.4)	42 (15.5)	360 (23.0)	277 (28.7)	85 (29.6)			
55–64	586 (37.6)	50 (18.5)	518 (33.2)	339 (35.1)	75 (26.1)			
Education (years)[a]								
Compulsory (≤9)	495 (31.8)	114 (42.1)	444 (28.4)	198 (20.5)	50 (17.4)	88.3 (< 0.001)	29.7 (< 0.001)	0.006
High school (10–12)	649 (41.7)	110 (40.6)	738 (47.2)	485 (50.3)	152 (53.0)			
University (> 12)	413 (26.5)	47 (17.3)	380 (24.3)	282 (29.2)	85 (29.6)			
Country of birth[a]								
Sweden	1171 (75.2)	219 (80.8)	1162 (74.4)	792 (82.1)	245 (85.4)	40.8 (< 0.001)	57.3 (< 0.001)	0.011
Other EU25 countries	106 (6.8)	12 (4.4)	95 (6.1)	55 (5.7)	10 (3.5)			
Rest of the world	280 (18.0)	40 (14.8)	305 (19.5)	118 (12.2)	32 (11.1)			
Type of living area[a,b]								
Big cities	683 (43.9)	97 (35.8)	586 (37.5)	375 (38.9)	111 (38.7)	21.9 (< 0.01)	20.6 (< 0.01)	0.004
Medium sized cities	485 (31.1)	95 (35.1)	553 (35.4)	353 (36.6)	90 (31.4)			
Small towns/villages	389 (25.0)	79 (29.2)	423 (27.1)	237 (24.6)	86 (30.0)			
Family situation[a]								
Married[c] living without children	250 (16.1)	32 (11.8)	248 (15.9)	168 (17.4)	45 (15.7)	91.9 (< 0.001)	27.1 (0.04)	0.005
Married[c] living with children	311 (20.0)	30 (11.1)	324 (20.7)	233 (24.1)	69 (24.0)			
Single[d] living without children	697 (44.8)	136 (50.2)	718 (46.0)	415 (43.0)	137 (47.7)			
Single[d] living with children	164 (10.5)	23 (8.5)	160 (10.2)	106 (11.0)	25 (8.7)			
Adolescents living with parents, < 20 years	135 (8.7)	50 (18.5)	112 (7.2)	43 (4.5)	11 (3.8)			
Medical characteristics								
Main DP diagnosis[a]								
Depressive disorders	630 (40.5)	117 (43.2)	727 (46.5)	521 (54.0)	155 (54.0)	140.7 (< 0.001)	75.5 (< 0.001)	0.015
Anxiety disorders	436 (28.0)	117 (43.2)	507 (32.5)	290 (30.1)	91 (31.7)			
Stress-related mental disorders	491 (31.5)	37 (13.7)	328 (21.0)	154 (16.0)	41 (14.3)			
Previous mental inpatient care[e]								
Yes	142 (9.1)	63 (23.2)	274 (17.5)	229 (23.7)	69 (24.0)	118.6 (< 0.001)	31.5 (< 0.001)	0.006
No	1415 (90.9)	208 (76.8)	1288 (82.5)	736 (76.3)	218 (76.0)			
Previous mental specialized outpatient care[e]								
Yes	630 (40.5)	183 (67.5)	942 (60.3)	691 (71.6)	228 (79.4)	336.5 (< 0.001)	244.7 (< 0.001)	0.048

Table 2 Distributions and associations of socio-demographic and medical characteristics in each trajectory group of antidepressants according to annual defined daily doses (DDDs), in individuals with disability pension (DP) due to common mental disorders granted in 2009–2010 ($N = 4642$) in Sweden *(Continued)*

Characteristics	Low constant *n* (%) 1557(33.54)	Low increasing *n* (%) 271(5.84)	Middle constant *n* (%) 1562(33.65)	High constant *n* (%) 965(20.79)	High increasing *n* (%) 287(6.18)	Pearson's Chi-Square (*p*-value)[f]	Log-likelihood test Chi-Square (*p*-value)[g]	Diff. in R^2 *
No	927 (59.5)	88 (32.5)	620 (39.7)	274 (28.4)	59 (20.6)			
Previous somatic inpatient care[e]								
Yes	416 (26.7)	90 (33.2)	458 (29.3)	299 (31.0)	86 (30.0)	8.3 (0.08)	4.5 (0.4)	0.001
No	1141 (73.3)	181 (66.8)	1104 (70.7)	666 (69.0)	201 (70.0)			
Previous somatic specialized outpatient care[e]								
Yes	1153 (74.1)	203 (74.5)	1144 (73.2)	723 (74.9)	213 (74.2)	1.02 (0.91)	1.7 (0.8)	0.000
No	404 (25.9)	68 (25.1)	418 (26.8)	242 (25.1)	74 (25.8)			

*Difference in Nagelkerke pseudo R^2 between model including tested variable and model without tested variable. Nagelkerke pseudo R^2 for full model is 0.172
[a]Measured at t0
[b]Type of living area: big cities: Stockholm, Gothenburg and Malmö; medium sized cities: cities with more than 90,000 inhabitants within 30 km distance from the centre of the city; small cities/villages
[c]Married includes all living with partner; cohabitant
[d]Single includes divorced, separated, or widowed
[e]Measured during t-3 to t0
[f]Crude model
[g]Mutually adjusted model

and 24.3% vs 20.8%, respectively) and smaller proportions of 'middle constant' trajectory groups (24.1% vs 33.7%), and received lower levels of ADs. Multinomial regression suggested similar associations of covariates with trajectory groups as in the whole study population (data not shown).

Discussion

Main findings

In this explorative study, we identified five different trajectories of DDDs of ADs over a 6-year period among all 4642 individuals granted DP due to CMDs during 2009–2010. For the vast majority of individuals (89%), DDDs of ADs – though on different levels – varied only slightly before and after granting of a DP. Out of them about a third of the individuals, who more often had stress-related DP diagnoses and less psychiatric care, received very low levels or no ADs during the years around the time of DP grant. Two smaller groups (6% each) registersshowed increases of DDDs up to granting of the DP, in one group DDDs levelled off afterwards and in the other group they kept increasing. Individuals in this latter group tended to be younger and were more likely to have an anxiety disorder as a DP diagnosis.

Methodological considerations

To the best of our knowledge, this is the first study attempting to disentangle different groups of trajectories related to the amount of ADs during the years before and after being granted DP due to CMD. Previous studies have not discriminated between specific DP mental diagnoses and have used other statistical methods, which are not capable to identify groups with varying trajectories [18, 19].

Main strengths of this study include the use of high quality population-based nationwide registers [33–37] with longitudinal data linked at individual level. Further strengths result from the use of a large study group which comprised all individuals aged 18–64 from whole Sweden who were granted DP due to CMD during the studied exposure years (2009–2010). This means the study is not merely based on a sample. The register data also means that the study was not affected by recall bias regarding exposure and outcome measures. Moreover, there was no loss to follow up and DP diagnoses were set by the treating and certifying physician through thorough assessments of the patients' disease, functioning, and work incapacity. An additional advantage is that a wide range of socio-demographic and medical factors could be included as potential confounders. Another important strength of our study is that a potential social gradient for AD purchase can be considered negligible. First, drug purchase is considerably subsidised in Sweden and the level of these subsidies did not change much during study period. Moreover, analyses were controlled for socio-economic factors.

Regarding limitations, the validity of sick-leave and DP diagnoses is often discussed; however, few related studies are carried out so far. A Swedish study from 1991 concluded that sick-leave diagnoses have high validity when compared to the diagnoses from medical records [38]. Additionally, granting of DP is preceded by a long process of medical evaluation and work-capacity assessments [3]. Moreover, due to the stigma around mental diagnoses [39, 40], we assume that a mental diagnosis is given as a main DP diagnosis only when the patient actually has a mental disorder and when the main reason of work disability cannot be attributed to a somatic diagnosis [41]. On the other hand, this implies that some people with CMD might not have been given CMD as the main DP diagnosis on the DP certificate. Thus, they would not be included in this study. This can also be seen as a strength, as our cohort of individuals with DP due to CMD is more strictly defined. Another limitation is that, as in all studies using drug registers, we have no information on whether the individual actually used the dispensed AD. However, as the AD cannot be prescribed for more than 3 months at a time, it is plausible that the patient would not repeatedly have bought medication not used.

A point to be noted is, that we did not have the possibility to measure formally the severity of CMD, we have rather used information on in- or specialized outpatient healthcare use as a proxy of severity. Concerning the possibility of returning to work after DP granting, it should be noted that DP is a permanent measure for individuals aging from 30 to 64 years (around 75% of the study population). Moreover, as we have considered only the individuals who were on DP during the whole follow-up, it is unlikely for even the younger individuals (with temporal DP) to have returned to work. However, we do not have the information if some have returned to work after the follow-up period. Also, looking at the role of employers would have given further insight, but unfortunately, we do not have data on different aspects of employers.

Discussions of findings

The study revealed heterogeneity between the five groups identified based on the amounts of ADs. A third of the individuals in our study population had either no or very low annual DDDs of ADs during the 6 years of observation. This finding is surprising and may suggest that there is a possibility that these individuals might not have received optimal pharmacological treatment by ADs before being granted DP, which is in line with previous reports [16]. On the other hand, the individuals, if treated without pharmacotherapy, e.g., psychotherapy only, or other occupational therapy during some years of observation and later with ADs, might show low DDDs during the study period. Moreover, some in the cohort were prescribed other psychotropic drugs than ADs. Around 8–11% (depending upon the trajectory group) of the individuals in this cohort were prescribed anxiolytics or sedatives, separately or along with AD (data not shown). There is also a possibility of poor compliance to ADs due to their potential side effects, e.g., weight gain, decreased libido, diarrhoea, agitation etc. [42–44], which might have led to low annual DDDs. Finally, one should also consider that individuals might have improved clinically through AD treatment, but not regarding their work capacity [45–47].

Our analyses showed that most trajectory groups had relatively stable annual DDDs of AD around the time when granted DP. This is in contrast to findings from a Finnish project, where use of AD substantially increased before and decreased immediately after granted DP, especially among those with a mental DP diagnosis [18, 19]. These discrepancies in findings might arise from the differences in DP diagnoses, i.e. in our study the focus was on CMDs, while other previous studies included all mental disorders. One group differed considerably from the patterns of the other trajectory groups, i.e., the 'low increasing' group which showed a steep increase in DDDs of AD since the beginning of the study period (t-3) up to DP granting and continued to increase after that.

The study findings also indicate heterogeneity regarding socio-demographics and medical factors between the trajectory groups. Among the socio-demographic variables, age had the strongest association with trajectory groups in the full model. There were also observable differences in educational level and family situation between the trajectory groups. Differences in educational level or in the family status in the 'low increasing' trajectory group might have been due to the younger age distribution in that group. Regarding the level of education, individuals with higher educational level are likely to have more employment security regarding a current job, or even a greater choice of alternative jobs if they are not able to remain at the present one due to health reasons [48]. It is further not unlikely that these individuals may remain longer time at work with a later pensionary age despite a higher clinical severity and higher AD doses than their low educated peers.

Depressive disorders were the most common DP diagnosis in all the trajectory groups. However, anxiety disorders contributed equally much in the 'low increasing' group. This may be because many of them were young, and anxiety disorders usually have an earlier onset and they are detected earlier in life [49–51]. Previous mental inpatient or specialized outpatient healthcare was proportionate to the amount of AD, i.e., the highest AD purchases were found in the constant 'high group' and the lowest in the 'low constant' group. It might be necessary to pay special attention to the 'low increasing' group because they also had a high use of previous mental healthcare. As this includes the youngest among all trajectory groups, we expected that they would less frequently be using healthcare [52, 53]. Thus, our results suggest that individuals belonging to this group might have suffered from severe mental disorders several years before granted DP, and that the disorders worsened with time leading to DP. Notably, this group also had the highest level of previous somatic inpatient care. Such high use of previous healthcare suggests that further research should also focus on somatic comorbidity. On the other hand, 20–60% of the individuals, depending on the trajectory groups, did not receive any specialized mental healthcare during 3 years prior to DP. This is not in accordance with the Swedish sick-leave guidelines [54], stating that all patients on sickness absence due to depression for more than 6 months, should be referred to a specialist. This may indicate that these individuals might have not received optimal treatment during the pre-DP years, leading to further worsening of work capacity and later resulting in exclusion from the labour market by being granted DP [16].

A large proportion of the study population (41%), who were more often granted DP due to stress-related mental disorders, did not receive psychiatric in- or specialized outpatient care during the 3 years before being granted DP. This is consistent with previous research suggesting that individuals with work disability due to stress-related mental disorders have a lower proportion of specialized health care than individuals with other common mental disorders e.g., depressive disorders [55].

Conclusion

The study identified five different groups according to the annual DDDs of ADs among individuals granted DP due to CMD. The five groups were heterogeneous regarding socio-demographics and medical factors, particularly regarding age, the severity of the mental disorder and the DP diagnoses. In the majority of the individuals within a trajectory group, the levels of DDDs of ADs varied only marginally before and after being granted DP. The study also posts a query regarding optimal pharmacological treatment for CMD during the pre-DP years, which in turn may contribute in prevention of premature exit from the labour market due to common mental disorders.

Abbreviations

AD: Antidepressant; ATC: Anatomical therapeutic chemical; BIC: Bayesian information criterion; CMD: Common mental disorder; DDD: Defined daily dose; DP: Disability pension; ICD: International classification of diseases; LISA: Longitudinal integration database for health insurance and labour market studies; MiDAS: Micro-data for analyses of social insurance; OECD: Organisation for Economic Co-operation and Development

Acknowledgements

Not applicable.

Funding

Swedish Research Council for Health, Working Life and Welfare, the Swedish Research Council (Project numbers: K2009-61P-21304-04-4; K2009-61X-21305-01-1; K2011-80P-21782-01-4), and the Karolinska Institutet's funding for doctoral students.

Authors' contributions

SR- planning, data management and analyses, interpreting results and writing. MW- data management and analyses, interpreting results and writing. KA- planning, interpreting results and writing. JJ- planning, interpreting results and writing. AT- planning, interpreting results and writing. EM- planning, interpreting results and writing. All authors read and approved the final manuscript.

Consent for publication

Not applicable

Competing interests

The authors declare that they have no competing interests.

Author details

[1]Department of Clinical Neuroscience, Division of Insurance Medicine, Karolinska Institutet, SE-171 77 Stockholm, Sweden. [2]Department of Clinical Neuroscience, Division of Psychiatry, Karolinska Institutet, Karolinska University Hospital, Stockholm, Sweden. [3]Department of Clinical Sciences, Division of Psychiatry, Umeå University, Umeå, Sweden. [4]National Institute for Health and Welfare, Helsinki, Finland. [5]Department of Analysis and Forecast, Swedish Social Insurance Agency, Stockholm, Sweden.

References

1. Järvisalo J, Anderson B, Boedeker W. Houtman I (eds.): mental disorders as a major challenge in prevention of work disability: experiences in Finland, Germany, the Netherlands and Sweden. Helsinki: Kela; 2005.
2. Alexanderson K, Norlund A. Swedish council on technology assessment in health care (SBU). Chapter 1. Aim, background, key concepts, regulations, and current statistics. Scand J Pub Health Suppl. 2004;63:12–30.
3. Social Insurance in Figures 2015. In. Sweden: The Social Insurance Agency; 2015.
4. OECD: Sickness, Disability and Work: Breaking the Barriers. A synthesis of findings across OECD countries. In. Paris; 2010.
5. OECD. Sick on the job? Myths and realities about mental health and work. In. Paris: OECD Publishing; 2012.
6. OECD. Mental health and work: Sweden. Paris: OECD Publishing; 2013.
7. Adler DA, McLaughlin TJ, Rogers WH, Chang H, Lapitsky L, Lerner D. Job performance deficits due to depression. Am J Psychiatry. 2006;163(9):1569–76.
8. Knudsen AK, Harvey SB, Mykletun A, Overland S. Common mental disorders and long-term sickness absence in a general working population. The Hordaland health study. Acta Psychiatr Scand. 2013;127(4):287–97.
9. Knudsen AK, Overland S, Aakvaag HF, Harvey SB, Hotopf M, Mykletun A. Common mental disorders and disability pension award: seven year follow-up of the HUSK study. J Psychosom Res. 2010;69(1):59–67.
10. Kupfer DJ, Frank E, Phillips ML. Major depressive disorder: new clinical, neurobiological, and treatment perspectives. Lancet. 2012;379(9820):1045–55.
11. Rhebergen D, Batelaan NM, de Graaf R, Nolen WA, Spijker J, Beekman AT, Penninx BW. The 7-year course of depression and anxiety in the general population. Acta Psychiatr Scand. 2011;123(4):297–306.
12. Simon GE, Barber C, Birnbaum HG, Frank RG, Greenberg PE, Rose RM, Wang PS, Kessler RC. Depression and work productivity: the comparative costs of treatment versus nontreatment. J Occup Environ Med. 2001;43(1):2–9.
13. Apfel T, Richer-Rossler A. Delay of diagnosis and treatment in psychiatric patients applying for a disability pension - a challenge for all of us. Swiss Med Wkly. 2008;138(23–24):348–54.
14. Beck A, Crain LA, Solberg LI, Unutzer J, Maciosek MV, Whitebird RR, Rossom RC. The effect of depression treatment on work productivity. Am J Manag Care. 2014;20(8):e294–301.
15. OECD: Mental health, disability and work: issues for discussion. In. Paris; 2010.
16. Honkonen TI, Aro TA, Isometsa ET, Virtanen EM, Katila HO. Quality of treatment and disability compensation in depression: comparison of 2 nationally representative samples with a 10-year interval in Finland. J Clin Psychiatry. 2007;68(12):1886–93.
17. Hartvig P. Untreated psychiatric disability. A study of disabled persons with major psychiatric health impairment, having never received psychiatric treatment. Scand J Soc Med. 1978;6(3):117–24.

18. Laaksonen M, Metsa-Simola N, Martikainen P, Pietilainen O, Rahkonen O, Gould R, Partonen T, Lahelma E. Trajectories of mental health before and after old-age and disability retirement: a register-based study on purchases of psychotropic drugs. Scand J Work Environ Health. 2012;38(5):409–17.
19. Leinonen T, Lahelma E, Martikainen P. Trajectories of antidepressant medication before and after retirement: the contribution of socio-demographic factors. Eur J Epidemiol. 2013;28(5):417–26.
20. Oksanen T, Vahtera J, Westerlund H, Pentti J, Sjosten N, Virtanen M, Kawachi I, Kivimaki M. Is retirement beneficial for mental health?: antidepressant use before and after retirement. Epidemiology (Cambridge, Mass). 2011;22(4):553–9.
21. Deverill C KM: Common Mental Disorders. In: Adult psychiatric morbidity in England. edn. Edited by McManus S MH, Brugha T, Bebbington P,, R J. London: The NHS Information Centre for health and social care; 2009: 25–27.
22. Koopmans PC, Bultmann U, Roelen CA, Hoedeman R, van der Klink JJ, Groothoff JW. Recurrence of sickness absence due to common mental disorders. Int Arch Occup Environ Health. 2011;84(2):193–201.
23. Rahman S, Alexanderson K, Jokinen J, Mittendorfer-Rutz E. Risk factors for suicidal behaviour in individuals on disability pension due to common mental disorders - a nationwide register-based prospective cohort study in Sweden. PLoS One. 2014;9(5):e98497.
24. Rahman SG, Alexanderson K, Jokinen J, Mittendorfer-Rutz E. Disability pension due to common mental disorders and subsequent suicidal behaviour: a population-based prospective cohort study. BMJ Open. 2016;6(4):e010152.
25. WHO: International Statistical Classification of Diseases and Related Health Problems, 10 revision (ICD 10). In.; 2010.
26. WHO Collaborating Centre for Drug Statistics Methodology (WHOCC). ATC/DDD Index 2016. http://www.whocc.no/atc_ddd_index/ . Accessed 7 Feb 2016.
27. WHO Collaborating Centre for Drug Statistics Methodology. Definition and general consideration 2016. http://www.whocc.no/ddd/definition_and_general_considera/ . Accessed 7 Feb 2016.
28. Mutual Information System on Social Protection. Social protection in the Member States of the European Union (MISSOC), European Economic Area and Switzerland. http://www.missoc.org/MISSOC/INFORMATIONBASE/COMPARATIVETABLES/MISSOCDATABASE/comparativeTableSearch.jsp. Accessed 1 June 2016.
29. The Dental and Pharmaceutical Benefits Agency (Tandvård- och Läkemedelsförmånsverket) http://tlv.se/lakemedel/hogkostnadsskyddet/sa-fungerar-hogkostnadsskyddet/. Accessed 1 June 2016.
30. Jones BL, Nagin DS, Roeder K. A SAS procedure based on mixture models for estimating developmental trajectories. Sociol Methods Res. 2001;29(3):374–93.
31. Cote S, Tremblay RE, Nagin D, Zoccolillo M, Vitaro F. The development of impulsivity, fearfulness, and helpfulness during childhood: patterns of consistency and change in the trajectories of boys and girls. J Child Psychol Psychiatry Allied Discip. 2002;43(5):609–18.
32. Jones BL. 'traj' group-based modeling of longitudinal data https://www.andrew.cmu.edu/user/bjones/index.htm . Accessed 3 Feb 2016.
33. Quality and content of Patient registry. In. Sweden: The National Board of Health and Welfare; 2009.
34. Ludvigsson JF, Andersson E, Ekbom A, Feychting M, Kim JL, Reuterwall C, Heurgren M, Olausson PO. External review and validation of the Swedish national inpatient register. BMC Public Health. 2011;11:450.
35. Cause of Death 2014. In. Sweden: The National Board of Health and Welfare; 2015.
36. Ludvigsson JF, Almqvist C, Bonamy AK, Ljung R, Michaelsson K, Neovius M, Stephansson O, Ye W. Registers of the Swedish total population and their use in medical research. Eur J Epidemiol. 2016;31(2):125–36.
37. Wettermark B, Hammar N, Fored CM, Leimanis A, Otterblad Olausson P, Bergman U, Persson I, Sundstrom A, Westerholm B, Rosen M. The new Swedish prescribed drug register–opportunities for pharmacoepidemiological research and experience from the first six months. Pharmacoepidemiol Drug Saf. 2007;16(7):726–35.
38. Ljungdahl LO, Bjurulf P. The accordance of diagnoses in a computerized sick-leave register with doctor's certificates and medical records. Scand J Soc Med. 1991;19(3):148–53.
39. Shrivastava A, Johnston M, Bureau Y. Stigma of mental Illness-1: clinical reflections. Mens Sana Monogr. 2012;10(1):70–84.
40. Lauber C. Stigma and discrimination against people with mental illness: a critical appraisal. Epidemiologia e Psichiatria Sociale. 2008;17(1):10–3.
41. Hensing G, Wahlstrom R. Swedish council on technology assessment in health care (SBU). Chapter 7. Sickness absence and psychiatric disorders. Scand J Pub Health Suppl. 2004;63:152–80.
42. Masand PS. Tolerability and adherence issues in antidepressant therapy. Clin Ther. 2003;25(8):2289–304.
43. David DJ, Gourion D. Antidepressant and tolerance: determinants and management of major side effects. L'Encephale. 2016;42(6):553–61.
44. Hung CI. Factors predicting adherence to antidepressant treatment. Curr Opin Psychiatry. 2014;27(5):344–9.
45. Trivedi MH, Morris DW, Wisniewski SR, Lesser I, Nierenberg AA, Daly E, Kurian BT, Gaynes BN, Balasubramani GK, Rush AJ. Increase in work productivity of depressed individuals with improvement in depressive symptom severity. Am J Psychiatry. 2013;170(6):633–41.
46. Hensing G, Bertilsson M, Ahlborg G, Jr., Waern M, Vaez M: Self-assessed mental health problems and work capacity as determinants of return to work: a prospective general population-based study of individuals with all-cause sickness absence. BMC Psychiatry 2013, 13:259.
47. Bertilsson M, Love J, Ahlborg G, Jr., Hensing G: Health care professionals' experience-based understanding of individuals' capacity to work while depressed and anxious. Scand J Occup Ther 2015, 22(2):126–136.
48. Clark A, Postel-Vinay F. Job security and job protection. Oxf Econ Pap. 2009; 61(2):207–39.
49. Kessler RC, Berglund P, Demler O, Jin R, Merikangas KR, Walters EE. Lifetime prevalence and age-of-onset distributions of DSM-IV disorders in the National Comorbidity Survey Replication. Arch Gen Psychiatry. 2005;62(6):593–602.
50. Copeland WE, Angold A, Shanahan L, Costello EJ. Longitudinal patterns of anxiety from childhood to adulthood: the great Smoky Mountains study. J Am Acad Child Adolesc Psychiatry. 2014;53(1):21–33.
51. Merikangas KR, He JP, Burstein M, Swanson SA, Avenevoli S, Cui L, Benjet C, Georgiades K, Swendsen J. Lifetime prevalence of mental disorders in U.S. adolescents: results from the National Comorbidity Survey Replication–Adolescent Supplement (NCS-A). J Am Acad Child Adolesc Psychiatry. 2010; 49(10):980–9.
52. Eisenberg D, Golberstein E, Gollust SE. Help-seeking and access to mental health care in a university student population. Med Care. 2007;45(7):594–601.
53. Burns BJ, Ryan Wagner H, Gaynes BN, Wells KB, Schulberg HC. General medical and specialty mental health service use for major depression. Int J Psychiatry Med. 2000;30(2):127–43.
54. Skaner Y, Nilsson GH, Arrelov B, Lindholm C, Hinas E, Wilteus AL, Alexanderson K. Use and usefulness of guidelines for sickness certification: results from a national survey of all general practitioners in Sweden. BMJ Open. 2011;1(2):e000303.
55. Mittendorfer-Rutz E, Alexanderson K, Kjeldgård L, Wikman A. Sjukskrivning och risk för framtida sjuk- och aktivitetsersättning bland kvinnor och män [Report in Swedish]. Sickness absence and risk for future Disability pension among women and men [Translation]. Stockholm. Division of Insurance Medicine, Deaprtment of Clinical Neurosciencew, Karolinska Institutet. http://ki.se/sites/default/files/delrapport_3_hela_1.pdf . Accessed 23 Dec 2017.

6

Body image in patients with somatoform disorder

M. Scheffers[1*†], H. Kalisvaart[1,2†], J. T. van Busschbach[1,3], R. J. Bosscher[1], M. A. J. van Duijn[4], S. A. M. van Broeckhuysen-Kloth[2], R. A. Schoevers[3,5] and R. Geenen[2,6]

Abstract

Background: Although body-related problems are common in patients with somatoform disorder, research focusing on how patients with somatoform disorder perceive and evaluate their body is scarce. The present study compared differences in body image between patients with somatoform disorder and respondents from a general population sample. It also examined differences within the somatoform disorder group between men and women and between the diagnostic subgroups conversion disorder, pain disorder and undifferentiated somatoform disorder.

Methods: Data were obtained from 657 patients (67.5% female) with somatoform disorder (DSM-IV-TR 300.7, 300.11, 300.81, 300.82) and 761 participants (58.6% female) from the general population. The Dresden Body Image Questionnaire (DBIQ) was used to assess body image in five domains: body acceptance, vitality, physical contact, sexual fulfilment, and self-aggrandizement. Confirmatory factor analysis and analyses of variance were performed. Since differences in age and sex were found between the somatoform disorder sample and the comparison sample, analyses were done with two samples of 560 patients with somatoform disorder and 351 individuals from the comparison sample matched on proportion of men and women and age.

Results: Patients scored significantly lower than the comparison sample on all DBIQ domains. Men scored higher than women. Patients with conversion disorder scored significantly higher on vitality and body acceptance than patients with undifferentiated somatoform disorder and pain disorder.

Conclusions: The mostly large differences in body image between patients with somatoform disorder and the comparison sample as well as differences between diagnostic subgroups underline that body image is an important feature in patients with somatoform disorder. The results indicate the usefulness of assessing body image and treating negative body image in patients with somatoform or somatic symptom disorder.

Keywords: Body image, Somatoform disorder, Somatic symptom disorder, Dresden body image questionnaire

Background

Somatoform disorder (SFD), the precursor diagnostic category of "somatic symptom disorder" [1], is characterized by persistent physical symptoms that suggest the presence of a medical condition, but cannot be adequately explained by such a medical condition, nor by the direct effects of substance use or by a mental condition [2]. A core feature of somatoform disorder and somatic symptom disorder is the problematic relation of patients with their body. Patients perceive their body as dysfunctional [3] and have difficulty not only to acknowledge and understand bodily signals in an adequate manner, but also to adapt their behavior according to these signals [4–7]. Core problems of SFD include distrust and non-acceptance of the body, intimacy problems, changed physical identity, loss of vitality, as well as lack of awareness and incorrect interpretation of bodily signals [6, 8–10]. All of these aspects may have substantial consequences for an individual's development and quality of life [11]. Patients with SFD have been suggested to be impaired in "embodied mentalization", described as "the capacity to see the body as the seat of emotions, wishes,

* Correspondence: wjscheffers@gmail.com; wj.scheffers@windesheim.nl
†M. Scheffers and H. Kalisvaart contributed equally to this work.
[1]Windesheim University of Applied Sciences, School of Human Movement and Education, Campus 2-6, 8017 CA Zwolle, the Netherlands
Full list of author information is available at the end of the article

and feelings and the capacity to reflect on one's own bodily experiences and sensations and their relationships to intentional mental states in the self and others" ([12], p3).

Although body-related problems are common in patients with SFD, research focusing on how patients with SFD perceive and evaluate their body is scarce. A first condition for research is the possibility to assess the complex relation with their body in patients with SFD. This is important to acquire knowledge about the specificity and severity of body-related problems in patients with SFD as compared to reference groups. Moreover, specific symptoms such as pain, fatigue, or dissociation differ among diagnostic categories of SFD, and it could be studied whether their impact on the relation with one's body differs as well [13, 14]. Finally, body-related assessment is needed as an evaluation tool when body-oriented interventions are part of the combined treatment package offered to patients with SFD [15, 16]. Thus, an adequate instrument to assess and evaluate the severity and scope of problems related to body image in people with SFD is a necessity.

In general, the term 'body image' has been used to describe and assess a variety of body-related phenomena, including perceptions, cognitions, and affects with regard to the body [17, 18]. However, most questionnaires measuring body image either emphasize physical appearance and weight or shape-related themes or specifically evaluate body image problems in eating disorders or body dysmorphic disorder, which makes them not particularly suitable for patients with SFD (for an overview, see [17]). Questionnaires directed at the general population mostly focus on a specific aspect of body image, such as satisfaction with body parts and processes [19, 20] or sociocultural attitudes towards appearance [21, 22]. Other questionnaires, developed for clinical use, focus on physical symptoms [23–25] or body awareness [26–28]. In SFD patients, however, all of these body-related aspects are important [5] and a self-report questionnaire addressing a broad range of body-related aspects is needed for both research and clinical practice.

For this purpose, the present study employed the Dresden Body Image Questionnaire (DBIQ) to measure a broad range of body-related self-perceptions in five domains: body acceptance, vitality, physical contact, sexual fulfilment, and self-aggrandizement [29, 30]. Especially the incorporation of physical contact and sexual fulfilment, often reported by patients as problematic topics but rarely included in questionnaires, makes the DBIQ a suitable instrument for the SFD population. One of the present study's aims was to obtain more information on the severity of disturbances in these domains by comparing patients with SFD with a sample matched on sex and age from the general population described in an earlier study [31].

Studies of body image in the general population indicate that men and women appreciate their body image differently [32–34]. Women are generally more preoccupied and dissatisfied with their body than men [35], which may be explained by sociocultural values, genetic differences and differences in bodily development and experiences like trauma [36]. We expect these differences to be also present in the group of patients with SFD.

Body image may also differ between patients with different diagnostic categories conversion disorder, pain disorder and undifferentiated somatoform disorder. With no previous studies available, we base our expectation that patients with pain and undifferentiated somatoform disorder score lower on vitality than patients with conversion disorder on clinical observation.

In order to obtain insight into the significance of body image assessments for patients with SFD, the present study aimed to evaluate differences in body image as measured with the DBIQ between patients with SFD and a sample from the general population. It also aimed to evaluate, within the patient group, differences between women and men and between the diagnostic categories conversion disorder, pain disorder, and undifferentiated somatoform disorder. Prior to the evaluation of differences, measurement invariance across clinical and non-clinical samples and across sex in the somatoform sample was tested, in order to affirm whether comparisons are valid.

Methods

Participants

Participants were patients with severe SFD referred to Altrecht Psychosomatic Medicine, a tertiary care centre for psychosomatic medicine that is specialized in the treatment of patients with severe SFD. This centre is located in Zeist, the Netherlands. On average, patients admitted to this institution have had medically unexplained symptoms for 10 years and have, received five previous treatments for somatoform disorder in primary or secondary care. In about half of the cases, patients have comorbid disorders; mainly other somatoform diagnoses but also mood and anxiety disorders, substance dependence and personality disorder [37]. The main treatment criterion applied by the institution is the presence of a diagnosis of SFD (pain disorder, conversion disorder or undifferentiated SFD) as the primary disorder, in line with the criteria described in the Diagnostic and Statistical Manual of Mental Disorders (DSM-IV-TR) [2], diagnosed by a trained psychologist, and confirmed by the resident psychiatrist. Exclusion criteria applied by the treatment centre were people with (a) a diagnosis of hypochondriasis or body dysmorphic disorder, (b) a diagnosis of addiction, bipolar disorder, or psychosis, and (c) a crisis situation requiring immediate attention (e.g., high suicidality); and (d) patients under treatment by a specialized physician outside the center.

In an intensive intake procedure, all patients consecutively referred in the period 2011–2014 were assessed for eligibility for treatment. Treatment inclusion was based on an initial diagnostic assessment and on the patient's informed consent to accept the treatment offered. All patients eligible for treatment were included in the study unless informed consent to participate in the study was not obtained.

Data were gathered from 657 patients with SFD between 24 and 69 years of age (Mean = 43.3, *SD* = 10.8), 443 women and 214 men with mean ages of 42.7 (*SD* = 11.0) and 44.5 (*SD* = 10.3) years. Table 1 shows the primary diagnoses according to DSM-IV-TR. The number of patients with conversion disorder was relatively high (22.4%) since the treatment centre is the only institute in the Netherlands with clinical facilities that admits patients that are difficult to treat in secondary care.

A convenience sample from the general population [31] was used as comparison. This sample consisted of 761 adults (433 women, 326 men, two persons with sex unknown), with a mean age of 30.9 years (SD = 13.6, range 18–65). Details about recruitment of participants, data collection, and measurements used can be found in [31].

Measures

The Dresden Body Image Questionnaire (DBIQ) [29, 30] is a 35-item questionnaire with positively and negatively worded statements across five subscales: body acceptance (e.g., "I wish I had a different body"), vitality (e.g., "I am physically fit"), physical contact (e.g., "Physical contact is important for me to express closeness"), sexual fulfilment (e.g., "I am very satisfied with my sexual experiences"), and self-aggrandizement (e.g., "I use my body to attract attention"). The level of agreement with items is scored on a 5-point Likert scale ranging from 1 (= not at all) to 5 (= fully).

In a German non-clinical sample [30] Cronbach's α for the subscales varied from $\alpha = .81$ for self-aggrandizement to $\alpha = .94$ for vitality. Correlations between the subscales varied from $r = .37$ (sexual fulfilment and self -aggrandizement) to $r = .65$ (body acceptance and vitality). The five-factor structure of the non-clinical sample was replicated using a confirmatory factor analysis in a clinical psychiatric sample of 560 patients, of whom 45% had somatoform complaints (CFI = .90; RMSEA = .06) [29]. In this clinical sample Cronbach's α for the subscales varied from $\alpha = .83$ for self-aggrandizement to $\alpha = .92$ for sexual fulfilment. Correlations between the subscales varied between $r = .31$ (vitality and physical contact) to $r = .65$ (physical contact and sexual fulfilment).

Confirmatory factor analyses of the Dutch version of the DBIQ (DBIQ-35-NL) in the sample that was used in the present study for comparison showed a five-factor structure in accordance with the original scale, where model fit was improved significantly by moving one item from the subscale body acceptance to the subscale self-aggrandizement [31]. The equivalence of the measurement model across sex and age was evaluated in this study as well, demonstrating partial strong invariance. Internal consistency of the subscales in this Dutch version was good: Cronbach's α varied from $\alpha = .74$ for the subscale physical contact to $\alpha = .91$ for the subscale sexual fulfilment. The correlations between the subscales varied from $r = .17$ for vitality and physical contact to $r = .53$ for acceptance and sexual fulfilment. Temporal stability over 2 weeks was satisfactory, varying from an intra-class correlation coefficient (ICC) of .64 for physical contact to .82 for vitality (see Additional file 1: Table S1 for DBIQ items in English).

Table 1 Primary diagnoses of participants with somatoform disorder

Diagnoses[a]	*n* (%)	% men
Conversion Disorder (300.11)	147 (22.4)	37.4
Pain Disorder (307.80, 307.89)	185 (28.2)	38.9
Undifferentiated SFD (300.82)	325 (49.5)	27.4
Total	657 (100)	32.5

[a] Diagnosis according to DSM-IV-TR

Procedure

Patients completed the Dutch version of the DBIQ as part of a routine initial diagnostic screening and provided written informed consent for the use of the data for scientific purposes. This part of the study protocol was approved by the institutional review board (CWO) of Altrecht, Zeist, the Netherlands (CWOnr 1419).

The study in the general population used as a comparison sample was conducted in agreement with the VU University Amsterdam guideline for research for educational purposes, allowing students to collect data with the use of questionnaires in healthy groups of respondents when participation is voluntary and data are analyzed anonymously. The Medical Ethics Review Committee of VU University waived the requirement for formal ethical approval of the procedures used (for more details see [31]).

Data analysis

The factor structure of the clinical sample was evaluated using confirmatory factor analysis with maximum likelihood estimation robust to non-normality (MLR). Moreover, measurement invariance was examined across the two groups (somatoform disorder and general population) and across sex within the somatoform group, to ensure meaningful comparisons between scores in these groups [38–40]. We used the procedures and fit indices used in the study of the comparison sample [31]: model selection was performed by testing invariance by the Scaled Difference in Chi-Squares (SDCS) test [41] for nested models estimated with MLR. Because little consensus exists with regard to recommended fit indices [38], standardized root mean square residual (SRMR) and Tucker Lewis index (TLI) are reported, in addition to the comparative fit index (CFI) and root mean square error of approximation (RMSEA). Analyses were conducted with Mplus Version 5.1 [42].

SPSS 20.00 for Windows was used to compare group differences in the clinical sample with analysis of variance. Because of the differences in sample size in the diagnostic categories, Hochberg's GT2 test was used for post hoc analyses [43]. Mean differences between subgroups were expressed in Cohen's d and considered large if ≥0.80, moderate between 0.50 and 0.80 and small between 0.20 and 0.50 [44].

For comparison of the DBIQ scores across samples, the clinical sample was matched to the comparison sample on sex and age (see Additional file 2: Figure S1 for age distribution of males and females in the clinical sample and in the comparison sample). The exact matching procedure from the R package MatchIt [45] was used to make 72 groups with respondents of both groups with equal age and proportion of men and women. A total of 580 patients from the somatoform sample (387 women; 193 men) were matched to 341 respondents in the comparison sample (201 women, 140 men), with appropriate weights [46]. The weighted mean ages were 44.8 for men (range 25–65) and 42.8 for women (range 24–64) in both matched samples, with almost equal (weighted) standard deviations of 10.4 and 10.9 for men and women respectively across the two samples. Note that the matching procedure led to discarding the older respondents in the somatoform sample, whereas the younger respondents from the comparison sample were not included in the matched sample.

Results

Measurement invariance

CFA in the somatoform sample showed the earlier found five-factor structure, with the same item shifted as in the general population sample [31]. Evaluation of measurement invariance for the somatoform sample and the comparison sample showed a model with partial strong measurement invariance, with different loadings across the groups for items 1 ("I move gracefully") of the subscale self-aggrandizement and item 7 ("There are lots of situations in which I feel happy about my body") of the subscale body acceptance estimated freely, as best fit (RMSEA (90% CI) = .061 (.059–.063), SRMR = .074, CFI = .828, TLI = .823).

In the evaluation of the somatoform sample for measurement invariance with sex as a grouping variable, item 15 of the subscale body acceptance ("I choose clothing that hides the shape of my body") was the only item not showing invariance (RMSEA (90% CI) = .061 (.058–.064), SRMR = .073, CFI = .832, TLI = .828). This item was also identified as non-invariant in the general population sample [31]. For detailed analysis of measurement invariance see Additional file 3: Table S2. Based on these analyses and based on comparisons of the scores with and without the items that are not invariant across groups, which led to only marginally different (sub)-scale scores (for details see Additional file 4: Table S3), we concluded that use of the full scale ensures meaningful comparisons within this study and with results of other studies.

Internal consistency and correlations between subscales

In the group of patients with SFD, Cronbach's α for the subscales were .78 for physical contact and self-aggrandizement, .80 for vitality, .84 for acceptance and .92 for sexual fulfilment. Correlations between the subscales varied from $r = .14$ (vitality and physical contact) to $r = .50$ (self-aggrandizement and sexual fulfilment).

Differences between SFD diagnostic categories

Table 2 shows means of the diagnostic categories for the total score and all subscales of the DBIQ. Analysis of variance of the three diagnostic categories (conversion disorder, undifferentiated SFD and pain disorder) showed statistically significant higher scores for patients with conversion disorder on overall body image, vitality and body acceptance than for patients with undifferentiated SFD and pain disorder. Differences were largest for vitality.

Differences between women and men

In Table 3 means of women and men with SFD on DBIQ total score and on all subscales are presented. Analysis of variance showed that men scored significantly higher than women on total DBIQ, body acceptance, sexual fulfilment and self-aggrandizement. No such differences were apparent for vitality and physical contact.

Comparisons of the matched samples

Table 4 presents means of DBIQ total score and subscales in the clinical and comparison sample matched on age and sex. Patients with SFD scored significantly lower ($p < .001$) than the comparison sample on DBIQ total mean score and on all subscales, with the largest differences for sexual fulfilment (1.2 point) and vitality (1.6

Table 2 Means (*M*) and standard deviations (*SD*) of scores on the Dresden Body Image Questionnaire (DBIQ) in subgroups of patients in three diagnostic categories of somatoform disorder, test of the difference between diagnostic categories

	Conversion Disorder ($n = 147$)	Pain Disorder ($n = 185$)	Undifferentiated SFD ($n = 325$)		
(sub) scale	*M (SD)*	*M (SD)*	*M (SD)*	*F(2)*	*p*
total score	$2.78_{a,b}$ (0.65)	2.55_{b} (0.54)	2.60_{a} (0.56)	7.32	.001
vitality	$2.56_{a,b}$ (0.84)	2.21_{b} (0.67)	2.07_{a} (0.62)	25.08	<.001
body acceptance	$3.25_{a,b}$ (0.97)	2.86_{a} (0.83)	2.99_{b} (0.98)	7.00	.001
sexual fulfilment	2.61 (1.18)	2.42 (0.97)	2.49 (0.98)	1.44	.24
physical contact	3.32 (0.82)	3.19 (0.79)	3.31 (0.82)	1.47	.23
self-aggrandizement	2.31 (0.67)	2.20 (0.63)	2.27 (0.63)	1.19	.43

[a, b]Means in a row sharing subscripts are significantly different based on Hochberg's GT2 test

point). Cohen's d was large (≥ 0.80) for all (sub)scales but physical contact.

Discussion

The aim of the current study was to gain more detailed insight into body image in patients with SFD. To this end, we compared DBIQ scores in patients with SFD and people from the general population. In addition, we compared DBIQ scores in patients with different SFD diagnoses and scores demonstrated by women and men with SFD. After measurement invariance was confirmed across the clinical sample and the comparison sample as well as across sex in the clinical sample, the most prominent finding was that body image scores of patients with SFD were substantially lower than body image scores in the general population, showing large differences between groups on all domains of body image.

With respect to diagnostic categories of SFD, patients with conversion disorder scored higher on vitality, body acceptance and the total DBIQ score than patients with undifferentiated SFD and pain disorder. This difference in vitality scores is in accordance with our clinical impression that fatigue is less prevalent in conversion disorder. The higher score in body acceptance of patients with conversion disorder were unexpected. Patients with conversion disorder still scored substantially lower than the comparison group on all body image domains.

As hypothesized on the basis of results in non-clinical samples [35], women in the SFD sample scored lower than men on total DBIQ, body acceptance, sexual fulfilment and self-aggrandizement. No differences between women and men for vitality and physical contact were measured, which for vitality is in agreement with observations in chronic fatigue syndrome [47]. Overall, our study confirms that account should be taken of differences between men and women when assessing body image.

When tentatively comparing our findings with studies of the DBIQ in patients with mixed mental disorders [48], women with childhood trauma [49], and patients with depressive disorder [50], especially the relatively low scores on vitality for patients with somatoform disorder are noteworthy. Scores on sexual fulfilment and self-aggrandizement tend to be lower than those of the mental disorders group [48] but higher than the scores of the childhood trauma group [49], while scores on body acceptance and physical contact are about the same as in the mixed mental disorders group. Overall, body image scores appear to be about similar to scores of a sample of patients with mixed mental disorders, with lower vitality scores as the most distinct main outstanding feature in patients with somatoform disorder, especially in patients with pain disorder and undifferentiated somatoform disorder. While body-oriented psychotherapy is considered important in both severe somatoform disorder [51] and other severe mental disorders [52], the

Table 3 Means (*M*) and standard deviations (*SD*) of scores on the Dresden Body Image Questionnaire (DBIQ) of women and men, test of the difference between women and men in the SFD sample

	women ($n = 443$)	men ($n = 214$)			
(sub) scale	*M (SD)*	*M (SD)*	*t*	*p*	Cohen's *d*
total mean score	2.55 (0.56)	2.73 (0.61)	4.69	<.001	0.31
vitality	2.18 (0.68)	2.29 (0.78)	1.85	.07	0.15
body acceptance	2.88 (0.98)	3.12 (0.89)	5.50	<.001	0.26
sexual fulfilment	2.39 (0.99)	2.71 (1.06)	3.79	<.001	0.31
physical contact	3.25 (0.80)	3.33 (0.84)	1.08	.29	0.10
self-aggrandizement	2.20 (0.63)	2.39 (0.65)	3.70	<.001	0.30

Table 4 Means (M), standard deviations (*SD*), test of the difference (*t*), and effect size (Cohen's *d*) of scores on the Dresden Body Image Questionnaire in age and sex matched samples of patients with somatoform disorder ($n = 580$) and comparison sample ($n = 341$)

	Somatoform	Comparison sample		
(sub)scale	*M (SD)*	*M (SD)*	*t*	Cohen's *d*
total mean score	2.62 (0.58)	3.59 (0.42)	−29.3*	− 1.9
vitality	2.20 (0.71)	3.79 (0.58)	−36.9*	− 2.4
body acceptance	3.00 (0.94)	3.81 (0.66)	−15.2*	− 1.0
sexual fulfilment	2.48 (1.02)	3.71 (0.67)	−22.1*	− 1.4
physical contact	3.28 (0.82)	3.73 (0.58)	−9.7*	− 0.6
self-aggrandizement	2.26 (0.65)	3.00 (0.54)	−18.9*	− 1.2

*$p < .001$

current study adds that a focus on body image might be an important aspect of these therapies.

The DBIQ covers five body-related aspects, that all proved to be substantially affected in patients with SFD. This finding, together with the evidence for partial strong measurement invariance across the comparison group and the SFD group, leads to the conclusion that the DBIQ is a suitable instrument to evaluate the broad scope of body-related problems in patients with SFD [5]. However, it should be acknowledged that the DBIQ does not cover all body-related themes. For example, body awareness, the sensory awareness that originates from the body's physiological states, processes, actions and functions [27], is considered pivotal in the development and progress of SFD [53, 54] because lack of body awareness may undermine healthy behavior [55]. Furthermore, a self-report questionnaire such as the DBIQ does not address behavioural aspects, such as movement patterns and levels of activity [56]. Notwithstanding these restrictions, the large differences between patients with SFD and the general population comparison group on a broad range of body-related topics as well as the differences between diagnostic categories indicate the relevance of the DBIQ for patients with SFD.

Because data on the validity of the DBIQ scales are still scarce, comparisons with other assessments may be useful to support validity. The subscale vitality has an effect size (d = 2.5) comparable with that of the fatigue scale of the Checklist Individual Strength (CIS-20R) that has been used to compare patients with chronic fatigue syndrome (CFS) and a healthy reference group ($d = 3.0$) [47]. Furthermore, symptoms measured with the Symptom Checklist (SCL-90, [57]) in a severe SFD group have shown, when compared with a general population group, effect sizes that are comparable with or even smaller than those found for some DBIQ subscales (0.9 for anxiety, 1.2 for depression, 1.6 for somatization and 1.3 for overall psychopathology [51].

Future studies must establish the clinical relevance of using DBIQ scales for patients with SFD by examining the effects of treatment on body image (sensitivity to change) as well as the prognostic value of the DBIQ for treatment outcome in patients with SFD. Treatment for patients with SFD aims at goals such as reducing or coping with physical complaints, enhancing body acceptance, and ameliorating quality of life, all depending on individual situations and patient preferences. With respect to these goals, vitality and body acceptance seem to be the most relevant subscales of the DBIQ, but the current study shows that domains of self-aggrandizement, physical contact, and sexual fulfilment should not be overlooked in the assessment, treatment and evaluation of patients with SFD. In addition to its potential diagnostic importance and use in treatment evaluation, measuring body image with the DBIQ may also be valuable in clinical practice to recognize body-related themes underlying symptom presentation [58] and to enhance communication between patient and therapist about body-related experiences. Sexual fulfilment, for example, may be hampered by physical complaints [59] and is in fact, as the current study indicates, a prevalent problem for SFD patients. Because sexuality is a sensitive subject to discuss for patients as well as therapists, incorporating the domain of sexuality into a questionnaire may shed further light on possible problems with sexuality and enhance communication about this subject [60].

One of the present study's strengths lies in the fact that its sample of patients with a certified diagnosis of severe and chronic SFD was large: this enabled us to compare body image between different SFD diagnoses as well as between patients and a sample from the general population. A limitation with respect to generalizability is that the results apply to a group that was referred to tertiary care; results cannot be generalized to patients with somatoform disorder who present themselves in secondary and primary care. The relatively high amount of comorbid disorders may have confounded the results but comorbid mental disorders are a characteristic of this group with severe somatoform disorders.

Conclusion

The observed mostly large differences in body image between patients with somatoform disorder and the comparison sample as well as differences between diagnostic subgroups underline that body image is an important feature in patients with somatoform disorder. The results indicate the usefulness of assessing body image and treating negative body image in patients with somatoform or somatic symptom disorder.

Abbreviations

CFA: Confirmatory Factor Analysis; CFI: Comparative Fit Index; CFS: Chronic Fatigue Syndrome; CI: Confidence Interval; CIS: Checklist Individual Strength; CWO: Commissie Wetenschappelijk Onderzoek (institutional review board); DBIQ: Dresden Body Image Questionnaire; DSM-IV-TR: Diagnostic and Statistical Manual of Mental Disorders, Text Revision; M: Mean; RMSEA: Root Mean Square Error of Approximation; SCL: Symptom Checklist; SD: Standard Deviation; SDCS: Scaled Difference in Chi-Squares; SFD: Somatoform Disorder; SRMR: Standardized Root Mean square Residual (SRMR); TLI: Tucker Lewis Index

Funding

Not applicable.

Authors' contributions

All authors participated in the writing of the manuscript. The study design and ethical supervision was provided by RS, MvD, JvB, SvB, and RG. Data collection was conducted by HK, RB, and SvB. Data analysis was performed by HK, MS, RG and MvD. Interpretation of data was performed by HK, MS, RG, MvD, JvB, and SvB. All authors approved the final version of the manuscript.

Consent for publication

Not applicable.

Competing interests

The authors declare that they have no competing interests.

Author details

[1]Windesheim University of Applied Sciences, School of Human Movement and Education, Campus 2-6, 8017 CA Zwolle, the Netherlands. [2]Altrecht Psychosomatic Medicine, Vrijbaan 2, 3705 WC Zeist, the Netherlands. [3]Department of Psychiatry, University of Groningen, University Medical Center Groningen, P.O. Box 30.001, CC72, 9700, RB Groningen, the Netherlands. [4]Department of Sociology, University of Groningen, Grote Rozenstraat, 31 9712 TG Groningen, the Netherlands. [5]Research School of Behavioural and Cognitive Neurosciences (BCN), Interdisciplinary, Center for Psychopathology and Emotion regulation (ICPE), P.O. Box 30.001, CC72, 9700, RB Groningen, the Netherlands. [6]Department of Psychology, Utrecht University, Heidelberglaan 1, 3584CS, Utrecht, the Netherlands.

References

1. American Psychiatric Association. Diagnostic and statistical manual of mental disorders. 5th ed. Arlington: American Psychiatric Association; 2013.
2. American Psychiatric Association. Diagnostic and statistical manual of mental disorders DSM-IV-TR (text revision). Washington, DC: American Psychiatric Association; 2000.
3. Röhricht F. Das theoretische Modell und die therapeutischen Prinzipien/ Mechanismen einer integrativen Körperpsychotherapie (KPT) bei somatoformen Störungen. Psychother-Wiss. 2011;1:5–13.
4. Creed F, Henningsen P, Fink P. Medically unexplained symptoms, somatisation and bodily distress. Developing better clinical services. Cambridge: University Press; 2011.
5. Henningsen P, Zipfel S, Herzog W. Management of functional somatic syndromes. Lancet. 2007;369:946–55.
6. Kalisvaart H, van Broeckhuysen S, Buhring M, Kool MB, van Dulmen S, Geenen R. Definition and structure of body-relatedness from the perspective of patients with severe somatoform disorder and their therapists. PLoS One. 2012;7:e42534.
7. Lind AB, Delmar C, Nielsen K. Searching for existential security: a prospective qualitative study on the influence of mindfulness therapy on experienced stress and coping strategies among patients with somatoform disorders. J Psychosom Res. 2014;77:516–21.
8. Bakal D, Coll P, Schaefer J. Somatic awareness in the clinical care of patients with body distress symptoms. Biopsychosoc Med. 2008;2:6.
9. Gard G. Body awareness therapy for patients with fibromyalgia and chronic pain. Disabil Rehabil. 2005;27:725–8.
10. McWhinney IR, Epstein RM, Freeman TR. Rethinking somatization. Ann Intern Med. 1997;126:747–50.
11. Cash TF. Body image: past, present, and future. Body Image. 2004;1:1–5.
12. Luyten P, van Houdenhove B, Lemma A, Target M, Fonagy P. Vulnerability for functional somatic disorders: a contemporary psychodynamic approach. J Psychother Integr. 2013;23:12.
13. Sertoz OO, Doganavsargil O, Elbi H. Body image and self-esteem in somatizing patients. Psychiatry Clin Neurosci. 2009;63:508–15.
14. Afrell M, Biguet G, Rudebeck CE. Living with a body in pain - between acceptance and denial. Scand J Caring Sci. 2007;21:291–6.
15. Joraschky P, Pöhlmann K. Schatten im Körperbild. Die Bedeutung von Traumatisierungen und strukturellen Störungen. Psychodyn Psychother. 2014;13:27–40.
16. Zipfel S, Herzog W, Kruse J, Henningsen P. Psychosomatic medicine in Germany: more timely than ever. Psychother Psychosom. 2016;85:262–9.
17. Cash TF, Smolak L. Body image: a handbook of science, practice and prevention. New York: Guilford Press; 2011.
18. Röhricht F, Seidler KP, Joraschky P, Borkenhagen A, Lausberg H, Lemche E, Loew T. Consensus paper on the terminological differentiation of various aspects of body experience. Psychother Psychosom Med Psychol. 2005;55: 183–90.
19. Mendelson BK, Mendelson MJ, White DR. Body-esteem scale for adolescents and adults. J Pers Assess. 2001;76:90–106.
20. Secord PF, Jourard SM. The appraisal of body-cathexis: body-cathexis and the self. J Consult Psychol. 1953;17:343–7.
21. Fisher E, Dunn M, Thompson JK. Social comparison and body image: an investigation of body comparison processes using multidimensional scaling. J Soc Clin Psychol. 2002;21:566–79.
22. Heinberg LJ, Thompson JK, Stormer S. Development and validation of the sociocultural attitudes towards appearance questionnaire. Int J Eat Disord. 1995;17:81–9.
23. de Waal MW, Arnold IA, Spinhoven P, Eekhof JA, Assendelft WJ, van Hemert AM. The role of comorbidity in the detection of psychiatric disorders with checklists for mental and physical symptoms in primary care. Soc Psychiatry Psychiatr Epidemiol. 2009;44:78–85.
24. Kerns RD, Turk DC, Rudy TE. The west haven-Yale multidimensional pain inventory (WHYMPI). Pain. 1985;23:345–56.
25. Vercoulen JH, Swanink CM, Fennis JF, Galama JM, van der Meer JW, Bleijenberg G. Dimensional assessment of chronic fatigue syndrome. J Psychosom Res. 1994;38:383–92.
26. Kolk AM, Hanewald GJ, Schagen S, Gijsbers van Wijk CM. A symptom perception approach to common physical symptoms. Soc Sci Med. 2003;57: 2343–54.
27. Mehling WE, Gopisetty V, Daubenmier J, Price CJ, Hecht FM, Stewart A. Body awareness: construct and self-report measures. PLoS One. 2009;4: e5614.
28. Price CJ, Thompson EA. Measuring dimensions of body connection: body awareness and bodily dissociation. J Altern Complement Med. 2007;13:945–53.
29. Pöhlmann K, Roth M, Brahler E, Joraschky P. The Dresden body image inventory (DKB-35): validity in a clinical sample. Psychother Psychosom Med Psychol. 2014;64:93–100.
30. Pöhlmann K, Thiel P, Joraschky P. Development and validation of the Dresden body image questionnaire. In: Joraschky P, Lausberg H, Pöhlmann K, editors. Body oriented diagnostics and psychotherapy in patients with eating disorders. Gießen: Psychosozial-Verlag; 2008. p. 57–72.

31. Scheffers M, van Duijn MAJ, Bosscher RJ, Wiersma D, Schoevers RA, van Busschbach JT. Psychometric properties of the Dresden body image questionnaire: a multiple-group confirmatory factor analysis across sex and age in a Dutch non-clinical sample. PLoS One. 2017;12:e0181908.
32. Abbott BD, Barber BL. Embodied image: gender differences in functional and aesthetic body image among Australian adolescents. Body Image. 2010; 7:22–31.
33. Davison TE, McCabe MP. Relationships between men's and women's body image and their psychological, social, and sexual functioning. Sex Roles. 2005;(7–8):463–75.
34. Tylka TL, Wood-Barcalow NL. The body appreciation Scale-2: item refinement and psychometric evaluation. Body Image. 2015;12:53–67.
35. Algars A, Santtila P, Varjonen M, Witting M, Johansson A, Jern P. The adult body: how age, gender, and body mass index are related to body image. J Aging Health. 2009;21:1112–32.
36. Sack M, Boroske-Leiner K, Lahmann C. Association of nonsexual and sexual traumatizations with body image and psychosomatic symptoms in psychosomatic outpatients. Gen Hosp Psychiatry. 2010;32:315–20.
37. Van der Boom KJ, Houtveen JH. Psychiatric comorbidity in patients in tertiary care suffering from severe somatoform disorders. Tijdschrift voor psychiatrie. 2014;56:743–7.
38. Brown TA. Confirmatory factor analysis for applied research. 2th ed. New York: Guilford Press; 2015.
39. Gregorich SE. Do self-report instruments allow meaningful comparisons across diverse population groups? Testing measurement invariance using the confirmatory factor analysis framework. Med Care. 2006;44:S78–94.
40. Rusticus SA, Hubley AM, Zumbo BD. Measurement invariance of the appearance schemas inventory-revised and the body image quality of life inventory across age and gender. Assessment. 2008;15:60–71.
41. Satorra A, Bentler PM. Corrections to test statistics and standard errors in covariance structure analysis. In: Eye AV, Clogg CC, editors. Latent variables analysis: applications for developmental research. Thousand Oaks: Sage; 1994. p. 399–419.
42. Muthén LK, Muthén BO. Mplus User's Guide. 5th ed. Los Angeles: Muthén & Muthén; 2007.
43. Field AP. Discovering statistics using SPSS. London: Sage; 2009.
44. Cohen J. A power primer. Psychol Bull. 1992;112:155–9.
45. Ho DE, Imai K, King G, Matchlt SEA. Nonparametric preprocessing for parametric causal inference. J Stat Softw. 2011;42:1–28 URL http://www.jstatsoft.org/v42/i08/.
46. Jacobson NS, Truax P. Clinical significance: a statistical approach to defining meaningful change in psychotherapy research. J Consult Clin Psychol. 1991; 59:12–9.
47. Schulte-van Maaren YW, Giltay EJ, van Hemert AM, Zitman FG, de Waal MW, Van Rood YR. Reference values for the body image concern inventory (BICI), the whitely index (WI), and the checklist individual strength (CIS-20R): the Leiden routine outcome monitoring study. J Affect Disord. 2014;164:82–9.
48. Scheffers M, van Busschbach JT, Bosscher RJ, Aerts LC, Wiersma D, Schoevers RA. Body image in patients with mental disorders: characteristics, associations with diagnosis and treatment outcome. Compr Psychiatry. 2017;74:53–60.
49. Scheffers M, Hoek M, Bosscher RJ, van Duijn MAJ, Schoevers RA, van Busschbach JT. Negative body experience in women with early childhood trauma: associations with trauma severity and dissociation. Eur J Psychotraumatol. 2017;8:1322892.
50. Scheffers M, van Duijn MAJ, Beldman M, Bosscher RJ, van Busschbach JT, Schoevers RA. Body attitude, body satisfaction and body awareness in a clinical group of depressed patients: an observational study on the associations with depression severity and the influence of treatment. J Affect Disord. 2019;242:22–8.
51. Houtveen JH, van Broeckhuysen-Kloth S, Lintmeijer LL, Bühring MEF, Geenen R. Intensive multidisciplinary treatment of severe somatoform disorder. A prospective evaluation. J Nerv Ment Dis. 2015;203:141–8.
52. Rohricht F. Body psychotherapy for the treatment of severe mental disorders - an overview. Body Mov Dance Psychother. 2015;10:51–67.
53. Price C, Mehling WE. Body awareness and pain. In: Thompson DL, Brooks M, editors. Integrative pain management. Williston: Handspring publishing; 2016. p. 235–51.
54. Schaefer M, Egloff B, Witthoft M. Is interoceptive awareness really altered in somatoform disorders? Testing competing theories with two paradigms of heartbeat perception. J Abnorm Psychol. 2012;121:719–24.
55. van der Maas LC, Koke A, Pont M, Bosscher RJ, Twisk JW, Janssen TW. Improving the multidisciplinary treatment of chronic pain by stimulating body awareness: a cluster-randomized trial. Clin J Pain. 2015;31:660–9.
56. Körperschema LH. Körperbild und Bewegungsmuster - Bewegungsanalyse in der Diagnostik von Körperschema und Körperbildstörungen. In: Joraschky P, Loew T, Röhricht F, editors. Körpererleben und Körperbild. Ein Handbuch zur Diagnostik. Stuttgart: Schattauer; 2009. p. 125–33.
57. Derogatis LR. SCL-90-R: symptom Checklist-90-R. Minnesota: NCS Pearson; 1994.
58. Porcelli P, Guidi J. The clinical utility of the diagnostic criteria for psychosomatic research: a review of studies. Psychother Psychosom. 2015; 84:265–72.
59. Prins MA, Woertman L, Kool MB, Geenen R. Sexual functioning of women with fibromyalgia. Clin Exp Rheumatol. 2006;24:555–61.
60. de Boer MK, Castelein S, Bous J, van den Heuvel ER, Wiersma D, Schoevers RA. The antipsychotics and sexual functioning questionnaire (ASFQ): preliminary evidence for reliability and validity. Schizophr Res. 2013;150:410–5.

7

Predictors of medication adherence among patients with severe psychiatric disorders: findings from the baseline assessment of a randomized controlled trial (Tecla)

Ulrike Stentzel[1*†], Neeltje van den Berg[1†], Lara N. Schulze[2], Thea Schwaneberg[1,3], Franziska Radicke[1], Jens M. Langosch[4], Harald J. Freyberger[2,5], Wolfgang Hoffmann[1] and Hans-Jörgen Grabe[2]

Abstract

Background: Schizophrenia and bipolar disorder are characterized by a high disease burden. Antipsychotic medication is an essential part of the treatment. However, non-adherence is a major problem. Our aim was to examine potential determinants of non-adherence for patients with severe mental disorders.

Methods: Baseline data of the study "Post stationary telemedical care of patients with severe psychiatric disorders" (Tecla) were used. Medication adherence was assessed with the Medication Adherence Report Scale German version (MARS-D). A logistic regression was calculated with age, sex, education, employment status, level of global functioning, social support and intake of typical and atypical antipsychotics as predictors.

Results: $N = 127$ participants were included in the analysis ($n = 73$ men, mean age 42 years). The mean MARS-D Score was 23.4 (SD 2.5). The most common reason for non-adherence was forgetting to take the medicine. Significant positive determinants for adherence were older age (OR 1.02, 95% CI 1.011–1.024, $p < 0.0001$), being employed (OR 2.46, 95% CI 1.893–3.206, $p < 0.0001$), higher level of global functioning (overall measure of how patients are doing) (OR 1.02, 95% CI 1.012–1.028, $p < 0.0001$), having social support (OR 1.02, 95% CI 1.013–1.026, $p < 0.0001$), and intake of typical antipsychotics (OR 2.389, 95% CI 1.796–3.178, $p < 0.0001$). A negative determinant was (female) sex (OR 0.73, 95% CI 0. 625–0.859, $p = 0.0001$).

Conclusions: Especially employment, functioning and social support could be promising targets to facilitate adherence in patients with schizophrenia or bipolar disorder.

Keywords: Psychiatry, Mental health disorders, Schizophrenia, Psychotic disorders, Bipolar disorders, Adherence, Non-adherence, MARS-D

* Correspondence: ulrike.stentzel@uni-greifswald.de
†Ulrike Stentzel and Neeltje van den Berg contributed equally to this work.
[1]Institute for Community Medicine, University Medicine Greifswald, Ellernholzstraße 1-2, 17487 Greifswald, Germany
Full list of author information is available at the end of the article

Background

Schizophrenia as well as other psychotic disorders and bipolar disorders are serious mental diseases. In Germany, 19 new schizophrenia-cases per 100,000 people per year are diagnosed. In Germany, the 12-month-prevalence of schizophrenia and other psychotic disorders is estimated 2.6% and of bipolar disorders 1.5% [1]. The disease burden is high for mental disorders. The number of days with limitations is 3 times higher for people with mental disorders compared to healthy persons [1] and schizophrenia is one of the ten diseases with the highest number of years of life lived with disability (YLD) [2].

Medication is an essential part of the treatment of schizophrenia and bipolar disorders; both in acute episodes and in long-term management. Several studies showed that the relapse rate is significantly lower with drug therapy [2–5], provided that the patient is adherent. Adherence is defined by the WHO as "the extent to which a person's behavior – taking medication, following a diet, and/or executing lifestyle changes – corresponds with agreed recommendations from a health care provider" [6]. Non-adherent behavior increases the risk of relapses and rehospitalization [7–9]. However, non-adherence is one of the major problems in patients with schizophrenia and bipolar disorders [10]. The prevalence of non-adherence to antipsychotics ranges from 20 to 89% for patients with schizophrenia or bipolar disorders [11–13]. Dolder et al. examined adherence in an outpatient setting using prescription fill rates. Their results showed an adherence of 55% after 12 months among patients taking atypical antipsychotics (second generation) [14].

To reduce non-adherence in patients with severe mental disorders, it is necessary to know more about the reasons for non-adherence und to determine factors that influence adherence positively or negatively. A few studies have addressed specific factors determining adherence of patients with schizophrenia or with bipolar disorders [15–20]. However, the results of these studies often differ [16, 19, 20] and non-adherence is considered a multi-causal phenomenon [16].

The aim of this analysis is to identify possible determinants for non-adherence of patients with schizophrenia, other psychotic disorders and bipolar disorders, including age, sex, education, the status of employment, the level of functioning, presence of social support, adverse drug effects.

Methods

Patient sample and data

The data for this analysis were taken from the baseline assessment from an intervention study to evaluate telemedical care for patients with severe psychiatric disorders ("Post stationary telemedical care of patients with severe psychiatric disorders" (Tecla)). The goal of this project is to improve medication adherence for patients with severe psychiatric disorders on the basis of regular, individualized telephone calls and short-text-messages. Tecla is designed as a prospective controlled randomized intervention study. All participants receive computer assisted baseline and follow-up interviews after 3 and 6 months. The participants are recruited from three psychiatric departments in Western-Pomerania in the very northeast of Germany. Participants were patients in day-care hospitals or in open or closed inpatient wards. The recruitment occurs shortly before discharge and is done by a study psychologist. Inclusion criteria are a medical diagnosis of any form of schizophrenia (ICD-10 F20), schizoaffective disorders (ICD-10 F25), or bipolar disorders (ICD-10 F31), and age ≥ 18 years. Exclusion criteria were scheduled inpatient treatments within the next 6 months and missing accessibility by telephone. A comprehensive description of the study protocol for the Tecla study is published elsewhere [21].

Additionally, data from participants of the IMeS study (Approaches of individualized medicine in psychiatric disorders) were included. The aim of this study is to identify biomarkers from genetic material, and to examine metabolic processes and bodily protein in blood samples. The recruitment of the patients, the inclusion criteria and the baseline assessment of the IMeS-study are identical with the Tecla study. Both samples were collected at the same recruitment sites.

All participating patients gave their written informed consent. The data assessment and documentation were conducted based on eCRFs and an IT-supported documentation system [22].

Measures

Medication adherence was measured with the Medication Adherence Report Scale, German version (MARS-D) that detects non-adherent behavior by self-report [23]. It is a measure for non-adherence in general, not for mental disorders in particular. The scale considers also the frequency of non-adherent behavior. The questions are formulated in a non-threatening and non-judgmental way to minimize social desirability bias [24, 25]. The original Medication Adherence Report Scale (MARS-5, in English language) was developed because patients tend to overestimate their adherence [26–28] or to conceal non-adherent behavior [23]. The MARS-D has 5 items to assess how the drugs were taken. The 5 items are "I forget to take my medication", "I change the dose of my medication", "From time to time I stop taking my medication for a while", "I sometimes decide to skip the medication" and "I take less medication than I am instructed to." The questions provide 5 answer categories from "always" to "never" (scored 1 to 5) so that the total score is between 5 (no adherence) and 25 (complete adherence) [29].

The Global Assessment of Functioning (GAF) is an overall measure of how patients are doing from positive mental health up to severe psychopathology [30]. It is known, that functioning is low in people with current mental health disorders, so functioning can be used as an expression of the severity of illness [31]. The GAF-questionnaire measures the degree of mental illness by rating psychological, social and occupational functioning [30] on an ordinal scale from 1 to 100 [32]. The scale is divided into 10-point intervals. The lowest interval (score 1 to 10) represents severe illness, the highest interval (score 91 to 100) represents the healthiest condition [30].

Social support was assessed using the measure F-SozU (Social support, short form with 14 items) [33]. The authors defined social support as the result of cognitive-emotional processing and assessment of current and past social interactions. The concept is based on cognitive approaches and assesses the subjective conviction to get support from the subject's social network if necessary. This 14-item short form is appropriate for the assessment of a more generally perceived social support [33]. The statements refer to the fields of emotional support (to be liked and accepted by others, to share feelings, to experience participation), to provide practical assistance (practical help in everyday problems, for example to borrow things, getting practical advice, getting help with challenging tasks) and social integration (belonging to a circle of friends, doing joint ventures, knowing people with similar interests) and are assessed using a 5 category Likert-scale from "does not apply" (scored 1) to "applies exactly" (scored 5) [33].

Adverse drug effects were assessed using a 5 category Likert-scale including "no side effects", "little", "moderate", "strong" and "very strong" for each of the following side effects: movement disorders, muscle stiffness, involuntary shiver, motionlessness, muscle spasm, agonizing restlessness/problems to sit still (can't be suppressed at will), lack of sexual desire/loss of libido, increase in weight, increased appetite, heavy feeling of illness/chills/fever and milk flow [34].

To adjust for social desirability (defined as the "tendency to give overly positive self-descriptions" [35]), the Short Scale Social Desirability-Gamma (KSE-G) was used [36]. The KSE-G measures two aspects of social desirability: the exaggeration of positive qualities (PQ +), and the minimization of negative qualities (NQ-) [35]. Both aspects were assessed with three items each on a 5 category Likert-scale. The categories range from "does not apply" (score 0) to "fully applies" (score 4) [36].

The baseline assessment contained also a sociodemographic part to assess sex, age, education, and employment status. Patients' diagnoses were extracted from medical files.

Statistical analysis

To investigate determinants for medication adherence, a multivariate logistic regression approach was used. The MARS-D score was dichotomized in "adherent" and "non-adherent". Following recent literature, the cut-off was set at a MARS-D score of 24. Participants with a MARS-D score of 25 were seen as adherent (coded as 1), participants with a score < 25 were considered as non-adherent (coded as 0) [37, 38]. A multiple imputation (based on the EM algorithm [39]) was performed to deal with missing data. Fifty-nine percent of the records where complete. Thirty percent of the records missed one and 11% of the records missed two or more items. There were no missing items regarding the questionnaire of the primary endpoint. The data was missing at random. With the imputed data set a multivariate intension to treat analysis was performed. As independent variables age, sex, education, employment status, GAF, social support, the total number of strong and very strong adverse drug effects, the NQ-aspect of social desirability, and the intake of atypical and typical antipsychotics were included in the model. Data processing and statistical calculations were performed with SAS 9.4 (© 2002–2012 by SAS Institute Inc., Cary, North Carolina, USA.).

In a sensitivity analysis the MARS-D score was modelled as a continuous variable. Due to its discrete distribution a Poisson regression was performed in a generalized linear model (GLM). It was necessary to reverse the MARS-D-variable for the Poisson regression because of the left skewed distribution of the data.

Results

Of 135 participants recruited, 127 could be included in the analyses (Fig. 1).

The participants had a mean age of 42 years (SD 12.9), 57% were men. Eighty-four percent were unemployed and 28% had an education of less than 10 years. One hundred and-six participants had a diagnosis of schizophrenia, schizotypal and delusional disorders (F20 – F29), thereof 72 paranoid schizophrenia (F20), 1 Persistent delusional disorders (F22), 8 acute and transient psychotic disorders (F 23) and 25 schizoaffective disorders (F25). Thirty participants had a diagnosis of mood (affective) disorders (F30 – F39), thereof 27 bipolar affective disorder (F31) and 3 depressive episode (F32). Nine participants had both a diagnosis of schizophrenia, schizotypal and delusional disorders as well as mood (affective) disorders. Atypical antipsychotics were prescribed to 85 participants. Typical antipsychotics were prescribed to 27 participants. Fifteen participants had no prescription for antipsychotics but for drugs of other drug types. Table 1 shows the descriptive results for adherence, global functioning, social support, the number of strong to very strong adverse drug effects, and social desirability. The adherence showed a left skewed distribution

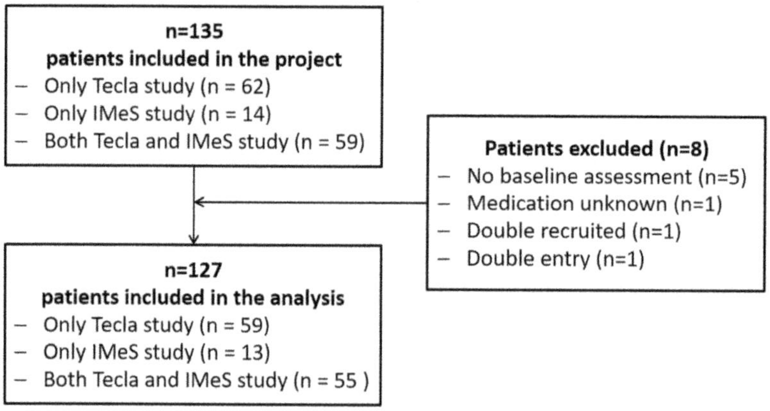

Fig. 1 Number of patients included in the analysis

(Fig. 2), 54% of the participants reported some kind of non-adherence (MARS-D score < 25).

Figure 3 shows the reasons for non-adherence. To forget to take the medicine is the most frequent reason for non-adherent behavior. Active deviation from the prescribed medication scheme (change the dose, stop taking medicines for a while, skip a dose, take less than instructed) were each reported at prevalence of less than 20%.

The results of the logistic regression are shown in Table 2. Higher age, being employed in full time, part time or vocational training, a higher level of global functioning, having more social support and intake of typical antipsychotics have a significant positive influence on adherence. Being female is a negative determinant for adherence. The level of education, the number of strong and very strong adverse drug effects and intake of atypical antipsychotics have no statistically significant effect on adherence.

A Poisson regression model was performed and used as a sensitivity analysis. The reversal of the MARS-D for the linear Poisson regression also leads to a reversal in the direction of the results. The results (Table 3) are similar to the findings of the primary analysis except for sex and employment status. Patients with lower education, patients

Table 1 Descriptive statistics of the measured variables (Tecla baseline assessment)

	Mean (SD)	Median	Range
Adherence (MARS-D)	23.4 (2.5)	24	13–25
Global functioning (GAF)	54.8 (10.9)	55	30–85
Social support (score)	48.6 (12.9)	51	14–70
Social desirability			
positive qualities (PQ+)	2.7 (0.8)	2.7	0–4
minimize negative qualities (NQ-)	1.1 (0.8)	1	0–4
Number of strong to very strong adverse drug effects	2.6 (1.5)	2	1–10

SD standard deviation

that are not or just marginally employed and a lower level of global functioning (GAF) are associated with lesser adherence. Having social support showed no significant impact on medication adherence. The intake of atypical antipsychotics is significantly associated with higher non-adherence whereas the intake of typical antipsychotics is associated with higher adherence.

Discussion

The MARS-5 was designed to evaluate reasons and prevalences for non-adherent behavior, [23, 40] rather than to measure exact values of the medication use [25, 41, 42]. In the patient group with severe mental disorders, both the primary and the sensitivity analyses showed a positive influence of the global functioning level, of having social support and being employed on adherence.

Medication adherence of patients with severe psychiatric diseases is generally low. The patients in this study were treated in hospitals or day clinics, data assessment was performed shortly before their discharge. However, the proportion of non-adherent patients was relatively high (54%). Stange et al. compared the adherence of patients during the hospital stay with the situation 6 weeks after discharge and found that non-adherence was lower during hospital stay (37.6% vs. 61.2% after 6 weeks) [37]. Hence long-term non-adherence is likely underestimated in our analysis.

Jonsdottir et al. examined medication adherence in patients with severe mental disorders in an ambulant setting [8]. The MARS-5 mean score in this study (22.0) was slightly lower than in our analysis. These authors also found a statistically significant correlation with provider rated medication adherence which supports the validity of the self-rated score used in our study.

In two studies (Mahler et al. [43] and Huther et al. [38]) the adherence of chronically ill patients with

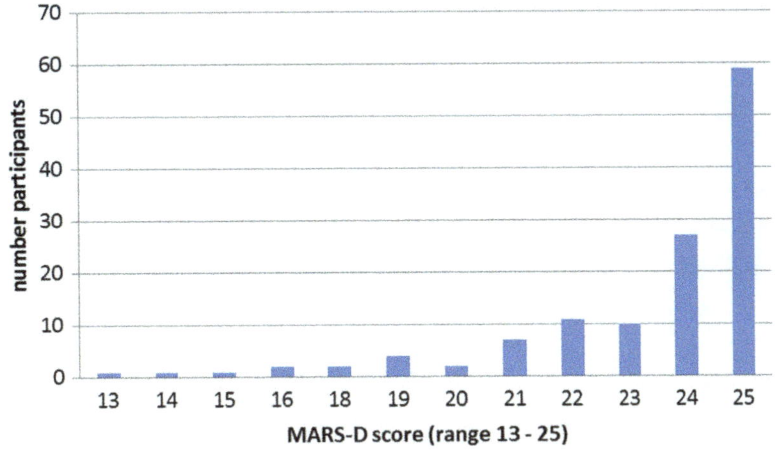

Fig. 2 Histogram of the MARS-D score (MARS-D score 25 means complete adherence, < 25 some kind of non-adherence, the lower the MARS-D score the higher is non-adherence)

MARS-D in primary care settings in Germany was examined. The average MARS-D scores were similar in both studies (mean 23.6 (SD 2.17) [43] and mean 23.5 (SD 2.7) [38]). Mahler et al. reported 'forget the medication intake' as the most common cause of non-adherence [43]. These findings correspond with our results. However, Huther et al. found no significant determinants for medication adherence in a subsequent multivariate analysis [38].

Tommelein et al. investigated the accuracy of the MARS-5 for patients with chronic obstructive pulmonary disease (COPD) [40]. The mean adherence for COPD patients was 23.5 (SD = 2.6). 52.9% of patients recorded complete adherence (MARS-5 sum score = 25). Further testing of the MARS-5 showed low sensitivity, specificity, and positive predictive value (PPV). Hence the authors assessed the MARS-5 as inaccurate in identifying non-adherent users of inhalation medication in patients with COPD [40].

Menckeberg et al. used the MARS-5 in a study about inhaled corticosteroids (ICS) in asthma control [41]. In their patient group the mean score value was 19.4 (SD 4.4). Compared to our and others' findings this score is rather low. However, with 79% scoring above the scale midpoint Menckeberg's results showed a skewed distribution too. The study showed that many patients were skeptical about the benefits of ICS [41]. This might be one cause for the discrepancy between their results and results of other studies.

In many cases, medication adherence is overestimated based on self-report questionnaires [23, 26–28]. Ose et al. examined the concordance in rating medication adherence among multimorbid patients and their general practitioners (GPs) [44]. Patients often rated their adherence higher than their GPs and only for 20% of the patients medication adherence was rated concordantly. An inherent limitation of self-report questionnaires is that

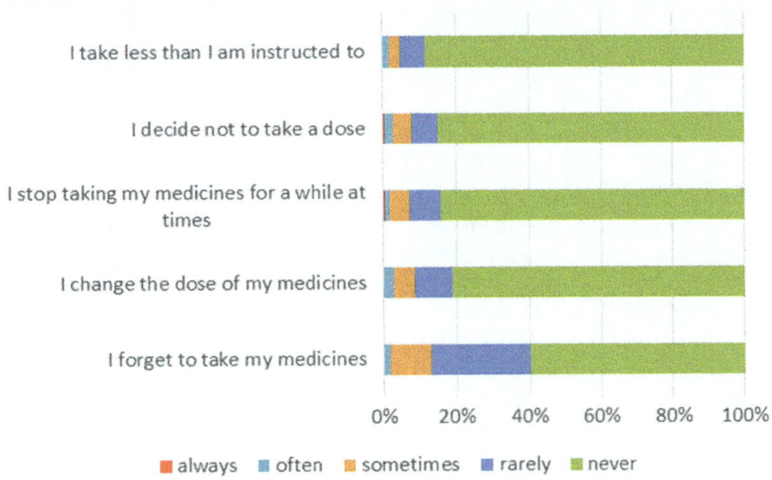

Fig. 3 Relative frequencies for reasons of non-adherent behavior assessed with MARS-D

Table 2 Results of the multivariate logistic regression (dependent variable: dichotomized adherence (MARS-D), cut-off score = 24), (being adherent vs. being non-adherent)

	regression coefficient	standard error	*p*-value (α 0.05)	OR	95% CI
Age in years	0.0170	0.0033	< 0.0001	1.017	1.011–1.024
Sex (female vs male)	−0.1557	0.0406	0.0001	0.732	0.625–0.859
Education (≥ 10 years of education vs. < 10 years of education)	0.0026	0.0448	0.9531	1.005	0.843–1.198
Employment status (being employed[a] vs. not or marginally employed)	0.4507	0.0672	< 0.0001	2.463	1.893–3.206
Global assessment of functioning (GAF)	0.0198	0.0039	< 0.0001	1.02	1.012–1.028
Social desirability (NQ-)	−0.6507	0.0562	< 0.0001	0.522	0.467–0.582
Social support	0.0193	0.0032	< 0.0001	1.02	1.013–1.026
Adverse drug effects	0.0382	0.0255	0.1341	1.039	0.988–1.092
Atypical antipsychotics (atypical drugs vs. other drug types)	−0.1036	0.0627	0.0987	0.813	0.636–1.039
Typical antipsychotics (typical drugs vs. other drug types)	0.4355	0.0728	< 0.0001	2.389	1.796–3.178

OR odds Ratio, *CI* confidence interval
[a] full time, part time, vocational training

unintentional non-adherence is commonly not assessed [40, 42].

Besides self-reports, adherence can be measured by directly observing the patients while taking their medication, using pill counts, Medication Event Monitoring Systems (MEMS), medical records, medication dispensing records, and pharmacological and biochemical markers [42, 45]. Some of these methods are costly and require increased effort or can only be used for certain drugs. Due to the importance of non-adherent behavior, a simple tool is needed that can easily be implemented in various study settings [8]. Self-reporting questionnaires are more patient-friendly, less expensive and easier to conduct. Jonsdottir et al. validated self-report measures with serum concentrations and found self-report questionnaires a valid method for measuring adherence [8]. The original MARS-5 in English as well as the German version MARS-D are reliable and valid self-report measures of non-adherence [23, 46].

In the literature, predictors for adherence or non-adherence differ. Sendt et al. gives a comprehensive overview [19]. As possible predictors were indicated marriage status, higher education, status of employment, gender, higher subjective well-being, later stage of illness, absence of cannabis use, lower rates of illicit substances and alcohol use, lower rates of medication refusal in early stages of treatment, better therapeutic alliance and higher trust in the physicians [19]. In our findings, higher education showed no significant results but being employed versus not or just marginally being employed showed a strong influence on adherence. Inconsistent predictors were symptom severity, insight, positive

Table 3 Results of the generalized linear Poisson regression. Dependent variable: MARS-D score

	Regression coefficient	Standard error	*p*-value (α 0.05)	beta estimate	95% CI
Age	0,0018	0,0012	0,1321	1,0018	0,9994–1,0042
sex (female vs male)	−0,0873	0,0295	0,0031	0,9164	0,8649–0,9711
Education (≥ 10 years of education vs. < 10 years of education)	−0,2761	0,0321	< 0.0001	0,7587	0,7125–0,8079
Employment status (being employed[a] vs. not or marginally employed)	−0,2793	0,0523	< 0.0001	0,7563	0,6826–0,8380
Global functioning (GAF)	−0,0246	0,0014	< 0.0001	0,9757	0,9731–0,9784
Social desirability (NQ-)	0,3951	0,0181	< 0.0001	1,4846	1,4329–1,5381
social support	0,0018	0,0012	0,1336	1,0018	0,9995–1,0041
adverse drug effects	0,0152	0,0084	0,0721	1,0153	0,9986–1,0323
Atypical antipsychotics (atypical drugs vs. other drug types)	0,2339	0,0245	< 0.0001	1,2635	1,2043–1,3257
Typical antipsychotics (typical drugs vs. other drug types)	−0,2533	0,0313	< 0.0001	0,7762	0,7300–0,8254

CI confidence interval
[a] full time, part time, vocational training

attitudes and social support [19]. An Israeli study showed better adherence with having more social support [47]. A majority of studies did not found associations between side effects and adherence [19, 48, 49]. This corresponds to our findings.Our results showed that participants taking typical antipsychotics had a significantly better adherence whereas the intake of atypical psychotics was associated with lower adherence. That result differs from other studies, where adherence was higher in patients taking atypical antipsychotics [14, 49, 50].

In summary, this suggests that adherence apparently is a complex issue [49]. Further research that also considers longitudinal analysis is intended.

Conclusions

Medication adherence is a complex problem that is influenced by many different parameters [45]. An important finding of this study is that also parameters that are influenceable by interventions like the functioning level or the degree of social support have an effect on adherence. These results can specifically be used for the development of adherence-promoting interventions. For example, knowledge, understanding and support for drug treatment should be strengthened also in the patient's social environment, among family members and caregivers.

Abbreviations

CI: Confidence interval; COPD: Chronic obstructive pulmonary disease; eCRF: Electronic Care Report Forms; F-SozU: Social support questionnaire; GAF : Global Assessment Functioning; GP: General practitioner; ICS: inhaled corticosteroids; IMeS: Study "Approaches of individualized medicine in psychiatric disorders"; KSE-G: Short scale Social desirability-gamma questionnaire; MARS: Original Medication Adherence Report Scale in English language; MARS-D: Medication Adherence Report Scale, German version; MEMS: Medication Event Monitoring Systems; NQ-: Minimization of negative qualities (social desirability); OR: Odds ratio; PPV: positive predictive value; PQ +: Exaggeration of positive qualities (social desirability); SD: Standard deviation; Tecla: Study "Post stationary **tele**medical **ca**re of patients with severe psychiatric disorders"; YLD: years of life lived with disability

Acknowledgments

We would like to thank the Department of General Practice and Health Services Research and Department of Internal Medicine VI, Clinical Pharmacology and Pharmacoepidemiology, University Hospital Heidelberg, Heidelberg, Germany for providing the German version of the Medication Adherence Rating Scale (MARS-D).

Funding

This study is funded by the Damp Foundation (Damp Stiftung c/o NGEG mbH) after a peer review process. The Damp Foundation fosters medical research and teaching, social projects and the education of young professionals in the medical profession in the German federal states Schleswig-Holstein, Hamburg and Western-Pomerania. The Damp Stiftung only financed the study. The study design, data collection, analysis, data interpretation and the writing of the manuscript was performed independently from the funder.

Authors' contributions

NvdB, HJG, WH and HJF designed the study. LNS, HJG, JML and NvdB participated in the coordination of the patient recruitment. US and LNS coordinate the study. US conducted the statistical calculation with support from TS and FR. US and NvdB drafted the manuscript. All authors read and approved the final manuscript.

Competing interests

The authors declare that they have no competing interests.

Author details

[1]Institute for Community Medicine, University Medicine Greifswald, Ellernholzstraße 1-2, 17487 Greifswald, Germany. [2]Department of Psychiatry and Psychotherapy, University Medicine Greifswald, Ellernholzstraße 1-2, 17487 Greifswald, Germany. [3]Department of Vascular Medicine, University Heart Center Hamburg, University Medical Center Hamburg-Eppendorf (UKE), Martinistraße 52, 20246 Hamburg, Germany. [4]Bethanien Hospital for Psychiatry, Psychosomatics and Psychotherapy, Gützkower Landstraße 69, 17489 Greifswald, Germany. [5]HELIOS Hanseklinikum Stralsund, department for psychiatry and psychotherapy, Rostocker Chaussee 70, 18437 Stralsund, Germany.

References

1. Jacobi F, Höfler M, Strehle J, Mack S, Gerschler A, Scholl L, Busch MA, Maske U, Hapke U, Gaebel W, et al. Mental disorders in the general population. Study on the health of adults in Germany and the additional module mental health (DEGS1-MH). In: Nervenarzt; 2014. p. 77–87.
2. Gaebel W, Wölwer W. Schizophrenie. Berlin: Robert Koch-Institut; 2010.
3. Hogarty GE, Goldberg SC, Schooler NR. Drug and sociotherapy in the aftercare of schizophrenic patients. III Adjustment of nonrelapsed patients. Arch Gen Psychiatry. 1974;31(5):609–18.
4. Loebel A, Lieberman J, Alvir J. Time to treatment response in successive episodes of early onset schizophrenia. Schizophrenia. 1995;1–2:158.
5. Davis JM, Schaffer CB, Killian GA, Kinard C, Chan C. Important issues in the drug treatment of schizophrenia. Schizophr Bull. 1980;6(1):70–87.
6. Burkhart PV, Sabate E. Adherence to long-term therapies: evidence for action. J Nurs Scholarsh. 2003;35(3):207.
7. Law MR, Soumerai SB, Ross-Degnan D, Adams AS. A longitudinal study of medication nonadherence and hospitalization risk in schizophrenia. J Clin Psychiatry. 2008;69(1):47–53.
8. Jonsdottir H, Opjordsmoen S, Birkenaes AB, Engh JA, Ringen PA, Vaskinn A, Aamo TO, Friis S, Andreassen OA. Medication adherence in outpatients with severe mental disorders: relation between self-reports and serum level. J Clin Psychopharmacol. 2010;30(2):169–75.
9. Ascher-Svanum H, Faries DE, Zhu B, Ernst FR, Swartz MS, Swanson JW. Medication adherence and long-term functional outcomes in the treatment of schizophrenia in usual care. J Clin Psychiatry. 2006;67(3):453–60.
10. Kane JM. Review of treatments that can ameliorate nonadherence in patients with schizophrenia. J Clin Psychiatry. 2006;67(Suppl 5):9–14.
11. Barkhof E, Meijer CJ, de Sonneville LMJ, Linszen DH, de Haan L. Interventions to improve adherence to antipsychotic medication in patients with schizophrenia–a review of the past decade. European Psychiatry. 2012;27(1):9–18.
12. Lindenmayer JP, Liu-Seifert H, Kulkarni PM, Kinon BJ, Stauffer V, Edwards SE, Chen L, Adams DH, Ascher-Svanum H, Buckley PF, et al. Medication nonadherence and treatment outcome in patients with schizophrenia or schizoaffective disorder with suboptimal prior response. J Clin Psychiatry. 2009;70(7):990–6.
13. Cramer J, Rosenheck R. Compliance with medication regimes for mental and physical disorder. Psychiatr Serv. 1998;49(2):196–201.
14. Dolder CR, Lacro JP, Dunn LB, Jeste DV. Antipsychotic medication adherence: is there a difference between typical and atypical agents? Am J Psychiatry. 2002;159(1):103–8.
15. Chakrabarti S. Treatment-adherence in bipolar disorder: a patient-centred approach. World J Psychiatry. 2016;6(4):399–409.

16. Leclerc E, Mansur RB, Brietzke E. Determinants of adherence to treatment in bipolar disorder: a comprehensive review. J Affect Disord. 2013;149(1–3):247–52.
17. McCann TV, Lu S. Medication adherence and significant others' support of consumers with schizophrenia in Australia. Nurs Health Sci. 2009;11(3):228–34.
18. San L, Bernardo M, Gomez A, Pena M. Factors associated with relapse in patients with schizophrenia. Int J Psychiatry Clin Pract. 2013;17(1):2–9.
19. Sendt KV, Tracy DK, Bhattacharyya S. A systematic review of factors influencing adherence to antipsychotic medication in schizophrenia-spectrum disorders. Psychiatry Res. 2015;225(1–2):14–30.
20. Shuler KM. Approaches to improve adherence to pharmacotherapy in patients with schizophrenia. Patient Prefer Adherence. 2014;8:701–14.
21. van den Berg N, Grabe HJ, Baumeister SE, Freyberger HJ, Hoffmann W. A telephone- and text message-based telemedicine concept for patients with mental health disorders: results of a randomized controlled trial. Psychother Psychosom. 2015;84(2):82–9.
22. Meyer J, Fredrich D, Piegsa J, Habes M, van den Berg N, Hoffmann W. A mobile and asynchronous electronic data capture system for epidemiologic studies. Comput Methods Prog Biomed. 2013;110(3):369–79.
23. Mahler C, Hermann K, Horne R, Ludt S, Haefeli WE, Szecsenyi J, Jank S. Assessing reported adherence to pharmacological treatment recommendations. Translation and evaluation of the medication adherence report scale (MARS) in Germany. J Eval Clin Pract. 2010;16(3):574–9.
24. Haynes RB, Taylor DW, Sackett DL, Gibson ES, Bernholz CD, Mukherjee J. Can simple clinical measurement detect patient noncompliance? Hypertension. 1980;2(6):757–64.
25. Horne R, Weinman J. Patients' beliefs about prescribed medicines and their role in adherence to treatment in chronic physical illness. J Psychosom Res. 1999;47(6):555–67.
26. Kelin K, Lambert T Jr, Brnabic AJ, Newton R, Ye W, Escamilla RI, Chen KP, Don L, Montgomery W, Karagianis J, et al. Treatment discontinuation and clinical outcomes in the 1-year naturalistic treatment of patients with schizophrenia at risk of treatment nonadherence. Patient Prefer Adherence. 2011;5:213–22.
27. DiMatteo MR. Variations in patients' adherence to medical recommendations: a quantitative review of 50 years of research. Med Care. 2004;42(3):200–9.
28. Garber MC, Nau DP, Erickson SR, Aikens JE, Lawrence JB. The concordance of self-report with other measures of medication adherence: a summary of the literature. Med Care. 2004;42(7):649–52.
29. Mahler C, Hermann K, Horne R, Jank S, Haefeli WE, Szecsenyi J. Patients' beliefs about medicines in a primary care setting in Germany. J Eval Clin Pract. 2012;18(2):409–13.
30. Aas IHM. Global Assessment of Functioning (GAF): properties and frontier of current knowledge. Ann General Psychiatry. 2010;9:20.
31. Wells KB, Stewart A, Hays RD, Burnam MA, Rogers W, Daniels M, Berry S, Greenfield S, Ware J. The functioning and well-being of depressed patients. Results from the medical outcomes study. Jama. 1989;262(7):914–9.
32. Jones SH, Thornicroft G, Coffey M, Dunn G. A brief mental health outcome scale-reliability and validity of the Global Assessment of Functioning (GAF). Br J Psychiatry. 1995;166(5):654–9.
33. Fydrich T, Sommer G, Tydecks S, Brähler E. Social support questionnaire (F-SozU): standardization of short form (K-14). Z Med Psychol. 2009;18:43–8.
34. Stentzel U, Grabe HJ, Strobel L, Penndorf P, Langosch J, Freyberger HJ, Hoffmann W, van den Berg N. Tecla: a telephone- and text-message based telemedical concept for patients with severe mental health disorders - study protocol for a controlled, randomized, study. BMC Psychiatry. 2015; 15(1):273.
35. Paulhus DL, Braun HI, Jackson DN, Wiley DE. Socially desirable responding: the evolution of a construct. The role of constructs in psychological and educational measurement. 2002;49459
36. Kemper CJ, Beierlein C, Bensch D, Kovaleva A, Rammstedt B. Eine Kurzskala zur Erfassung des Gamma-Faktors sozial erwünschten Antwortverhaltens: Die Kurzskala Soziale ERwünschtheit-Gamma (KSE-G). GESIS-Working Papers. 2012;25:1–27.
37. Stange D, Kriston L, von Wolff A, Baehr M, Dartsch DC. Medication complexity, prescription behaviour and patient adherence at the interface between ambulatory and stationary medical care. Eur J Clin Pharmacol. 2013;69(3):573–80.
38. Huther J, von Wolff A, Stange D, Harter M, Baehr M, Dartsch DC, Kriston L. Incomplete medication adherence of chronically ill patients in German primary care. Patient Prefer Adherence. 2013;7:237–44.
39. Dempster AP, Laird NM, Rubin DB. Maximum likelihood from incomplete data via EM algorithm. J Roy Stat Soc Series B Methodol. 1977;39(1):1–38.
40. Tommelein E, Mehuys E, Van Tongelen I, Brusselle G, Boussery K. Accuracy of the Medication Adherence Report Scale (MARS-5) as a quantitative measure of adherence to inhalation medication in patients with COPD. Ann Pharmacother. 2014;48(5):589–95.
41. Menckeberg TT, Bouvy ML, Bracke M, Kaptein AA, Leufkens HG, Raaijmakers JA, Horne R. Beliefs about medicines predict refill adherence to inhaled corticosteroids. J Psychosom Res. 2008;64(1):47–54.
42. Garfield S, Clifford S, Eliasson L, Barber N, Willson A. Suitability of measures of self-reported medication adherence for routine clinical use: a systematic review. BMC Med Res Methodol. 2011;11:149.
43. Mahler C, Jank S, Hermann K, Haefeli WE, Szecsenyi J. Information on medications - how do chronically ill patients assess counselling on drugs in general practice? Dtsch Med Wochenschr. 2009;134(33):1620–4.
44. Ose D, Mahler C, Vogel I, Ludt S, Szecsenyi J, Freund T. Let's talk about medication: concordance in rating medication adherence among multimorbid patients and their general practitioners. Patient Prefer Adherence. 2012;6:839–45.
45. Stange D, Kriston L, von Wolff A, Baehr M, Dartsch DC. Reducing cardiovascular medication complexity in a German university hospital: effects of a structured pharmaceutical management intervention on adherence. J Manag Care Pharm. 2013;19(5):396–407.
46. Russell J, Kazantzis N. Medication beliefs and adherence to antidepressants in primary care. N Z Med J. 2008;121(1286):14–20.
47. Baloush-Kleinman V, Levine SZ, Roe D, Shnitt D, Weizman A, Poyurovsky M. Adherence to antipsychotic drug treatment in early-episode schizophrenia: a six-month naturalistic follow-up study. Schizophr Res. 2011;130(1–3):176–81.
48. Jonsdottir H, Opjordsmoen S, Birkenaes AB, Simonsen C, Engh JA, Ringen PA, Vaskinn A, Friis S, Sundet K, Andreassen OA. Predictors of medication adherence in patients with schizophrenia and bipolar disorder. Acta Psychiatr Scand. 2013;127(1):23–33.
49. Vassileva I, Milanova V, Asan T. Predictors of medication non-adherence in Bulgarian outpatients with schizophrenia. Community Ment Health J. 2014; 50(7):854–61.
50. Velligan DI, Lam F, Ereshefsky L, Miller AL. Psychopharmacology: perspectives on medication adherence and atypical antipsychotic medications. Psychiatr Serv. 2003;54(5):665–7.

8

Excited catatonia in a patient with fatal pulmonary embolism and a successful treatment strategy

Wei-Ting Tseng and Tiao-Lai Huang*

Abstract

Background: Patients with psychiatric disorders in critical condition are difficult to treat. In this study, we report on a patient with underlying schizoaffective disorder who developed catatonia, cardiac arrest, and pulmonary embolism, as well as a successful treatment strategy.

Case presentation: The inpatient is a 41-year-old morbidly obese male with schizoaffective disorder whose clozapine dosage was titrated from 100 mg to 175 mg due to auditory hallucination and agitation. The patient abruptly developed acute cardiopulmonary symptoms associated with an elevated troponin-I level. He was transferred to a cardiac intensive care unit, where he remained for 3 days. He was also found to have excited catatonic symptoms, and the lorazepam-diazepam protocol was initiated to quickly relieve the catatonia. Once the coronary angiogram was read as normal, the patient was transferred back to the psychiatric ward. However, the patient then suffered from in-hospital cardiac arrest. He was resuscitated and again transferred to the medical intensive care unit. Computed tomography confirmed the diagnosis of a pulmonary embolism. The patient was treated with Rivaroxaban 30 mg/d for the first 21 days, followed by 20 mg daily for 3 months. To control his severe and refractory psychotic symptoms, the patient was re-prescribed clozapine. During the 15-month follow-up period, the patient demonstrated a fair response and tolerability to clozapine 150 mg without symptoms relapse and no thromboembolic event.

Conclusion: This report can serve to remind psychiatrists and physicians to be aware of fatal conditions in patients with psychiatric diseases and physical illnesses.

Keywords: Catatonia, Schizoaffective disorder, Cardiac arrest, Pulmonary embolism, Benzodiazepine

Background

Previous studies have reported that antipsychotic (AP) drugs may increase the risk of developing pulmonary embolism (PE), especially clozapine and low-potency first-generation APs [1]. A potentially fatal and complicated medical emergency in patients with psychiatric disease, pulmonary embolisms are frequently missed at first, resulting in a high mortality rate. Early detection and aggressive management are important in patients with psychiatric diseases, catatonia, and critical physical problems.

* Correspondence: a540520@adm.cgmh.org.tw
Department of Psychiatry, Kaohsiung Chang Gung Memorial Hospital and Chang Gung University College of Medicine, No. 123, Dapi Road, Niaosong District, Kaohsiung City 833, Taiwan

In this report, we present a 41-year-old male inpatient with schizoaffective disorder that developed acute cardiopulmonary symptoms and catatonic symptoms. The patient had two intensive care unit (ICU) stays, with an intra-hospital cardiac arrest in between them. A pulmonary embolism was eventually confirmed. After intensive treatments for PE and a benzodiazepine prescription to relieve the catatonia, he had a full recovery. The patient continued to be well during the 15-month follow-up, despite re-introducing clozapine.

Case presentation

Mr. T, a 41-year-old Taiwanese man, with educational level of 12 years, suffering from schizoaffective disorder for more than 10 years, ever hospitalized to psychiatric wards for 7 times due to disease relapses, despite of more than 2 antipsychotic trials. Before this episode, he had been treated with clozapine 100 mg and lithium 900 mg daily with fair compliance and no remarkable side effects for 2 years. He was obese (body mass index, 39 kg/m^2), but a lifelong non-smoker with no alcohol or substance abuse, no systemic disease in his medical history and no other comorbid psychiatric disease like personality disorder. He lived with his parents, was unemployed, and was capable of doing simple housework at home.

One day, the patient was sent to the emergency room of a medical center because he had been hearing voices for more than one week. Initial examinations indicated stable vital signs and normal laboratory results, electrocardiogram, and plain chest film. The patient was admitted to the psychiatric unit.

After admission, he was observed to be talking to himself and to have an elevated mood, auditory hallucinations of commanding voices, referential and persecutory delusions, and the hyperactive and agitated behaviors of squatting, standing up, crawling on the ground, and violently attacking others. Some excited catatonic symptoms were also noted, including restlessness, stereotypy, impulsivity, and combativeness. With regard to controlling his agitation and violence symptoms, he was managed with protective restraints and injected lorazepam 2 mg 1 ampule and haloperidol 5 mg 1 ampule intramuscularly, a total of six doses in the first week. A primary regimen of lithium 900 mg/d and clozapine 100 mg/d was used and titrated up to 175 mg/d. Two days after clozapine titration, the patient developed acute cardiopulmonary symptoms, including cold sweats, chest tightness, orthopnea, and tachycardia. Lab results showed elevated cardiac enzymes of CK-MB 37.7 ng/mL, troponin I 3.328 ng/mL, increased WBC 16500/mm^3, and increased creatine kinase 8045 U/L with 100% MM form. Electrocardiogram showed sinus tachycardia and ST-segment depression in V1–V4. Due to suspected acute non-ST elevation myocardial infarction, the patient was transferred to the cardiac care unit (CCU), where he was managed with enoxaparin subcutaneously and dual antiplatelet agents (DAPT), and the antipsychotics and lithium were discontinued.

His catatonia symptoms persisted, and the patient scored a 20 on the Bush–Francis Catatonia Rating Scale (BFCRS) [2]. A diazepam intravenous drip (10 mg/ 500 ml infused in normal saline at a rate of 1.25 mg/h) and oral-form lorazepam 4 mg/d were administered [3]. With this treatment, the BFCRS score became 0. After staying 3 days in the CCU, the coronary angiography was reported as being normal, and the enoxaparin and DAPT were discontinued. With a relatively stable physical condition, the patient was transferred back to the psychiatric unit.

However, 3 days after discontinuing enoxaparin and DAPT, the patient suddenly collapsed after defecating in the psychiatric ward. He was resuscitated for 5 min, regaining his pulse, and presented with hypoxia with 80% saturation under Ambu bagging. Laboratory testing showed an elevated d-dimer level > 35 mg/L FEU. The electrocardiogram showed sinus tachycardia and ST depressed at precordial leads V1 -V4. The patient was immediately intubated and once again transferred to the medical ICU. During the second ICU stay, which lasted 7 days, the patient gradually improved and was extubated. While the chest computed tomography reported multifocal filling defects in the bilateral pulmonary arteries, which is in line with a pulmonary embolization, oral rivaroxaban 30 mg/d was given, and the patient was sent back to the psychiatric ward. Since the patient presented with refractory psychotic symptoms and severely agitated behaviors, which may have disturbed his physical recovery, clozapine was prescribed again with an initial dose of 50 mg/d, and the dosage was carefully titrated up to 150 mg as of his discharge approximately 2 weeks later, when he fully recovered physically and mentally. The patient was managed with rivaroxaban 30 mg/d for the first 2 weeks and then 20 mg/d for 3 months.

During the outpatient follow-up period of 15 months, at which point this report was prepared, the patient remained free of any further psychotic, mood, or thromboembolic episodes.

Discussion

Timely identifying and relieving catatonia in physically ill patients is crucial, as delayed treatment may lead to a prolonged diagnosis and then recovery of underlying physical problems or serious complications, like venous thromboembolism (VTE) [4, 5]. Catatonia is considered a risk factor of deep vein thrombosis, which has a higher incidence rate of 25.3% in catatonic patients, particularly in patients with the retarded form of catatonia rather than the excited form of catatonia [6]. With regard to treating catatonia, the lorazepam-diazepam protocol has been reported to be a rapid and effective strategy for relieving catatonia in patients with schizophrenia, mood disorders, and general medical conditions [3, 7–9]. In this case, we noticed the excited catatonia episode when the patient was sent to the CCU and prescribed a continuous diazepam intravenous drip and oral-form lorazepam 4 mg/d. The benzodiazepine rapidly relieved the patient's catatonic symptoms so that he could be properly engaged in the intensive medical treatments.

PE, which is among the most life threatening medical emergencies, occurs when clotted blood enters the pulmonary arterial circulation [10]. Patients with similar comorbidities and clot burdens may experience drastically different clinical presentations, ranging from none to sudden death. A retrospective observation study reported that approximately one-third (33.5%) of patients who presented to the emergency department with an acute PE were undiagnosed before being sent home or hospitalized [11].

The risk factors of PE have been well documented in previous studies and include such factors as obesity, pregnancy, malignancy, thrombophilia, recent surgery or major trauma, immobility, smoking, and the use of estrogen-containing medications. Recently, atypical APs such as clozapine ware also reported to be associated with mortality due to PE. The estimated rate of PE in patients treated with clozapine is about 27.5 times higher than in the general population (95% CI 17.1–42.2) [12]. Other evidence has indicated that PE should be suspected in any APs users, even if recently discontinued or decreasing the dose, and particularly with any comorbid risks of thromboembolism, such as immobility [13].

The bio-mechanism of the relationship between clozapine use and PE remains largely unknown, but several hypotheses have been proposed, such as drug induced sedation, obesity, increased levels of antiphospholipid antibodies, hyperhomocysteinemia, hyperprolactinemia, aggregation of platelets antibodies and venous stasis exacerbated by sedation, and immobility secondary to sedation or restraint [1, 13–15]. Based on this patient's clinical course, in addition to his clozapine use, other risk factors may have also contributed to the PE, including obesity, temporary immobility under restraints, and catatonia symptoms. The patient had no smoking history, immobility or bed rest for more than 72 h, previous thromboembolism history, or family history of thromboembolism. Wells' score for PE on the cardiac arrest episode was 4.5, which was among the moderate risk group (27.8%) [16].

Conclusion

In this report, we present a complicated patient with underlying schizoaffective disorder that developed excited catatonia symptoms and cardiac arrest and was diagnosed with a pulmonary embolism. We further provided a successful management strategy with use of lorazepam-diazepam protocol for such critical conditions. We hope that this report will serve as a reminder to psychiatrists and physicians to be aware of fatal conditions in patients with psychiatric diseases and medical illnesses.

Abbreviations

AP: antipsychotic; BFCRS: Bush–Francis Catatonia Rating Scale; CCU: cardiac care unit; DAPT: dual antiplatelet agents; ICU: intensive care unit; PE: pulmonary embolism; VTE: venous thromboembolism

Acknowledgements

This work was supported by a clinical research grant (CMRPG8F1461) from Chang Gung Memorial Hospital in Taiwan. We did not receive financial support from any drug companies.

Authors' contributions

WT was the primary clinician involved in the assessment, management, and follow-up of the patient and wrote the manuscript with assistance from TH, who was involved in the management of the patient and provided overall supervision of this case, including patient care and manuscript preparation. Both authors contributed to the literature review and manuscript preparation and approved the final manuscript.

Consent for publication

Written informed consent was obtained from the patient for the publication of this case report.

Competing interests

The authors declare that they have no competing interests.

References

1. Hagg S, Jonsson AK, Spigset O. Risk of venous thromboembolism due to antipsychotic drug therapy. Expert Opin Drug Saf. 2009;8(5):537–47.
2. Bush G, Fink M, Petrides G, Dowling F, Francis A. Catatonia. I. Rating scale and standardized examination. Acta Psychiatr Scand. 1996;93(2):129–36.
3. Lin CC, Hung YY, Tsai MC, Huang TL. The lorazepam and diazepam protocol for catatonia due to general medical condition and substance in liaison psychiatry. PLoS One. 2017;12(1):e0170452.
4. Gross AF, Smith FA, Stern TA. Dread complications of catatonia: a case discussion and review of the literature. Prim Care Companion J Clin Psychiatry. 2008;10(2):153–5.
5. Lachner C, Sandson NB. Medical complications of catatonia: a case of catatonia-induced deep venous thrombosis. Psychosomatics. 2003;44(6):512–4.
6. Ishida T, Sakurai H, Watanabe K, Iwashita S, Mimura M, Uchida H. Incidence of deep vein thrombosis in catatonic patients: a chart review. Psychiatry Res. 2016;241:61–5.
7. Huang YC, Lin CC, Hung YY, Huang TL. Rapid relief of catatonia in mood disorder by lorazepam and diazepam. Biom J. 2013;36(1):35–9.
8. Lin CC, Huang TL. Lorazepam-diazepam protocol for catatonia in schizophrenia: a 21-case analysis. Compr Psychiatry. 2013;54(8):1210–4.
9. Lin CC, Lee CT, Lo YT, Huang TL. Brain-derived neurotrophic factor protein and mRNA levels in patients with bipolar mania - a preliminary study. Biom J. 2016;39(4):272–6.
10. Tapson VF. Acute pulmonary embolism. N Engl J Med. 2008;358(10):1037–52.
11. Torres-Macho J, Mancebo-Plaza AB, Crespo-Gimenez A, Sanz de Barros MR, Bibiano-Guillen C, Fallos-Marti R, Calderon-Parra J, de Miguel-Yanes JM. Clinical features of patients inappropriately undiagnosed of pulmonary embolism. Am J Emerg Med. 2013;31(12):1646–50.
12. Kortepeter C, Chen M, Knudsen JF, Dubitsky GM, Ahmad SR, Beitz J. Clozapine and venous thromboembolism. Am J Psychiatry. 2002;159(5):876–7.
13. Gami RK, Mishra P, Sedlak T. Pulmonary embolism and clozapine use: a case report and literature review. Psychosomatics. 2017;58(2):203–8.
14. Thomassen R, Vandenbroucke JP, Rosendaal FR. Antipsychotic medication and venous thrombosis. Br J Psychiatry. 2001;179:63–6.

9

A community-based peer support service for persons with severe mental illness in China

Yunge Fan[1], Ning Ma[1*], Liang Ma[2], Wei Xu[2], J. Steven Lamberti[3] and Eric D. Caine[3]

Abstract

Background: Peer support services for patients with severe mental illness (SMI) originated from Western countries and have become increasingly popular during the past twenty years. The aim of this paper is to describe a peer service model and its implementation in China, including the model's feasibility and sustainability.

Methods: A peer support service was developed in four Chinese communities. Implementation, feasibility and sustainability were assessed across five domains: Service process, service contents, peer training and supervision, service satisfaction, and service perceived benefit.

Results: *Service process*: 214 peer support activities were held between July 2013 and June 2016. No adverse events occurred during three years. Each activity ranged from 40 to 120 min; most were conducted in a community rehabilitation center or community health care center. *Service content*: Activities focused on eight primary topics—daily life skills, social skills, knowledge of mental disorders, entertainment, fine motor skill practice, personal perceptions, healthy life style support, emotional support. *Peer training and supervision*: Intensive training was provided for all peers before they started to provide services. Regular supervision and continued training were provided thereafter; online supervision supplemented face to face meetings. *Service satisfaction*: Nineteen consumers (79.2%) ($\chi^2(1) = 12.76$, $p < 0.001$) were satisfied with the peers and 17 consumers (70.8%) ($\chi^2(1) = 8.05$, $p = 0.005$) expressed a strong desire to continue to participate in the service. Fourteen caregivers (93.3%) ($\chi^2(1) = 11.27$, $p = 0.001$) wanted the patients to continue to organize or participate in the service. *Service perceived benefit:* Six peers (85.7%) ($\chi^2(1) = 3.57$, $p = 0.059$) reported an improvement of working skills. Ten consumers (41.7%) ($\chi^2(1) = 0.05$, $p = 0.827$) reported better social communication skills. Six caregivers (40%) ($\chi^2(1) = 1.67$, $p = 0.197$) observed patients' increase in social communication skills, five (33.3%) ($\chi^2(1) = 1.67$, $p = 0.197$) found their own mood had been improved.

Conclusions: Peer support services for patients with SMI can be sustainably implemented within Chinese communities without adverse events that jeopardize safety and patient stability. Suggestions for future service development include having professionals give increased levels of support to peers at the beginning of a new program. A culturally consistent peer service manual, including peer role definition, peer training curriculum, and supervision methods, should be developed to help implement the service smoothly.

Keywords: Severe mental illness, Peer support, Community, China

* Correspondence: maning@bjmu.edu.cn

[1]Peking University Sixth Hospital; Peking University Institute of Mental Health; Key Laboratory of Mental Health, Ministry of Health (Peking University); National Clinical Research Center for Mental Disorders (Peking University Sixth Hospital), Beijing, China

Full list of author information is available at the end of the article

Background

Peer support services are designed to bring together people with similar life experiences, culture, living environments, social status, concerns, and daily challenges [1]. This commonality promotes mutual respect, and it enables sharing of information, practical strategies and ongoing support that are critical to sustained behavior change [1]. Within the field of mental health services, peer service providers are individuals who have lived experience with mental illness, and who are willing to provide modeling and support to other individuals with mental illness [2]. Now regarded as a hallmark of recovery-oriented care [3], peer support services emphasize the importance of personal interests and strengths as foundations of recovery, rather than psychopathology and treatment considerations [4].

The benefits of peer support service are multifaceted, including benefits for peers (providers of peer support), consumers (receivers of peer support), the healthcare system, and society as a whole [5, 6]. Peers' benefits include self-efficacy resulting from the experience of helping others [7], and earning money [8]. In addition, providing peer support services can promote peers' communication skills, improve emotional and verbal expression, and increase social functioning [9]. All of these benefits contribute directly to the recovery process. The effects upon consumers with severe mental illness (SMI) are broad and include not only clinical benefits, such as fewer hospitalizations or psychiatric symptoms, but also personal and emotional benefits such as feelings of understanding, respect and trust [10, 11]. Peer support can also improve consumers' social functioning and quality of life [12]. Peer support services are able to benefit healthcare systems and society as a whole. Peers, as healthcare service providers, can enrich mental health service teams while providing additional support to clinicians. In addition, since peers communicate with patients more often, they can function as important bridges between doctors and patients [13]. Peer support can also reduce social discrimination against persons with SMI. By demonstrating that people with SMI can recover and work, peer service providers are able to promote social understanding and acceptance, decrease social stigma and fear, and decrease patients' feelings of shame and isolation [14].

Many studies have reported the importance of peers as positive role models of recovery and hope for consumers, caregivers and professional staff members alike [9, 15, 16]. Consumers as well as their caregivers become more positive and confident about themselves and their future, while peers can also help consumers like themselves better, believe in their own potential more and achieve their goals [9]. With regard to professional staff, they are able to see things differently and use other approaches to clients in specific situations [15].

The World Health Organization (WHO) Consultation documents the promise of peer support as an effective approach to chronic disease management and health promotion [17]. However, there is no widely accepted or standardized model for the operation of peer support services [18]. For example, peer support services in Rochester, NY, USA, are usually provided for a long-term duration and their contents are flexible. However, in New Zealand, peer run recovery houses are widely developed. The recovery house is an alternative to inpatient care in an acute psychiatric unit. It provides 24-h support, supervision and treatment [19]. In Australia, there is a Certificate IV Mental Health Peer Work as the minimum entry requirement for employment in peer support services, and their training content is relatively fixed [19, 20].

As for the format of peer service among patients with SMI, Davidson summarized it into three types: informal (naturally occurring) peer support, peer-run programs, and the employment of service recipients as service providers within traditional mental health programs [21]. Service duration can be long or short, and services can be located in the community or in hospitals. The content is varied, including activities such as disease and health education, social communication and daily life skills, and vocational support. Peer positions are often voluntary, and peers are typically selected by professionals based upon their communication skills, understanding of mental illness, personal responsibility and compassion, and level of clinical stability. In addition, professionals generally supervise peers during the delivery of support services [22]. Peer services currently operate in several countries including the United States [23], the United Kingdom [24], Australia [25], Germany [4], Brazil [26], New Zealand, and Canada [27]. The experiences of these countries have also proved that the operation of peer services should be consistent with local customs, values, and resource availability [28].

China, with its population of 1.3 billion, has more than 13 million persons suffering from psychotic disorders (hereafter labeled serious mental illness; SMI), based on an estimated prevalence of mood disorders was 6.1%, anxiety disorders was 5.6%, substance abuse disorders was 5.9%, and psychotic disorders was 1.0% [29]. At the end of 2014, there were only 25,307 psychiatrists (1.85/100,000 population) and 51,571 psychiatric nurses (3.77 /100,000 population) [30], very few psychotherapists and social workers, and almost no mental health occupational therapist. Outpatient mental health services for persons with SMI are offered primarily in large psychiatric hospital clinics, where one psychiatrist often sees 50–100 patients per day, with pharmacotherapy being the primary mode of treatment. If peers joined the mental health workforce and assisted in providing rehabilitation services, this strategy could enrich the scope of service and be beneficial to maintain patients' good condition. It could also compensate for the lack of professional personnel in the long run.

This project was started in 2013 with the aim of establishing a community-based peer support service model for patients with SMI. No peer-based services existed in China at the time when we began the project. The project had the goal of demonstrating feasibility and sustainability, while also assessing whether the program would be associated with adverse patient events. In this paper, we described the implementation of a peer support service in China.

Methods

Participants

A peer support service was developed in four communities located in the Chaoyang district of Beijing: Tuanjiehu, Maizidian, Xiangheyuan, and Jinsong. Peer support was initiated in July 2013 in Tuanjiehu and Maizidian, and in the other two communities in August 2015.

All peer service providers were recommended by community doctors and evaluated by a research team psychiatrist. Peers who agreed to participate in were subsequently utilized if they met the following inclusion criteria: Diagnosed with schizophrenia or bipolar disorder which was recoded from their medical record provided by community doctors; age between 18 and 60 years old; stable at least 6 months, being adherent with medications according to patients' and family members' report, and having insight about their disease which was assessed through individual interviews conducted by psychiatrists; no drug or alcohol abuse; no severe medical illness; and having good social functioning which was assessed by the personal and social performance scale (PSP), more than 50 scores in PSP is required [31]. All participating peers were expected to be compassionate and willing to help others. Applicants with strong practical skills (e.g., cooking, drawing) were preferred.

All peers participated in intensive pre-service training. Once they finished training, posters were placed in diverse community locations to recruit patient-recipients (i.e., consumers); others came to the program based on the recommendation of community doctors. Each potential consumer was evaluated by the team psychiatrist, using the following inclusion criteria: diagnosed with schizophrenia or bipolar disorder; age 18–60 years old; stable at least 3 months; no drug or alcohol abuse; and no severe medical illness.

We recruited 12 peer providers and 50 consumers by 2016 (see Table 1). One peer in Tuanjiehu community quit in 2015, expressing concerns about too much pressure working as a peer. The caregivers of peers and consumers were also recruited if they were willing to be contacted for the follow-up evaluation. Fifteen caregivers

Table 1 Numbers of peers and consumers enrolled in each community by year

Role in each Community	Year				χ^2 test of difference
	2013	2014	2015	2016	
Peer					$\chi^2(9) = 10.30$, $p = 0.326$
Tuanjiehu	5	5	4	4	
Maizidian	2	2	2	2	
Xiangheyuan	–	–	4	4	
Jingsong	–	–	2	2	
Total	7	7	12	12	
Consumer					$\chi^2(9) = 27.73$, $p = 0.001$
Tuanjiehu	10	11	14	14	
Maizidian	13	13	14	15	
Xiangheyuan	–	–	10	11	
Jingsong	–	–	10	10	
Total	23	24	48	50	

(seven of peers, eight of consumers) from 15 families had been recruited in this study. The project proposal was reviewed and approved by Peking University Sixth Hospital Ethics Committee, and all peers and consumers provided written informed consent.

Procedure

After the recruitment of peers and consumers, pre-service interviews with peers, consumers and their caregivers were conducted by a research assistant. The pre-service interviews were aimed to find out consumers' needs in order to make our service contents meet their demands. As long as peers have received the intensive pre-service training, they were able to provide service. Apart from the intensive pre-service training that each peer was required to attend, peers were supervised during the whole service course. During the first year of the service, community doctors and clinical psychologists provided direction to peers before and after each peer support activity, and the psychiatrist provided guidance and support to community doctors and clinical psychologists. Beginning in July 2014 (the second year), community doctors offered non-scheduled "as needed" supervision which mainly depended on peers' needs, while the clinical psychologists and psychiatrist offered group supervision every six weeks. After they had accumulated a year of experience, peers were able to prepare and organize session and training activities themselves; their credibility as service providers was well-established among consumers. In addition, two social workers were involved in this program beginning in March 2016, and they provided assistance before and after activities upon requests by the peers. These social workers also participated in group supervision. Along with face to face supervision, we also provided online supervision. A WeChat group was built which included peers, community doctors, social workers, clinical psychologists and psychiatrists.

An evaluation had been conducted among the peers, consumers, and their caregivers from the first two communities in December 2014, the evaluation concluded the service satisfaction and effectiveness.

Measures

We examined implementation and feasibility of the community-based peer support service model for patients with SMI in China from five aspects – service process, service content, peer training and supervision, service satisfaction, and service perceived benefit.

Service process [32]

Measures of service process included the number of activities, frequency, average session time, and format of each activity. Peers were required to fill in a self-compiled form called "Activity Process Form" each time after the service being provided. The form included the date, start and end time of each activity, as well as the format of each activity. The forms had to be well-preserved by each peer and submitted to the project manager every six weeks.

Service content [33]

Measures of service content included the activity topics and the proportion of each. These were also tested by "Activity Process Form" which contained the aim and theme of each activity as well as consumers' feedback. It was also required to be filled in after each service and submitted every six weeks.

Peer training and supervision [9]

Multi-background supervisor group was constituted by community doctors and professionals including psychiatrists, clinical psychologists and social workers. The measures of peer training and supervision included the contents of issues identified which were summarized from the training schedule and textbooks, audio and literal supervision records.

Service satisfaction [9, 18]

Semi-structured face to face interviews were conducted by a research assistant to measure the service satisfaction from the perspectives of consumers and their caregivers. The consumers were asked if they were satisfied with the peers and if they were willing to continue to participate in the peer support service. The caregivers were asked if they wanted the patients to continue to organize (for peers' caregivers) or participate (for consumers' caregivers) in the service. All the questions were supposed to be answered with yes or no.

Service perceived benefit [9, 15]

Feedback on the perceived impact of providing or receiving service was collected through brief structured face to face interviews conducted by a research assistant with peers, consumers as well as their caregivers. The peers and consumers were asked if organizing and participating in the service had any benefit to their improvement of skills or mood. The caregivers were also asked if the peer support service could improve their own mood or quality of life. All the questions were supposed to be answered with yes or no.

Data analysis

All the forms as well as audio and literal records were recoded by three graduate students independently. Descriptive and inferential statistics analyses were used. Continuous variables were reported as means ± SD and were tested for normality with the Shapiro-Wilk test. Mean differences were tested by independent samples t-tests. Discrete variables were reported as N's and percentages. Chi-square tests were used to examine differences. Analyses were performed with SPSS 19.0 for Windows.

Results

Peer and consumer participants

The numbers of peers and consumers enrolled in each community by year are shown in Table 1. There was a significant increase in consumers while non-significant in peers. Demographic information pertaining to peers and consumers is shown in Table 2. The mean ages of peers and consumers were 40.2 and 48.3, respectively. All peers and consumers were patients with SMI, most of them were diagnosed with schizophrenia. There was no significant difference between peers and consumers apart from age, working status and diagnosis. Peers were younger, less likely to be unemployed than consumers, and less peers had diagnoses of schizophrenia.

Service process

A total of 214 peer support sessions were delivered from July 2013 to June 2016. One peer session means that peer met with consumers once and conduct activities or support service in groups. There was no report of violence, self-harm, or other potentially adverse events. The number of sessions for each community by every 6-month period is shown in Fig. 1. The numbers among different communities and time period yielded statistical significance ($\chi^2(15) = 48.75$, $p < 0.001$). During the first 6 months, only two communities developed peer support services and the peers were not yet proficient in running activities, which were organized about once every one or two months. During the second year, sessions were delivered about once every two weeks in

Table 2 The demographic information of consumers and peers

Characteristic	Peers		Consumers		t test or χ^2 test of difference
	N	%	N	%	
Age (M ± SD)	40.2 ± 8.9		48.3 ± 8.2		$t = -2.99$, $p = 0.004$
Sex					$\chi^2(1) = 2.37$, $p = 0.124$
Male	8	66.7	21	42.0	
Female	4	33.3	29	58.0	
Education level					$\chi^2(5) = 2.93$, $p = 0.711$
Primary school	0	0	2	4.0	
Junior high school	1	8.3	10	20.0	
Senior high school	8	66.7	22	44.0	
Junior college	1	8.3	8	16.0	
Undergraduate degree	2	16.7	7	14.0	
Postgraduate degree	0	0	1	2.0	
Marital Status					$\chi^2(3) = 1.32$, $p = 0.726$
Single/never married	7	58.3	29	58.0	
Married	4	33.3	11	22.0	
Divorced	1	8.3	9	18.0	
Widowed	0	0	1	2.0	
Working status					$\chi^2(1) = 5.53$, $p = 0.039$
Yes (all part-time)	4	33.3	4	8.0	
No	8	66.7	46	92.0	
Diagnosis					$\chi^2(1) = 10.61$, $p = 0.004$
Schizophrenia	6	50.0	45	90.0	
Bipolar Disorder	6	50.0	5	10.0	

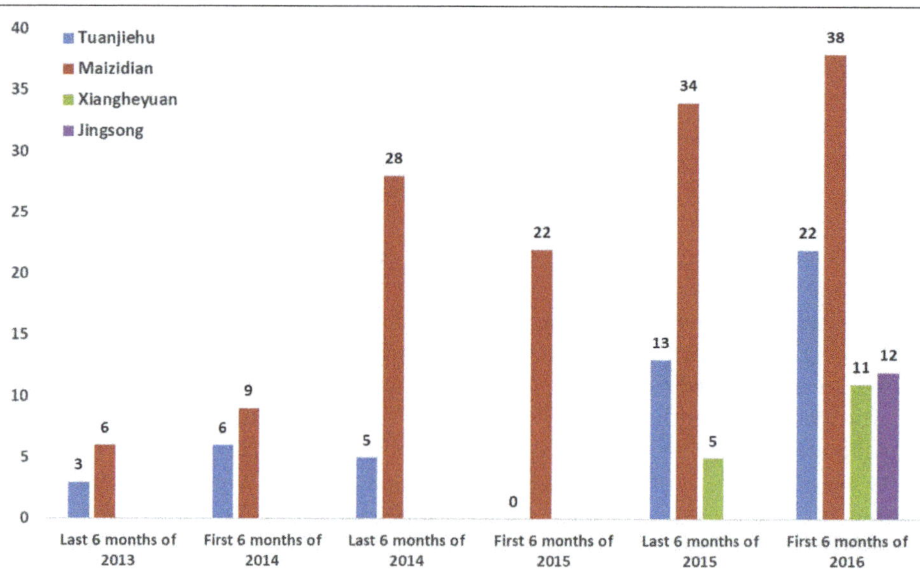

Fig. 1 The number of peer support activities in each communities by every 6 months

these two communities. During the first 6 months of 2015, one peer in Tuanjiehu quit and one peer in Maizidian asked for a temporary leave because of needing to assist his sick mother. In addition, Tuanjiehu had trouble in finding the service place because the old one could not be used anymore. Resulting in no session had been provided during this time period in Tuanjiehu community. Beginning in August 2015, peer support services were started in another two communities. In 2015 and 2016, the session frequency differed among communities. It occurred once or twice each week in the first two communities, and once every two weeks in the newer two communities. The duration of each session ranged from 40 min to 120 min, depending on the activity theme and format for the session. The format of each activity varied depending on the topics, including group discussion, role play, personal sharing, lecture, and outdoor exercises. Most sessions were held in community rehabilitation centers or community health care centers. Each session typically involved at least two peers, with one leading and the other one assisting with service delivery, record keeping, and documenting consumers' feedback.

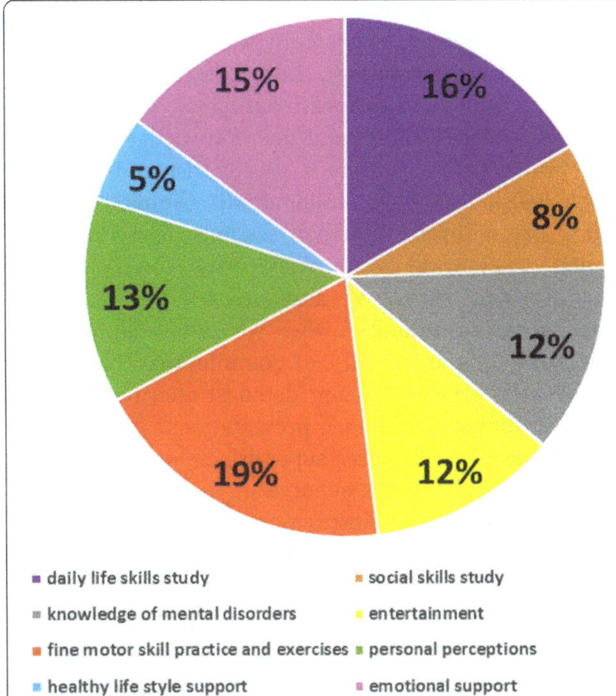

Fig. 2 The proportion of peer support activity categories

Service contents

On the basis of previous studies [34, 35], combining with the pre-service interviews, we summarized consumers' needs into eight categories: daily life skills, social interpersonal skills, knowledge of mental disorders, entertainment, fine motor skill practice and exercise, personal perceptions such as self-esteem and self-confidence, healthy life style, and emotional support. The eight categories had been provided to peers before the initiation of peer support sessions. Peers had freedom to choose which category and what specific contents they were going to afford.

Analyses of the service contents showed that each of the eight categories had been addressed during the three years' service. Some of the session contents examples are listed below: daily life skills study (e.g., cooking, how to use WeChat), social skills study (e.g., communicating with body language and facial expression, verbal communication skills), knowledge of mental disorders (e.g., treatments for schizophrenia, recognizing disease recurrence, medications, side-effects), entertainment (e.g., singing, watching movies), fine motor skill practice and exercises (e.g., handwriting, puzzles, physical exercise), personal perceptions (building self-esteem and self-confidence), healthy life style support (e.g., controlling your emotions, healthy diets), emotional support (e.g., sharing stories of childhood, building relationships with family members). The proportion of each category is shown in Fig. 2. The top three most popular activity categories were fine motor skill practice and exercise (19%), daily life skills study (16%) and emotional support (15%).

The program began by peers sharing the rules of this service with those consumers who were referred or who responded to our posters. Each was asked to review and sign an informed consent document as well as a service and group activity agreement before beginning the activities.

In addition, there were usually three parts for each session. First, there were brief warm up activities, such as icebreaking games or setting-up exercises. The main activities relating to each topic then were initiated. At the end, peer providers or consumers would summarize the activity, followed by reciting a poem or singing a song together. Peers were required to complete documentation for each session. Before one session's activities, they planned and completed an "Activity Plan Form". Upon completion of each session, peers completed the "Activity Process Form" and a "Participant List". If any adverse event or behavioral emergency (e.g., poorly controlled behavior, or problem that might require immediate attention) occurred during the session, peers were required to record the "Emergency Event Form" and to submit this report to the community doctors.

Peer training and supervision

Pre-service training was provided for all peers. Training contents included the concept and theory of peer support services, working principles and requirements (including confidentiality, boundaries, and relationships), how to design and implement group activities, effective listening and speaking skills, how to handle emergency situations, and how to complete the record forms. We developed the training curriculum with reference of USA and Australia experience [8], and integrated with extensive discussion with potential peers during the pre-service interviews to better understand their knowledge and needs. The primary trainers were a psychiatrist and a clinical psychologist. Pre-service training was completed in five half a day with six workshop sessions. The format included coursework, group sharing and discussion, role play, and storytelling. We also included the peers from our first two communities when we trained new peers in June 2015 for the second two communities. The former shared their experiences and demonstrated how to conduct activities as part of their presentations.

With regard to the peer supervision during the whole service course, while the supervision group initially functioned to provide basic instruction and support related to conducting activities, the group subsequently focused more upon addressing peers' difficulties and feelings of once they had accumulated service experience. For example, some peers might feel frustrated when they did not achieve their service goals, or when they encountered consumers who did not listen carefully or seemed bored. These experiences may undermine peers' confidence, even though they are related to factors other than the peers' level of skill or experience. The overall aim of supervision was to build peers' confidence as well as their work capacity, motivation, and self-satisfaction.

In addition, face to face supervisions were supplemented with the online supervision. According to unstructured interviews with peers and community doctors, online group provided timely and efficient input to support both peer and service development. Whenever the peers experienced challenging work situations, they could ask questions in the online WeChat group. This forum provided an opportunity for the professional staff to respond quickly, and it also provided an opportunity for the other peers to express support and to give suggestions. The success of our online supervision prompted peers to build additional online peer support services. Now, three communities have their own WeChat groups for peers and consumers in order to provide timely support for consumers.

Service satisfaction

Service satisfaction evaluation was only conducted among the first two communities (Tuanjiehu & Maizidian). Among the 24 consumers, three (12.5%) had not been assessed because of personal issues. Nineteen (79.2%) ($\chi^2(1) = 12.76$, $p < 0.001$) were satisfied with the peers and 17 (70.8%) ($\chi^2(1) = 8.05$, $p = 0.005$) expressed a strong desire to continue to participate in the service. Among the 15 caregivers, 14 (93.3%) ($\chi^2(1) = 11.27$, $p = 0.001$) wanted the patients to continue to organize or participate in the service.

Service perceived benefit

Service perceived benefit was only assessed among the first two communities (Tuanjiehu & Maizidian). For peers, six (85.7%) ($\chi^2(1) = 3.57$, $p = 0.059$) reported an improvement of working skills, four (57.1%) ($\chi^2(1) = 0.14$, $p = 0.705$) reported increase in social communication skills. For consumers, ten (41.7%) ($\chi^2(1) = 0.05$, $p = 0.827$) reported better social communication skills. For caregivers, six (40%) ($\chi^2(1) = 1.67$, $p = 0.197$) observed patients' increase of social communication skills, five (33.3%) ($\chi^2(1) = 1.67$, $p = 0.197$) found their own mood had been improved.

Discussion

The results of this evaluation suggest that peer support services for persons with SMI are feasible and sustainable in China. The peer service has been in operation for three years, and the number of communities that developed peer support services has increased from two to four with a significant increase of consumers. The service has received positive evaluation and satisfaction from consumers and caregivers of both peers and consumers. Our experience can serve as a point of reference for other areas of China where there is interest in developing peer support services within their respective communities. Although we did not establish a standardized model for the operation of peer support services, our work may provide a general framework upon which to build such services.

Several aspects of this framework are particularly important early in the course of service development and implementation. It is important to provide peers with extra help and support in figuring out the topic of activities and preparing for peer support sessions at the beginning of service delivery. It should be recognized that the role of peers is very new in China, the majority of them are lacking in experience and confidence. At the beginning of the project, both the caregivers and community workers were worried about the safety of service, they did not believe in peers. Even the peers did not believe in themselves and they tended to avoid telling stories about themselves or sharing their own life experiences because of the perceived stigma and the unfamiliar environment. Therefore, we guided peers to provide some entertainment or skill training activities at first. It is helpful to identify community workers, such as doctors, nurses and social workers, who are willing to guide peers in preparing activity materials, and in providing on-site support as peers assume their new roles. The early availability of supportive health professionals serves to alleviate stress that is commonly experienced by peers as they adopt the role of service provider. At the same time, it is important for community workers to give peers more autonomy as their proficiency increases. We came to understand, as well, that many community health workers, including physicians, frequently have scant knowledge about SMIs and their treatment, and about providing peer support services. Mental health professionals should provide more guidance for community health workers from the knowledge, skill training and supervision in helping peer providers. It should also be noted that the frequency of sessions was less during the first year in our first two communities. This slower initial pace allowed us to gradually develop the necessary procedures and practices to support peer service provision. Our pace increased during the third year period, especially as we opened a second set of services and as the peers' overall experience increased. In addition, after several months, the intimacy between peers and consumers also increased, then both the peers and community health workers became more positive about peer service.

It is essential to clarify the role of "peer." At the outset, peers reflected that they are patients too – that is, consumers – and they initially expressed doubt that other consumers would trust and listen to them. Community workers also commented that it was difficult for them to decide how closely they should work with the peers in providing support. Clear job descriptions and role clarification is necessary for both peers and community workers. We observed that the role of peer service providers can vary according to the characteristics and needs of consumers and the activities planned for each session. These roles can include being a professional assistant, an advocate, a supporter, and even a case manager. Despite this variability in roles, we found that their primary responsibility involved working as a role model and partner in recovery for other consumers. As such, peer providers should be prepared to provide emotional support, living and social skills development, education, sharing of experiences, and encouragement.

We recommend offering a range of service topics as part of the peer training curriculum. In this project, peers initially found it difficult to generate their own ideas for group activities, preferring that professionals would provide a list of topics. In the absence of such guidance from professionals, there is a risk that peer providers could become somewhat overwhelmed and demoralized. To minimize the risk, we recommend that peers first consider carrying out activities that relate to topics with which they are familiar. These can include daily life skills (e.g., cooking), basic social skills (e.g., introducing oneself), information about mental illness (e.g., early warning signs of relapse), entertainment suggestions (e.g., watching movies), and fine motor skill practice and exercises (e.g., Chinese calligraphy).

It is important to provide specific training and continuing supervision for peers through the use of multidisciplinary groups, including psychiatrists, psychological therapists, community workers (especially primary care doctors), and social workers, depending upon their local availability. Pre-service training is particularly important for peers and community doctors in order to clearly understand their roles and job requirements, and also for obtaining the necessary skills for providing services. The content of our pre-service training turned out to be consistent with the experience in Hong Kong, which proved to be practical in non-Western context [36]. One of our peer program's notable features is that we developed a group to provide supervision, an unusual feature in China. Several community doctors and peers mentioned that the supervision group effectively provided support for them. As for the format of supervision, we recommend combining both face-to-face and online formats. Face-to-face supervision is particularly helpful for affective interactions, while online supervision is more timely and efficient.

Finally, we recommend having at least two peers for each community, and to have both present at every session when possible. This level of peer staffing is particularly important for new programs. This team approach will better enable peers to monitor activities, and to adjust the peer role more effectively. Peer partners can support each other in a timely way before and after each session, discussing the plans and processes, sharing the job experiences, and identifying opportunities for improvement in future support and training activities. We received consistently positive feedback from peers and community doctors alike for having two peers working together by design.

There are some limitations in this study that need to be addressed. First, according to the results, although the service received positive evaluation and satisfaction from consumers and caregivers, the perceived benefit still not significant. This may because some of the effect have not been showed up by the evaluation or due to the small sample size, future researches are needed to replicate our study with larger sample size of peers, consumers as well as their caregivers. Secondly, based on our experience, at the initiate of peer service, peers tended to avoid telling stories about themselves or sharing their own life experiences because of the perceived stigma and the unfamiliar environment. However, the key idea of peer support service is that peer staff are trained to provide different services for which they are especially well suited based on their own life experiences and accumulated knowledge of how to live with a mental illness. So, although peers would adapt to their new roles eventually, future research could find more effective ways to speed up this process. We have also conducted follow-up evaluations with quantitative combined with qualitative measures among peers, consumers as well as their caregivers in the four communities, the results will be showed and discussed in another paper. Future research could also explore more long-term outcomes of peer support service in China.

Conclusions

Peer support service for patients with SMI can be sustainably implemented within Chinese communities without adverse events that jeopardize safety and patient stability. Suggestions for future service development include having professionals give increased levels of support to peer service providers at the beginning of a new program to minimize peers' anxiety and to promote rapid service model development. A culturally consistent peer support service manual, including information about peer role definition, the peer training curriculum, and supervision methods, should be developed to help peers implement the service smoothly.

Abbreviation

SMI: severe mental illness

Acknowledgements

The authors thank the research staff (Li Jing, Wei Guan, Chao Xv, Xingge Kang) of the four communities in Chaoyang District of Beijing for their assistance.

Funding

This research was supported by the grant from National Natural Science Foundation of China (71203003) and Beijing Health Development Research Project (2014-3-4111).

Authors' contributions

NM conceived of the study, oversaw data collection, supervised data analysis and wrote the manuscript. YGF conducted data analysis and wrote the manuscript draft. LM and WX helped in data collection. JSL and EDC contributed to writing of the manuscript. All authors read and approved the final manuscript.

Competing interests

The authors declare that they have no competing interests.

Author details

[1]Peking University Sixth Hospital; Peking University Institute of Mental Health; Key Laboratory of Mental Health, Ministry of Health (Peking University); National Clinical Research Center for Mental Disorders (Peking University Sixth Hospital), Beijing, China. [2]Beijing Chaoyang District Mental Disease Prevention and Control Center, The Third Hospital of Chaoyang District, Beijing, China. [3]Department of Psychiatry, University of Rochester Medical Center, Rochester, USA.

References

1. Boothroyd RI, Fisher EB. Peers for progress: promoting peer support for health around the world. Fam Pract. 2010;27(Suppl 1):i62–8.
2. Davidson L, Chinman M, Sells D, Rowe M. Peer support among adults with serious mental illness: a report from the field. Schizophr Bull. 2006;32(3):443–50.
3. Davidson L, Bellamy C, Guy K, Miller R. Peer support among persons with severe mental illnesses: a review of evidence and experience. World psychiatry. 2012;11(2):123–8.
4. Mahlke C, Heumann K, Ruppelt F, Meyer H-J, Rouhiainen T, Sielaff G, Lambert M, Bock T. Peer support for individuals with mental health problems and their relatives-background. Concept and Baseline Data Psychiatrische Praxis. 2015;42:S25–9.
5. Miyamoto Y, Sono T. Lessons from peer support among individuals with mental health difficulties: a review of the literature. Clinical practice and epidemiology in mental health: CP & EMH. 2012;8:22.
6. Repper J, Carter T. A review of the literature on peer support in mental health services. J Ment Health. 2011;20(4):392–411.
7. Ratzlaff S, McDiarmid D, Marty D, Rapp C. The Kansas consumer as provider program: measuring the effects of a supported education initiative. Psychiatric rehabilitation journal. 2006;29(3):174.
8. Yuen MS, Fossey EM. Working in a community recreation program: a study of consumer-staff perspectives. Aust Occup Ther J. 2003;50(2):54–63.
9. Lawn S, Smith A, Hunter K. Mental health peer support for hospital avoidance and early discharge: an Australian example of consumer driven and operated service. J Ment Health. 2008;17(5):498–508.
10. Chinman M, Lucksted A, Gresen R, Davis M, Losonczy M, Sussner B, Martone L. Early experiences of employing consumer-providers in the VA. Psychiatr Serv. 2008;59(11):1315–21.
11. Sells D, Davidson L, Jewell C, Falzer P, Rowe M. The treatment relationship in peer-based and regular case management for clients with severe mental illness. Psychiatr Serv. 2006;57(8):1179–84.
12. Yanos PT, Primavera LH, Knight EL. Consumer-run service participation, recovery of social functioning, and the mediating role of psychological factors. Psychiatr Serv. 2001;52(4):493–500.
13. Coleman R, Campbell J. Roads to recovery peer development project: the first year: Ongoing evaluation of the developmental process. Working to Recovery Publications; 2009.
14. Ochocka J, Nelson G, Janzen R, Trainor J. A longitudinal study of mental health consumer/survivor initiatives: part 3—a qualitative study of impacts of participation on new members. Journal of Community Psychology. 2006; 34(3):273–83.
15. Doherty I, Craig T, Attafua G, Boocock A, Jamieson-Craig R. The consumer-employee as a member of a mental health assertive outreach team. II. Impressions of consumer-employees and other team members. J Ment Health. 2004;13(1):71–81.
16. Mowbray CT, Moxley D, Thrasher S, Bybee D, Harris S. Consumers as community support providers: issues created by role innovation. Community Ment Health J. 1996;32(1):47–67.
17. Organization WH. Peer Support Programmes in Diabetes: Report of a WHO Consultation, 5–7 November 2007. Geneva: WHO; 2008.
18. Lloyd-Evans B, Mayo-Wilson E, Harrison B, Istead H, Brown E, Pilling S, Johnson S, Kendall T. A systematic review and meta-analysis of randomised controlled trials of peer support for people with severe mental illness. BMC psychiatry. 2014;14:39.
19. Health Workforce Australia. Mental Health Peer Workforce Literature Scan; 2014.
20. Franke CC, Paton BC, Gassner LA. Implementing mental health peer support: a south Australian experience. Australian journal of primary health. 2010;16(2):179–86.
21. Davidson L, Chinman M, Kloos B, Weingarten R, Stayner D, Tebes JK. Peer support among individuals with severe mental illness: a review of the evidence. Clin Psychol Sci Pract. 1999;6(2):165–87.
22. Morrell-Bellai TL, Boydell KM. The experience of mental health consumers as researchers. Can J Commun Ment Health. 2009;13(1):97–108.
23. Vayshenker B, Mulay AL, Gonzales L, West ML, Brown I, Yanos PT. Participation in peer support services and outcomes related to recovery. Psychiatric rehabilitation journal. 2016;39(3):274–81.
24. Collins R, Firth L, Shakespeare T. "very much evolving": a qualitative study of the views of psychiatrists about peer support workers. J Ment Health. 2016; 25(3):278–83.
25. Henderson AR, Kemp V. Australian consumer perceptions of peer support. Asia-Pacific psychiatry: official journal of the Pacific Rim College of Psychiatrists. 2013;5(3):152–6.
26. Magalhães CD, de Mendonça Moscoso JT, de Souza Mitkiewicz F, Wainstok MEB. Fernandes JdCS, Marcos GL, Tavares MC. " I am nuts, but networking": the qualification process for peer support work with mental health users in the psychosocial care network of Rio de Janeiro. Vertex (Buenos Aires, Argentina). 2013;24(112):445–54.

27. Trainor, J, Shepherd, M, Boydell, KM, Leff A, & Crawford E. Beyond the service paradigm: The impact and implications of consumer/survivor initiatives. Psychiatr Rehabil J. 1997;21(2):132–40.
28. Solomon P. Peer support/peer provided services underlying processes, benefits, and critical ingredients. Psychiatric rehabilitation journal. 2004;27(4):392.
29. Phillips MR, Zhang J, Shi Q, Song Z, Ding Z, Pang S, Li X, Zhang Y, Wang Z. Prevalence, treatment, and associated disability of mental disorders in four provinces in China during 2001-05: an epidemiological survey. Lancet. 2009; 373(9680):2041–53.
30. NHaFPCoC N. China Statistics Yearbook of Health and Family Planning. Beijing: Peking Union Medical College Press; 2015.
31. Morosini PL, Magliano L, Brambilla L, Ugolini S, Pioli R. Development, reliability and acceptability of a new version of the DSM-IV social and occupational functioning assessment scale (SOFAS) to assess routine social funtioning. Acta Psychiatr Scand. 2000;101(4):323–9.
32. Weissman EM, Covell NH, Kushner M, Irwin J, Essock SM. Implementing peer-assisted case management to help homeless veterans with mental illness transition to independent housing. Community Ment Health J. 2005; 41(3):267–76.
33. Cabassa LJ, Camacho D, Vélez-Grau CM, Stefancic A. Peer-based health interventions for people with serious mental illness: a systematic literature review. J Psychiatr Res. 2017;84:80–9.
34. Blixen C, Perzynski A, Kanuch S, Dawson N, Kaiser D, Lawless ME, Seeholzer E, Sajatovic M. Training peer educators to promote self-management skills in people with serious mental illness (SMI) and diabetes (DM) in a primary health care setting. Primary health care research & development. 2015;16(2):127–37.
35. Todd NJ, Jones SH, Lobban FA. What do service users with bipolar disorder want from a web-based self-management intervention? A qualitative focus group study. Clinical psychology & psychotherapy. 2013;20(6):531–43.
36. Yam KK, Lo WT, Chiu RL, Lau BS, Lau CK, Wu JK, Wan SM. A pilot training program for people in recovery of mental illness as vocational peer support workers in Hong Kong–job buddies training program (JBTP): a preliminary finding. Asian J Psychiatr. 2016; https://doi.org/10.1016/j.ajp.2016.10.002.

Experiences with the implementation of Individual Placement and Support for people with severe mental illness: a qualitative study among stakeholders

Miljana Vukadin[1,2*], Frederieke G. Schaafsma[1,2], Marjan J. Westerman[3], Harry W. C. Michon[4] and Johannes R. Anema[1,2]

Abstract

Background: Individual Placement and Support (IPS) is an evidence-based approach to help people with severe mental illness achieve competitive employment. This article provides insight into an organizational and a financial implementation strategy for IPS in the Netherlands by exploring the perceived facilitators and barriers among participating stakeholders. The goal of this multifaceted strategy was to improve IPS implementation by improving the collaboration between all organizations involved, and realising secured IPS funding with a 'pay for performance' element.

Methods: A qualitative, explorative study among practitioners ($n = 8$) and decision makers ($n = 7$) in mental health care and vocational rehabilitation was performed using semi-structured interviews to collect rich information about the possible facilitators and barriers with regard to the organizational and financial implementation strategy for IPS.

Results: Important perceived facilitators were the key principles of the IPS model, regular meetings of stakeholders in mental health care and vocational rehabilitation, stakeholders' experienced ownership of IPS and collaboration, the mandate and influence of the decision makers involved and secured IPS funding. Important perceived barriers included the experienced rigidity of the IPS model fidelity scale and lack of independent fidelity reviewers, the temporary and fragmented character of the secured funding, lack of communication between decision makers and practitioners and negative attitudes and beliefs among mental health clinicians. Changes in legislation were experienced as a facilitator as well as a barrier.

Conclusions: The results of this study suggest that the collaboration and IPS funding were experienced as improved by applying an organizational and a financial implementation strategy. However, considerable effort is still necessary to overcome the remaining barriers identified and to make the implementation of IPS a success in practice.

Keywords: Individual placement and support, Implementation, Strategy, Barriers, Facilitators

Background

Despite the importance of employment for people with severe mental illness (SMI) [1–4], their labour market participation is poor: in both the United States and Europe it does not exceed 20%. Although between 30 and 65% of these individuals report to desire some form of employment [5–7], they often rely on social assistance or disability benefits [4]. In the Netherlands, for example, up to 25% of the individuals who are granted a disability benefit have SMI [4, 8]. Until now, most vocational approaches for people with SMI have been stepwise, first training individuals before placing them in, often sheltered or volunteer, work ("train and place") [9, 10]. However, in the past few years, the focus has shifted to supported employment ("place and train"), aiming to place individuals in regular competitive jobs without prevocational training [9–11]. Several systematic reviews conclude that supported employment is more effective than other

* Correspondence: m.vukadin@vumc.nl
[1]Department of Public and Occupational Health, Amsterdam Public Health research institute, VU University Medical Center, Van der Boechorststraat 7, 1081 BT Amsterdam, the Netherlands
[2]Research Center for Insurance Medicine: collaboration between AMC–UMCG – UWV – VUmc, Amsterdam, the Netherlands
Full list of author information is available at the end of the article

interventions in obtaining and maintaining employment for people with SMI [12, 13].

Individual Placement and Support (IPS) is an evidence-based example of such an approach [14]. IPS includes the following key principles: eligibility based on client choice (zero-exclusion), a focus on competitive employment and clients' preferences, work incentives planning, systematic job development, rapid job search and placement with individualized job supports, and integration of mental health and employment services [5]. Fidelity to the IPS model is associated with greater effectiveness with regard to employment outcomes [12, 15].

Despite the strong evidence base for IPS, implementation of this model in the daily practice of mental health care and vocational rehabilitation institutes is difficult [16, 17]. Important barriers to implementation are insufficient collaboration between the organizations involved and inadequate, fragmented and bureaucratically complicated funding [5, 10, 17–20].

To improve IPS implementation, a Dutch mental health agency (MHA), the Dutch Social Security Institute: the Institute for Employee Benefits Schemes (UWV), the municipality of Amsterdam, and a health insurance company (HIC) started to collaborate since 2014. This collaboration included an organizational and a financial strategy to help remove the aforementioned barriers. The organizational implementation strategy consisted of regular meetings between the different stakeholders involved. The financial implementation strategy consisted of secured IPS funding with a 'pay for performance' element, rewarding the MHA for placing an IPS participant in a competitive job.

Although previous research has shown that some organizational and financial factors are important implementation barriers [5, 10, 17–20], no studies have provided in-depth understanding of whether strategies focusing on removing these barriers can actually be effective for IPS implementation in practice. The aim of the present study was to provide more insight into an organizational and a financial implementation strategy for IPS, by.

exploring the facilitators and barriers perceived by participating stakeholders.

Methods

Study design

A qualitative explorative study among stakeholders was performed using semi-structured interviews to collect rich information about the possible facilitators and barriers with regard to an organizational and a financial implementation strategy for IPS [21].

Context information

IPS before the start of the collaboration

Before this collaboration between the different organizations started, there were few mental health agencies in the Netherlands that provided IPS services according to the IPS model [5]. There were also no formal agreements related to the practical execution and funding of IPS. Depending on the mental health agency, IPS services were usually partly financed by health insurance companies or one of the benefit agencies. In practice, it was rather unclear which part was financed by which organization during an IPS trajectory. This became even more unclear when the client actually started working in a competitive job, and as a consequence lost (a part of) his benefits.

IPS within the collaboration

Any client with SMI who received treatment at the MHA and benefits from UWV or the municipality of Amsterdam, could express his desire to obtain a competitive job to his mental health clinician. The client then was referred to an IPS specialist who was part of the same specialized MHA treatment team and provided IPS services according to the IPS model [5]. In the first year of the collaboration each full-time IPS specialist involved had a caseload of 20 clients or fewer and worked within one or two specialized MHA treatment teams. At intake, the IPS specialist and the client decided within eight consultations whether IPS was the right intervention for the client. Then the IPS specialist discussed in a multidisciplinary meeting with vocational rehabilitation practitioners of UWV and the municipality whether the IPS applicant qualified for funding. This meeting and the funding were part of the organizational and financial implementation strategy, respectively.

Organizational implementation strategy

The organizational implementation strategy consisted of collaboration between the different organizations involved at two levels:

1) At the management level, there was a meeting every 8 weeks between the decision makers who were considered key leaders and had a managing or advising role within their organization. They initiated the collaboration and arranged the agreements related to the practical execution and funding of IPS. Their goal was to improve the collaboration and communication between the MHA, UWV, the municipality and the HIC, facilitate practitioners, create support within their own organization and ensure IPS sustainment.
2) At the practitioner level, there was a meeting every 6 weeks between the IPS specialists, the labour experts, the insurance physician and the case manager. In their meetings, these mental health care and vocational rehabilitation practitioners discussed whether new IPS applicants qualified for funding. They also discussed the progress of the

current IPS participants and any questions related to the participants' benefits.

Financial implementation strategy

The financial implementation strategy consisted of secured IPS funding with a 'pay for performance' element. A fair or good IPS fidelity score was a condition for this funding. The duration and amount of the funding (excluding intake and job coaching) depended on the type of benefits the client received.

For clients who received social assistance benefits, IPS was funded by the municipality conform regular responsibilities. The MHA received 900 euro at the start, 900 euro after 3 months and 900 euro after a maximum of 18 months. To stimulate a successful IPS trajectory, the MHA received an extra 1800 euro when placing a client within 9 months in a competitive job for at least 12 h a week during at least 1 month.

For clients who received disability benefits, IPS was funded by UWV conform regular responsibilities. The MHA received 2420 euro at the start and 2420 euro after a maximum of 36 months. To stimulate a successful IPS trajectory, the MHA received an extra 1210 euro when placing a client in a competitive job for at least 12 h at 35% of the minimum wage during at least 2 months.

All the IPS intakes were funded by the HIC for a maximum of 8 hours. All the job coaching was funded by UWV as usual.

Socio-political context: The participation act

Since 2015 a new law in the Netherlands, the so called Participation Act, replaced several older Acts for social assistance benefits and disability schemes [22, 23]. This new Act was introduced to stimulate more people with a distance to the labour market, such as people with a disability, into competitive employment. Municipalities were made fully responsible for the execution of the Participation Act. Following the implementation of this Act, both employers and the government guaranteed 125.000 additional jobs by 2026 for people with a disability or social assistance benefits.

Study participants

All stakeholders involved in the first year of this collaboration were asked to participate in this qualitative study. These stakeholders were from the various organizations: one municipality, two different UWV front offices, two different locations of one MHA and one HIC.

Interviews

For the interviews ($n = 15$) a topic list was used, based on the theoretical framework of determinants of innovations [24–26]. The interview topics were related to the innovation, the professionals and the organizations involved, and the socio-political context [24–26]. In the present study, the innovation consisted of both IPS and the organizational and the financial implementation strategy. Additional file 1 provides an overview of the interview topics and questions.

The semi-structured interviews were conducted between October 2015 and June 2016 by one researcher (M.V.), trained in qualitative research methods. Participants were asked to tell the interviewer about their experiences with the collaboration with the stakeholders of the other organizations involved, the IPS funding, IPS within the context of this collaboration and the impact of laws and regulations. They were also asked about how the new strategy fitted within their own organization and their role in this collaboration. To elicit any information the participants deemed important, open narrations were encouraged .

Interviews lasted about 1 hour (range 30–95 min) and were voice-recorded. One interview was conducted by telephone; all others were face to face and took place at a location convenient for the participants, usually the participants' work location.

Analysis

All interviews were transcribed verbatim. Atlas.ti software was used to facilitate data management and analysis. All transcripts were read thoroughly and analysed. A summary of each interview was made and sent to each participant to determine whether the themes were appropriately described and matched their responses. This member checking was used to improve the credibility and validity of the data [21]. Ten participants responded, and five of them requested minor changes. Thematic content approach was used for data analysis [27].

The analyses were conducted iteratively allowing emerging themes to be explored in subsequent interviews.

All transcripts were coded by one researcher (M.V.). The five most information-rich interviews were coded independently by two researchers (M.V. and F.G.S.). A coding scheme was developed by these two researchers and consensus was reached by discussion. The themes, facilitators and barriers identified by these two researchers were discussed in meetings with a third researcher (M.J.W.), focusing on understanding the collected data and correct interpretation. After several research meetings, a thematic map was developed. Within the themes, facilitators and barriers were distinguished. The aforementioned theoretical framework was used to guide the analysis of the interviews [25]. In the last phase, the themes were refined and the facilitators and barriers identified were sorted and collated according to overarching themes by M.V. and F.G.S. Provisional and final results were critically discussed in the research team meetings with all authors.

The quotations in the Results section were translated from Dutch to English by M.V., and were also discussed with the other authors. Back translation was not performed.

Ethical considerations

The Medical Ethics Committee of the VU University Medical Center gave approval for the study. All procedures performed in this study were in accordance with the ethical standards of this institutional research committee and with the 1964 Helsinki declaration and its later amendments or comparable ethical standards.

Results

Participant characteristics

All invited stakeholders were willing to participate. Participant characteristics are presented in Table 1.

Table 1 Participant characteristics

Level (n) / Organization / Stakeholder	Experience in current role, years
Decision maker (*n* = 7)	
MHA	
Director	7
Policy adviser	8.5
IPS program leader	1
Staff member/ occupational therapist	36
UWV	
Manager	2.5
Municipality of Amsterdam	
Participation adviser	10
HIC	
Mental health care adviser	7
Practitioner (n = 8)	
MHA	
IPS specialist (a)	2
IPS specialist (b)	2
IPS specialist (c)	2
IPS specialist (d)	2
UWV	
Insurance physician	28
Labour expert (a)	15
Labour expert (b)	5
Municipality of Amsterdam	
Case manager	6

MHA Mental Health Agency, *UWV* Dutch Social Security Institute: the Institute for Employee Benefits Schemes, *HIC* Health Insurance Company

Experiences, facilitators and barriers

The participants shared their experiences on how they had perceived this first year of collaboration for IPS between the organizations and mentioned a large number of facilitators and barriers. The perceived facilitators and barriers were classified into different themes related to the innovation and the socio-political context [24–26, 28]. [Additional file 2: Table S2] provides a thematic overview of all perceived facilitators and barriers. A summary of these facilitators and barriers is shown in Table 2. The most discussed themes are reported below, along with quotations to illustrate some facilitators and barriers.

Innovation

IPS In general, IPS was considered to be an effective intervention for a difficult target group. The key principles of the IPS model were perceived as a facilitator. Several decision makers and MHA practitioners thought implementing IPS with high fidelity to the IPS model was important, because they expected high fidelity IPS services to be more effective.

However, the IPS model fidelity scale was experienced as a barrier by different decision makers, as some items of this scale were considered rigid; the item about integration of the IPS specialist in a specialized MHA treatment team, for example. These decision makers argued that IPS services should not be limited to specialized mental health care, which is now the case in the Netherlands.

> MHA decision maker (policy adviser): *"Our healthcare system is continuously changing. That's a good thing (...) I think you have to keep an open mind for these changes and should not stick to the model fidelity that rigidly."*

Some MHA decision makers and practitioners also thought it was inappropriate that the fidelity reviews were conducted by the same organization as where IPS specialists were trained. The fidelity reviewers of this organization were not considered independent.

Collaboration The collaboration between the organizations involved was experienced as successful. An important facilitator for this collaboration was having the regular meetings of stakeholders at management and practitioner level. Most participants pointed out that these meetings, particularly at practitioner level, provided designated and easy to reach contact persons. Both collaboration aspects (meetings, contact persons) facilitated short decision lines and fast responses of the stakeholders involved. Some participants also pointed out that regular meetings at both levels stimulated evaluation of new procedures. All participants agreed that regular meetings with stakeholders working within different organizations increased the trust

Table 2 Summary of perceived facilitators and barriers

Themes	Facilitators	Barriers
1. Innovation		
1.1 IPS		
Intervention	Evidence based effectiveness of IPS	Costs of IPS
	Key principles of the IPS model	IPS model fidelity scale and fidelity reviews
		Compatibility of IPS with existing work procedures
1.2 Collaboration		
Between organizations involved[a]	Regular meetings of stakeholders	Clients' privacy and medical confidentiality
	Sharing information, knowledge and expertise	Organization of the structural meetings
	Pre-existing relationships and collaboration between stakeholders	Lack of involvement of practitioners in vocational rehabilitation
	Shared interests, goals and vision of stakeholders	Lack of communication between decision makers and practitioners
Professionals involved		
Stakeholders characteristics	Mandate and influence of decision makers	
Attitude and beliefs	Ownership of IPS and collaboration	IPS not experienced as part of the mental health treatment
		Work not experienced as a achievable goal for people with SMI
1.3 IPS funding		
Secured funding[b]	Substantial funding for IPS	Fragmented funding
		Lack of clarity with regard to costs of IPS services
Ethics		
Pay for performance[b]	Pay for performance might encourage IPS specialists	Not appropriate to receive extra payments within health care setting
Sustainability	Covenant between involved organizations stimulates collaboration and funding	Lack of proven cost-effectiveness of IPS Temporary financial agreements between the organizations involved
2. Socio-political context		
Government	Support and funding of Ministry of Social Affairs and Employment New Participation Act provides sense of urgency regarding participation of people with SMI	Dutch social safety net does not stimulate participation in paid work New Participation Act has unwanted consequences Health insurance act limits IPS funding by health insurance company

[a]Part of the organizational implementation strategy. [b]Part of the financial implementation strategy

between these stakeholders, as they got to know each other better. This trust improved the perceived reliability of each other's judgement and facilitated open communication.

> MHA practitioner (IPS specialist (a)): *"I considered it a useful meeting (...) the lines of communication are short... and it's quite useful to have a contact person within those organizations."*

Most participants pointed out that the collaboration between the organizations was stimulated by stakeholders that experienced ownership of IPS and the collaboration, and were enthusiastic and passionate with regard to IPS. In addition, the mandate and the influence of the participating decision makers was mentioned as an important facilitator by several decision makers. They were seen as opinion leaders with an affinity for the target group, who create support within organizations, arrange funding and promote sustainment of IPS.

> MHA decision maker (staff member/ occupational therapist): *"You need people that are inspired (...) with an extreme level of involvement, because otherwise you won't make it; just procedures aren't enough. You need people that step up and say: I'm going to do this!"*

Communication between the decision makers and the practitioners was experienced as a barrier by several participants. Most practitioners were not aware of the decisions made during management meetings. Some decision makers also admitted they did not know what the obstacles for MHA practitioners were with regard to

IPS and the collaboration with the practitioners of the other organizations.

> UWV decision maker (manager): "No, *I don't know [how these regular meetings between practitioners work in practice] and I suppose that's strange, because I proposed to initiate these meetings [between practitioners] myself."*

Some participants, mostly practitioners, also mentioned that there was no formal, written information available about the responsibilities and the roles of the different practitioners involved in the collaboration. This lack of a clear protocol and written information about the agreements between the organizations involved, sometimes resulted in uncertainties and miscommunication among practitioners.

> MHA practitioner (IPS specialist (c)): *"I think the agreements between MHA and UWV (...) should be documented, because at the moment there is no written information available."*

An important barrier mentioned by several MHA decision makers and practitioners was the lack of support experienced within their own organization, based on negative attitudes and beliefs among professionals not directly involved in the collaboration. According to the MHA participants, the mental health clinicians within the specialized MHA treatment teams often did not refer clients to the IPS specialists, because these clinicians did not experience IPS as a part of the regular mental health treatment, and were not focused on recovery related to societal participation in work.

> MHA practitioner (IPS specialist (d)): *"Some managers and colleagues see things differently. They don't support recovery as much as we do within IPS and that is an obstacle (...). [Colleagues argue:] My clients can't work, my clients won't work (...). I simply don't believe that if a case manager has a caseload of 40 clients, none of them wants to work".*

IPS funding All participants recognized that the secured, substantial funding for IPS was an important facilitator. Several participants thought the pay for performance element of the IPS funding might encourage IPS specialists.

> UWV decision maker (manager): *"Maybe some see it as a perverse incentive, but it does provide a reason not to give up for a client if you get a fee for success. Therefore, all in all, I think it's a very good strategy."*

Some participants argued that the funding was not adequate, because it was still fragmented and applying for the funding was time consuming. One of the MHA decision makers was also concerned that the funding would not cover all costs of IPS.

> MHA decision maker (IPS program leader): *"(...) it's not just one financial agreement, of course that always creates issues. Ideally, there would be one all-in package [IPS funding] for three years."*

With regard to the pay for performance element, a MHA decision maker expressed concerns about increased financial risks for the MHA and pressure to place clients in a regular, paid job. A few MHA decision makers also argued it was not appropriate to receive extra payments for achieving goals to place clients in paid work within a health care setting. While some decision makers were afraid that the pay for performance element would be a perverse incentive, other participants were convinced that it had little influence on IPS specialists in daily practice. Most participants thought an important barrier was that the financial agreements between the organizations involved were only temporary.

> HIC decision maker (mental health care adviser): *"The municipality has ensured IPS financing for two years, but that means financing ends next year. The same goes for us, we have agreed on financing up to February 2018. In the period ahead, we will all have to discuss how we can ensure sustainable IPS funding."*

Another barrier mentioned by the decision makers of the benefit agencies and the HIC, was the lack of proven cost-effectiveness of IPS. They all agreed proven cost-effectiveness of IPS was necessary in order to decide whether to continue IPS funding.

Socio-political context

The socio-political context was experienced as favourable for the implementation of IPS, but also challenging because of the ongoing changes in laws and regulations regarding the IPS funding and participation of people with SMI. Most participants mentioned the new Participation Act as a facilitator, because it provided a sense of urgency regarding the participation of people with SMI among employers and within benefit agencies. This sense of urgency contributed to the realization of secured IPS funding.

Several participants thought the new Participation Act also had a few unwanted consequences, such as insecurity for people with SMI and organizations involved, and the increased influence of the municipalities regarding the participation policy (decentralization).

> MHA practitioner (IPS specialist (d)): *"I think the Participation Act is really complicated, because your access to [IPS] services depends on the municipality you live in. (...) you depend on the political orientation of your municipality, how rich your municipality is and what they want to spend money on. Well, I think that's insane."*

Discussion

The aim of the present study was to gain in-depth insight into an organizational and a financial implementation strategy for IPS by exploring the perceived facilitators and barriers among participating practitioners and decision makers in mental health care and vocational rehabilitation. Using a theoretical framework [24, 25], several perceived facilitators and barriers related to IPS, the implementation strategies and the socio-political context were identified. Important perceived facilitators were the key principles of the IPS model, regular meetings of stakeholders in mental health care and vocational rehabilitation, stakeholders' experienced ownership of IPS and collaboration, the mandate and influence of the decision makers involved and secured IPS funding. Important perceived barriers included the experienced rigidity of the IPS model fidelity scale and lack of independent fidelity reviewers, the temporary and fragmented character of the secured funding, lack of communication between decision makers and practitioners and negative attitudes and beliefs among mental health clinicians. Changes in legislation were experienced as a facilitator as well as a barrier.

Comparison with other studies

In the literature on multifaceted implementation strategies, financial and organizational implementation activities are underrepresented [29]. Grimshaw et al. showed that most strategies focused on professionals involved [30]. An important reason for that may be that professional-directed implementation strategies are easier to realise in the study practice than financial or organizational strategies [29]. There is, however, some literature on facilitators and barriers to the implementation and sustainment of supported employment [10, 20, 31], and to components of multifaceted implementation strategies for supported employment [32, 33]. For example, two studies evaluating implementation [10] and sustainment [20] of supported employment found that important facilitators to IPS implementation and sustainment were strong personal commitments by program leaders [10] and leadership [20], in line with the facilitators found in the present study. Unlike the present study, these studies [10, 20] focused only on the experiences of MHA and IPS stakeholders and did not include stakeholders from different organizations.

Regular meetings of professionals comparable to the meetings in this implementation study were also found to be important in the study by Holwerda et al. [34]. Using questionnaires to assess the collaboration between professionals in mental health care and vocational rehabilitation to support employment of individuals with mental disorders, they also found that collaborating in a structural way was essential for developing an effective collaboration between the organizations involved [34].

Although the secured IPS funding (including pay for performance) as a strategy was experienced as a facilitator, it was not perceived as adequate, as the funding itself was still rather fragmented, and the agreements about the funding were only temporary. Previous studies also identified inadequate funding as an important barrier to IPS implementation and sustainment [10, 19, 20, 31]. Noel et al. concluded that, within the context of an active learning community, secured funding was an important facilitator to IPS sustainment [20]. This learning community promotes dissemination, implementation, sustainment and expansion of IPS [19, 20].

The finding of limited consensus about the added value of pay for performance in the present study was also reported by McGrew et al. [32], who found that although some participating professionals where satisfied with the funding, others raised concerns about increased financial risks, pressure to achieve job placements and possible pressures for adverse client selection.

Strengths and limitations

A strength of this study is that it is one of the first studies to assess the experiences with a multifaceted implementation strategy for IPS among stakeholders. Another strength is that all decision makers and practitioners involved in the first year of the collaboration between the different organizations were interviewed. This helped to achieve an accurate and complete understanding of perceived facilitators and barriers among these different stakeholders. Furthermore, the participants provided feedback on their interview summary, which improves the credibility and validity of the data. The credibility of the analysis is also increased by coding five interviews independently and developing the coding scheme by two researchers, and discussing the results in research team meetings with all authors.

The use of a theoretical framework [24, 25] to develop a topic list and guide the interviews and their analysis, is both a strength and a limitation of this study. It is a strength because using a framework based on prior research enables a structured analysis and might improve the validity of the data; it is also a limitation because the framework [24, 25] focuses on innovations within health care organizations. The innovation in this study, however, consisted of a multifaceted implementation strategy, mainly focusing on improving the IPS implementation by collaboration between different types of organizations and secured IPS funding.

A limitation of this study is the limited generalizability of the findings due to the small number of participants within this qualitative study focusing on the Dutch social security context. However, similar facilitators and barriers to the implementation of IPS have been reported in other countries with a different social security system [19, 20, 31, 35].

Implications for practice and research

Important barriers were the ignorance of decision makers regarding obstacles for MHA practitioners, and a lack of formal written information about the responsibilities and the roles of the different practitioners involved. These findings suggest that communication between decision makers and practitioners, and information transfer with regard to the innovation, can be improved and therefore need more attention in future implementation strategies in order to make IPS a success in practice.

The perceived barriers related to the IPS funding suggest that there is a need for one, sustainable funding for all clients based on proven cost-effectiveness of IPS. Consequently, future research should focus on evaluating the cost-effectiveness of IPS. In addition, the.

experienced rigidity of the IPS model fidelity scale and lack of independent fidelity reviewers were perceived as barriers to providing IPS services and may need further evaluation in the European context, considering the dependence of IPS funding on the IPS fidelity score. However, it appears to be important to continue IPS fidelity monitoring, since ongoing fidelity monitoring may promote long-term sustainability of IPS [15, 19, 31].

An important barrier was the lack of support experienced within the MHA, based on negative attitudes and beliefs among mental health clinicians. Fortunately, these negative attitudes and beliefs of clinicians are likely to change over time, as they come to better understand the relevance of employment on health for everyone [36]. This process may be accelerated by increasing clinicians' involvement in the IPS trajectories and by presenting frequently examples of successful IPS candidates to them. However, not only were negative attitudes and beliefs among clinicians experienced as challenging for IPS implementation in the MHA by several MHA participants, the ongoing changes in laws and regulations regarding IPS funding and participation of people with SMI also seemed to complicate this process. It is therefore important to ensure ongoing support and continuity within all organizations involved, and to continue facilitating IPS specialists.

Conclusions

This qualitative study provides more insight into the perceived facilitators and barriers of an organizational and a financial implementation strategy for IPS in the Netherlands by exploring the experiences of stakeholders involved. Important perceived facilitators were the key principles of the IPS model, regular meetings of stakeholders in mental health care and vocational rehabilitation, stakeholders' experienced ownership of IPS and collaboration, the mandate and influence of the decision makers involved and secured IPS funding. Important perceived barriers included the experienced rigidity of the IPS model fidelity scale and lack of independent fidelity reviewers, the temporary and fragmented character of the secured funding, lack of communication between decision makers and practitioners and negative attitudes and beliefs among mental health clinicians. Changes in legislation were experienced as a facilitator as well as a barrier. These results suggest that the collaboration and IPS funding were experienced as improved by applying this implementation strategy. However, considerable effort is still necessary to overcome the remaining barriers identified and to make the implementation of IPS a success in practice.

Abbreviations

HIC: Health insurance company; IPS: Individual Placement and Support; MHA: Mental health agency; SMI: Severe mental illness; UWV: The Dutch Social Security Institute: the Institute for Employee Benefits Schemes

Funding

This study was funded by the Dutch Social Security Institute: the Institute for Employee Benefits Schemes (UWV) (funding number 2001170). The funding organization had no further role in analysis and interpretation of the data, in writing the paper and in the decision to submit the paper for publication.

Authors' contributions

M.V., F.G.S., H.W.C.M. and J.R.A. were involved in the conception and design of the study. M.V. conducted the interviews, analysed the data and drafted the first version of the manuscript. F.G.S. and M.J.W. were involved in the first phase of analysis. All authors were involved in the last phase of analysis, read, contributed to, and approved the final version of the manuscript.

Competing interests

Author M.V. is an employee of the Dutch Social Security Institute: the Institute for Employee Benefits Schemes (UWV). Author J.R.A is a shareholder of Evalua Nederland B.V. (www.evalua.nl) and holds a chair in Insurance Medicine on behalf of the Dutch Social Security Institute: the Institute for Employee Benefits Schemes (UWV). All authors declare that they have no conflict of interest in the analysis and interpretation of the data, in writing the paper and in the decision to submit the paper for publication.

Author details

[1]Department of Public and Occupational Health, Amsterdam Public Health research institute, VU University Medical Center, Van der Boechorststraat 7, 1081 BT Amsterdam, the Netherlands. [2]Research Center for Insurance

Medicine: collaboration between AMC– UMCG – UWV – VUmc, Amsterdam, the Netherlands. [3]Department of Health Sciences, Vrije Universiteit Amsterdam, De Boelelaan 1105, 1081 HV Amsterdam, the Netherlands. [4]Trimbos Institute, The Netherlands Institute of Mental Health and Addiction, Da Costakade 45, 3521 VS Utrecht, the Netherlands.

References

1. Bond GR, Resnick SG, Drake RE, Xie H, McHugo GJ, Bebout RR. Does competitive employment improve nonvocational outcomes for people with severe mental illness? J Consult Clin Psychol. 2001;69:489–501.
2. Burns T, Catty J, White S, Becker T, Koletsi M, Fioritti A, Rossler W, Tomov T, van Busschbach J, Wiersma D, et al. The impact of supported employment and working on clinical and social functioning: results of an international study of individual placement and support. Schizophr Bull. 2009;35:949–58.
3. Koletsi M, Niersman A, van Busschbach JT, Catty J, Becker T, Burns T, Fioritti A, Kalkan R, Lauber C, Rossler W, et al. Working with mental health problems: clients' experiences of IPS, vocational rehabilitation and employment. Soc Psychiatry Psychiatr Epidemiol. 2009;44:961–70.
4. OECD: Sick on the job?: myths and realities about mental health and work. 2012.
5. Bond GR, Drake RE. Making the case for IPS supported employment. Admin Pol Ment Health. 2014;41:69–73.
6. Marwaha S, Johnson S, Bebbington P, Stafford M, Angermeyer MC, Brugha T, Azorin JM, Kilian R, Hansen K, Toumi M. Rates and correlates of employment in people with schizophrenia in the UK, France and Germany. Br J Psychiatry. 2007;191:30–7.
7. Salkever DS, Karakus MC, Slade EP, Harding CM, Hough RL, Rosenheck RA, Swartz MS, Barrio C, Yamada AM. Measures and predictors of community-based employment and earnings of persons with schizophrenia in a multisite study. Psychiatr Serv. 2007;58:315–24.
8. UWV: UWV Kennisverslag-1. pp. 42; 2014:42.
9. Burns T, Catty J, Group E. IPS in Europe: the EQOLISE trial. Psychiatr Rehabil J. 2008;31:313–7.
10. van Erp NH, Giesen FB, van Weeghel J, Kroon H, Michon HW, Becker D, McHugo GJ, Drake RE. A multisite study of implementing supported employment in the Netherlands. Psychiatr Serv. 2007;58:1421–6.
11. Michon H, van Busschbach JT, Stant AD, van Vugt MD, van Weeghel J, Kroon H. Effectiveness of individual placement and support for people with severe mental illness in the Netherlands: a 30-month randomized controlled trial. Psychiatr Rehabil J. 2014;37:129–36.
12. Kinoshita Y, Furukawa TA, Kinoshita K, Honyashiki M, Omori IM, Marshall M, Bond GR, Huxley P, Amano N, Kingdon D. Supported employment for adults with severe mental illness. Cochrane Database Syst Rev. 2013;13: CD008297.
13. Suijkerbuijk YB, Schaafsma FG, van Mechelen JC, Ojajarvi A, Corbiere M, Anema JR. Interventions for obtaining and maintaining employment in adults with severe mental illness, a network meta-analysis. Cochrane Database Syst Rev. 2017;9:CD011867.
14. Becker DR, Drake RE. A working life: The Individual Placement and Support (IPS) program.: concord. NH: New Hampshire-Dartmouth Psychiatric Research Center; 1993.
15. Lockett L, Waghorn G, Kydd R, Chant D. Predictive validity of evidence-based practices in supported employment: a systematic review and meta-analysis. Ment Health Rev J. 2016;21:261–81.
16. Giesen F, van Erp N, van Weeghel J, Michon H, Kroon H. The implementation of individual placement and support in the Netherlands. Tijdschr Psychiatr. 2007;49:611–21.
17. van Hoof F, Knispel A, Meije D, van Wijngaarden B, Vijselaar J. Trendrapportage GGZ. Utrecht: Trimbos Instituut; 2010.
18. Bond GR, Becker DR, Drake RE, Rapp CA, Meisler N, Lehman AF, Bell MD, Blyler CR. Implementing supported employment as an evidence-based practice. Psychiatr Serv. 2001;52:313–22.
19. Bond GR, Drake RE, Becker DR, Noel VA. The IPS learning community: a longitudinal study of sustainment, quality, and outcome. Psychiatr Serv. 2016;67:864–9.
20. Noel VA, Bond GR, Drake RE, Becker DR, McHugo GJ, Swanson SJ, Luciano AE, Greene MA. Barriers and facilitators to sustainment of an evidence-based supported employment program. Admin Pol Ment Health. 2017;44: 331–8.
21. Britten N. Qualitative interviews in medical research. BMJ. 1995;311:251–3.
22. Asscher LF: Besluit van 11 december 2014 tot wijziging van het Besluit van 4 juli 2014 tot vaststelling van het tijdstip van inwerkingtreding van de Wet maatregelen Wet werk en bijstand en enkele andere wetten, de Wet hervorming kindregelingen en de Invoeringswet Participatiewet (Stb. 271). 's-Gravenhage: Staatsblad van het Koninkrijk der Nederlanden (Official Gazette); 2014.
23. LWM D. Realisatie van de participatiesamenleving. Hervorming van de verzorgingsstaat in Nederland: 2010–2015. Belgisch Tijdschrift voor Sociale Zekerheid. 2016;2015:771–6.
24. Fleuren MA, Paulussen TG, Van Dommelen P, Van Buuren S. Towards a measurement instrument for determinants of innovations. Int J Qual Health Care. 2014;26:501–10.
25. Fleuren M, Wiefferink K, Paulussen T. Checklist determinanten van innovaties in gezondheidszorgorganisaties. TSG. 2010;88:51–4.
26. Grol R, Wensing M. What drives change? Barriers to and incentives for achieving evidence-based practice. Med J Aust. 2004;180:S57–60.
27. Braun V, Clarke V. Using thematic analysis in psychology. Qualitative research in psychology. Qualitative Research in Psychology. 2006;3:77–101.
28. Fleuren M, Wiefferink K, Paulussen T. Determinants of innovation within health care organizations: literature review and Delphi study. Int J Qual Health Care. 2004;16:107–23.
29. Grol R, Wensing M. Implementatie: effectieve verbetering van de patiëntenzorg. Amsterdam: Elsevier Gezondheidszorg; 2012.
30. Grimshaw JM, Thomas RE, MacLennan G, Fraser C, Ramsay CR, Vale L, Whitty P, Eccles MP, Matowe L, Shirran L, et al. Effectiveness and efficiency of guideline dissemination and implementation strategies. Health Technol Assess. 2004;8:iii–v. 1-72
31. Bond GR, Drake RE, McHugo GJ, Peterson AE, Jones AM, Williams J. Long-term sustainability of evidence-based practices in community mental health agencies. Admin Pol Ment Health. 2014;41:228–36.
32. McGrew JH, Johannesen JK, Griss ME, Born DL, Katuin CH. Performance-based funding of supported employment for persons with severe mental illness: vocational rehabilitation and employment staff perspectives. J Behav Health Serv Res. 2007;34:1–16.
33. McGrew JH, Johannesen JK, Griss ME, Born DL, Katuin CH. Performance-based funding of supported employment: A multi-site controlled trial. Journal of Vocational Rehabilitation. 2005;23:81–99.
34. Holwerda A, Fokkens AS, Engbers C, Brouwer S. Collaboration between mental health and employment services to support employment of individuals with mental disorders. Disabil Rehabil. 2016;38:1250–6.
35. Schneider J, Akhtar A. Implementation of individual placement and support: the Nottingham experience. Psychiatr Rehabil J. 2012;35:325–32.
36. Drake RE, Becker DR, Bond GR, Mueser KT. A process analysis of integrated and non-integrated approaches to supported employment. Journal of Vocational Rehabilitation. 2003;18:51–8.

Psychopathological sequelae of female genital mutilation and their neuroendocrinological associations

Anke Köbach[1,2*], Martina Ruf-Leuschner[1,2] and Thomas Elbert[1,2]

Abstract

Background: Anecdotal evidence suggests the frequently traumatic nature of female genital mutilation (FGM). At present, systematic research on the psychological sequelae of this tradition has remained limited. The study provides preliminary, high-quality psychodiagnostic data on potential psychopathological consequences of FGM, with a focus on posttraumatic stress disorder (PTSD), shutdown dissociation and other stress-related variables.

Methods: We investigated a convenience sample of $N = 167$ women, supported by the women's affairs headquarters in Jijiga (capital of the Ethiopian Somali Region) and a local Ethiopian non-governmental organization. Our main outcome measures were PTSD (PSS-I) and shutdown dissociation (ShuD). We also assessed depression and anxiety (HSCL-25), major depression, substance abuse and dependence, suicidality and psychotic disorders (M.I.N.I.; sub-scales A., B., K., and L.). In addition, we collected hair samples to assess hair cortisol concentrations (HCC) as a neuroendocrinological measure.

Results: The majority of women endured FGM (FGM I: 36%, FGM II/III: 52%) and, regardless of the level of the physical invasiveness, almost all women reported having felt intense fear and/or helplessness. FGM II/III, the more invasive form, was associated with a greater vulnerability to PTSD symptoms ($p < .001$) and shutdown dissociation ($p < .001$). Symptoms of depression ($p < .05$) and anxiety ($p < .01$) were also elevated. Random forest regression with conditional inference trees revealed evidence of an alteration of the cortisol levels in relation to the age when FGM was experienced (< 1 year) and the invasiveness of the procedure.

Conclusion: More extensive forms of FGM are associated with more severe psychopathological symptoms – particularly with an increased vulnerability to PTSD. Higher hair cortisol levels in women who experienced FGM before their first year of age or had more severe forms of FGM indicate long-term neuroendocrinological consequences of FGM and trauma in general on the stress system.

Keywords: Female genital mutilation, FGM, Female genital cutting, Posttraumatic stress disorder (PTSD), Dissociation, Depression, Hair cortisol

Background

Female genital mutilation (FGM) refers to all procedures that intentionally alter or harm the female genital organs for non-medical reasons [1]. The World Health Organization (WHO) has classified four major types: (1) *Clitoridectomy* (in the following referred to as FGM I) *is the partial or total removal of the clitoris and, in very rare cases, only the prepuce.* (2) *Excision* (in the following referred to as FGM II) *is the partial or total removal of the clitoris and the labia minora, with or without excision of the labia majora,* while (3) *infibulation* (in the following referred to as FGM III) *is the narrowing of the vaginal opening through the creation of a covering seal. The seal is formed by cutting and repositioning the inner, or outer, labia, with or without removal of the clitoris.* Defibulation—which usually takes place before sexual intercourse or childbirth—is the opening of the formerly infibulated part. In cultures that traditionally practice

* Correspondence: anke.koebach@uni-konstanz.de
[1]Department of Clinical and Neuropsychology, University Konstanz, Universitätsstraße 10, 78457 Konstanz, Germany
[2]Vivo international e.V., Postfach 5108, 78430 Konstanz, Germany

infibulation, women enter into a cycle of defibulations and re-infibulations (e.g., natural adhesion of the injured labia, infibulation after birth). (4) *Other practices include all other harmful procedures to the female genitalia for non-medical purposes,* e.g. *pricking, piercing, incising, scraping and cauterizing the genital area* [1]. International institutions such as the United Nations (UN) or WHO follow unambiguous anti-FGM policies. Still, more than 200 million women from countries in Africa and the Middle East are affected [2]. Adverse obstetric outcomes increase alongside more extensive FGM [3].

Anecdotal evidence from women who have endured FGM provides insight into the traumatic nature of the tradition [4], and recent studies have confirmed that the majority of women with FGM reported having felt intense fear, helplessness and pain during the procedure [5]. Besides the subjective validation of FGM as traumatic event, within the DSM-5 classification system, FGM applies to the A-criterion (threatened death, serious injury and/or sexual violence) of posttraumatic stress disorder (PTSD) [6]. PTSD constitutes a psychiatric condition that typically develops in response to (repeated) exposure to serious threats [6], whereby cumulative exposure is a reliable predictor of the intensity of PTSD symptoms (also indicated as building block effect; e.g., [7, 8]). PTSD patients typically suffer from the cognitive, emotional, and physiological re-experiencing of their traumatic event(s) (B-criterion), avoidance of trauma reminders (C-criterion), an alteration of mood and cognition (D-criterion), and hyperarousal (E-criterion) [6]. Comorbidities with depression, substance dependency, dissociation and other psychological disorders are frequent [9]. To date, only a few scientific studies have investigated the relationship between FGM and PTSD. In fact, Mulongo et al. [10] reviewed more than 1 thousand articles on FGM, of which only ten reported psychological outcomes and only two original studies met high scientific standards. Behrendt and Moritz [5] compared 23 Senegalese women with FGM to 24 in the noFGM group. Compared to the noFGM group, the FGM group presented a higher prevalence of PTSD (30% vs. 0%) as well as an increased prevalence of other anxiety and affective disorders. Moreover, Knipscheer et al. [11] recently investigated a sample of 66 immigrant women in the Netherlands. More than one third of this group presented with clinically relevant symptoms of PTSD, anxiety and/or depression.

Psychoneuroendocrinological research reveals the important role of the Hypothalamus–Pituitary–Adrenal (HPA) axis in the regulation of stress reactions in trauma-exposed individuals with and without PTSD [12, 13]. Consequently, serious stressors, such as FGM and its associated lifelong sequelae of physical [3] and psychological pain [5, 9] may permanently alter the function of the HPA axis [14]. Especially early life stress has been linked with epigenetic (re)programming of the HPA axis (e.g. [15]). Hair cortisol concentration (HCC), measured in hair that has grown over the last month or more, quantifies long-term cortisol secretion patterns. With it, HCC serves as physiological marker for stress-related changes [13, 16, 17]. Specific associations of the HCC with FGM have not been investigated previously. Relevant earlier studies found higher HCC in patients suffering from chronic pain [18], who experienced a greater number of traumatic events [19–21], and for those reporting more major life stressors [22]. In contrast, Steudte-Schmiedgen et al. [23, 24] reported a negative association with the number of lifetime traumatic events, and Hinkelman et al. [25] found lower HCC in patients with depression than in healthy controls (both of whom were exposed to traumatic experiences during childhood). In a recent review, Steudte-Schmiedgen et al. [13] suggests a two-stage model hypothesizing an initial increase in cortisol after the traumatic event followed by a gradual attenuation as the event becomes more distant. With it, the authors emphasize the importance of the temporal aspect of trauma exposure and HPA axis regulation together with the current level of stress.

We conducted psychological interviews with women who live in Jijiga, the capital of the Ethiopian Somali Region. In this region, FGM is still widespread, despite the endorsement of legal provisions on behalf of the Ethiopian parliament to protect girls subject to the tradition. The *Ethiopian Demographic and Health Survey 2005* (EDHS 2005) [26] reported that 97.3% of women who live in the Somali region had endured FGM. Regarding the traumatic nature of the practice, we hypothesized FGM to be associated with a heightened risk of PTSD and trauma-related shutdown dissociation. We also take into account depression, anxiety, substance abuse and dependence, suicidality and psychosis. Focusing on PTSD severity, we expected FGM to exacerbate the cumulative effect of the number of potentially traumatic event types [8]. Furthermore, we aimed to explore the association between FGM and other stress-related variables with neuroendocrinological alterations by means of the HCC. To take all possible predictors into account, we approached this question in an explorative manner: First, we used a non-parametric machine learning technique (random forest regression embedded in a conditional inference framework [27]), allowing a large number of predictors to identify the most important predictors. Second, we computed a linear regression model predicting the HCC by identified variables, gaining information on the significance and the directions of associations as well as the general model fit.

Methods

Participants

In cooperation with the non-governmental organizations Norwegian Church Aid (NCA), EGLDAM and the

Women's Affairs headquarters in Jijiga, we recruited a convenience sample of 167 women living in various parts of the town. Two (1%) women did not know which FGM group they belonged to, and were therefore excluded in the analysis ($N = 165$). The local partners approached women from different districts in Jijiga and made appointments with those who had agreed to take part in an interview on their experience with FGM and their current mental wellbeing.

Table 1 shows the basic sociodemographic characteristics of the sample. On average, the participants were 30.7 years old ($SD = 12.6$, *range* 13–80) and the majority belonged to the Somali (59%, $n = 98$) or Amharic (30%, $n = 50$; other: 10%, $n = 17$) ethnic groups. In accord with the EDHS 2005 [28], a high percentage of women had endured FGM. During data assessment, we had difficulties finding uncircumcised women—the noFGM group in this study ultimately constitutes a small group ($n = 18$) of women with both manifold vulnerability and resilience characteristics. Therefore, the group cannot be interpreted as pseudo-experimental control group in the final analysis. Most of the participants reported FGM III (48%, $n = 79$) or FGM I (36%, $n = 60$). Only a minority reported FGM II (5%, $n = 8$) or being uncircumcised (11%, $n = 18$). Due to the small number of women reporting FGM II, the latter and FGM III were merged in the analysis. The age and type of FGM depended on the women's cultural background. Somali women were commonly circumcised according to FGM II/III at the age of 7.6 ($SD = 2.6$, 95% *CI* [7.1; 8.2]) years, with a secular trend towards circumcising girls at earlier ages: Somali women with FGM III aged 26 years and older reported an average circumcision age of 8.2 years ($SD = 2.7$, 95% *CI* [7.4; 9.0]), while the younger group (≤ 25 years) reported an average age of 6.9 years ($SD = 2.3$, 95% *CI* [6.1; 7.7]; $t(79) = -2.24$, $p < .05$).

Table 1 Basic information on sociodemographic characteristics, lifetime exposure to childhood familial violence, lifetime traumatic events and mental health outcome measures due to the FGM groups

	No FGM		FGM I		FGM II/III		
	$n = 18$		$n = 60$		$n = 87$		Statistics
Sociodemographic characteristics							
Age *(M ± SD [CI])*	24.8 ± 4.4	[22.6, 27.0]	30.6 ± 12.8	[27.3, 33.8]	32.1 ± 13.3	[29.2, 35.0][1]	$F_{(2,160)} = 2.59$
Years of education *(M ± SD [CI])*	10.3 ± 4.8	[8.0, 12.7]	8.1 ± 4.3	[7.0, 9.2][2]	4.1 ± 5.1	[3.0, 5.2]	$F_{(2,161)} = 19.55^{***}$
Ethnicity (%, *n*)							$Chi^2_{(4)} = 102.69^{***}$
Somali	5.6	(1)	23.3	(14)	95.4	(83)	
Amhara	77.8	(14)	58.3	(35)	1.1	(1)	
Other	16.7	(3)	18.3	(11)	3.4	(3)	
Marital status (%, *n*)							$Chi^2_{(6)} = 10.12$
Single	50.0	(9)	28.3	(17)	37.9	(33)	
Married	33.3	(6)	41.7	(25)	21.8	(19)	
Divorced	5.6	(1)	18.3	(11)	21.8	(19)	
Widowed	11.1	(2)	11.7	(7)	18.4	(16)	
CFV *(M ± SD [CI])*	5.4 ± 3.3	[3.7, 7.0]	6.2 ± 4.1	[5.1, 7.2]	5.6 ± 4.8	[4.5, 6.6][3]	$F_{(2,161)} = 0.34$
LTE *(M ± SD [CI])*	0.8 ± 1.2	[0.2, 1.43]	1.4 ± 1.5	[1.0, 1.8]	1.9 ± 1.9	[1.4, 2.3]	$F_{(2,162)} = 3.28^{*}$
Mental health measure							
HCC (pg/mol; *M ± SD [CI]*)	28.3 ± 19.7	[17.8, 38.8][4]	29.4 ± 18.3	[23.5, 35.2][5]	31.6 ± 13.2	[27.8, 35.4][6]	$F_{(2,103)} = 0.34$
PTSD score *(M ± SD [CI])*	1.2 ± 4.7	[−1.2, 3.5]	0.8 ± 2.6	[0.2, 1.5]	5.7 ± 10.6	[3.4, 7.9]	$Welch_{(2,43.94)} = 8.25^{***}$
PTSD diagnosis (%, *n*)	5.6	(1)	0	(0)	18.4	(16)	$Chi^2_{(2)} = 13.49^{***}$
ShuD Dissociation score *(M ± SD [CI])*	0.1 ± 0.3	[− 0.5, 0.3]	1.0 ± 3.1	[0.2, 1.8]	2.3 ± 5.3	[1.2, 3.4]	$Welch_{(2,98.07)} = 9.16^{***}$
Depression score *(M ± SD [CI])*	18.5 ± 6.7	[15.2, 21.8]	18.2 ± 6.0	[16.6, 19.7][2]	22.5 ± 11.0	[20.2, 24.9][1]	$Welch_{(2,51.20)} = 4.78^{*}$
Major Depression (%, *n*)	0	(0)	0 (0)[2]		12.6	(11)	$Chi^2_{(2)} = 10.44^{**}$
Anxiety score *(M ± SD [CI])*	11.7 ± 2.5	[10.51, 12.94]	11.6 ± 2.6	[11.0, 12.3]	14.1 ± 6.4	[12.7, 15.5][3]	$Welch_{(2,56.31)} = 5.30^{**}$
Substance dependence (%, *n*)	11.1	(2)	6.7	(4)	4.6	(4)	$Chi^2_{(2)} = 1.17$
Substance abuse (%, *n*)	0	(0)	1.7	(1)[2]	1.1	(1)	$Chi^2_{(2)} = 0.34$
Suicidal ideation (%, *n*)	0	(0)	8.3	(5)	10.3	(9)	$Chi^2_{(2)} = 2.06$
Psychotic disorder (%, *n*)	0	(0)	0	(0)	2.3	(2)	$Chi^2_{(2)} = 1.8$

CFV childhood familial violence, *LTE* lifetime traumatic events
$^{*}p \leq .05$, $^{**}p \leq .01$, $^{***}p \leq .001$; [1]$n = 85$, [2]$n = 59$, [3]$n = 86$, [4]$n = 16$, [5]$n = 40$, [6]$n = 50$

Somali women who underwent FGM I are a minority ($n = 14$, 14%), and have a younger average age (average age: $M = 24.5$, $SD = 13.9$, 95% CI [16.5; 32.5]). Amharic women typically endured the procedure shortly after birth ($n = 31$, 86%); only 5 women reported having undergone FGM later (one each at 3, 5, and 15 years of age, and two at 7 years of age). No particular pattern in terms of circumcision age was found for the FGM cases of the group of Oromo and other ethnicities ($N = 14$).

FGM procedural information

Table 2 provides a summary of information on FGM, presenting data on women without FGM and women who underwent FGM I, or FGM II/III, separately. The majority of women reported that they did not agree to their circumcision ($n = 101$, 69%) and that they were not informed prior to FGM as to what would happen ($n = 133$, 91%). During the procedure, 72 (65%) women were blindfolded, and 36 (33%) were gagged. Only a minor portion of women reported having received analgesics ($n = 36$, 25%), which were, however not necessarily effective. The procedure was usually performed using a razor blade ($n = 86$, 74%), or in a few cases, a knife ($n = 24$, 21%). One (1%) woman reported having been circumcised with broken glass and 4 (3%) with scissors. Almost all women ($n = 96$, 92%) who remembered the event reported having experienced intense fear and/or helplessness during the procedure; this did not differ according to the FGM type ($n_{FGM\ I} = 19$, 86.4%, $n_{FGM\ II/III} = 77$, 93.9%; $Chi^2_{(1)} = 1.39$, $p > .05$). In the aftermath of FGM II/III, 100% ($n = 83$) of the women reported having had their legs bound for 2 to 40 days ($M = 9.8$, $SD = 6.8$, 95% CI [8.3; 11.3]), 56 ($n = 64\%$) were isolated for several days ($M = 11.4$, $SD = 8.1$, 95% CI [9.2; 13.6]) and 83% ($n = 72$) were deprived of food or drink for up to 30 days ($M = 9.6$, $SD = 6.4$, 95% CI [8.1; 11.1]). This was less extensive for women who endured FGM I: 10 (17%) women reported having had their legs bound between 1 to 10 days ($M = 5.6$, $SD = 2.8$, 95% CI [3.6; 7.5]), 8 (13%) were isolated up to 20 days ($M = 11.0$, $SD = 4.8$, 95% CI [7.0; 15.1]) and 9 (15%) were deprived of food or drink for up to 12 days ($M = 6.9$, $SD = 3.1$, 95% CI [4.5; 9.2]).

The cycle of infibulation, defibulation, and re-infibulation

Menstruation, sexual intercourse and giving birth typically mean further stages of suffering in the aftermath of FGM—particularly following FGM II/III. In this subsample, 82 (94%) reported having been infibulated. This occurred by means of thorns ($n = 57$, 70%) or thread ($n = 24$, 30%). One woman did not know how she had been infibulated. During menstruation, 51 (62%) women reported having experienced severe pain, 52 (63%) had complications passing blood, and 32 (39%) had fever or infections. A total of 52 (60%) women had had sexual intercourse and were therefore able to answer questions on defibulation: 42 (82%) women were defibulated by a traditional circumciser or another person. For 9 (18%) women, the husband performed defibulation on the night of the wedding. After childbirth, a total of 21 (41%) women reported having been re-infibulated up to 10 times. On average, the vaginal opening had been closed up to 3.4 times ($SD = 2.7$, 95% CI [2.2; 4.6]) after childbirth.

Procedure

All interviews were conducted in a private office at the Women's Affairs headquarters in Jijiga in July, August and September 2010. Participants were asked to sign their informed consent prior to the interview; none of them refused. For minors (one was 13 years old, six were 16 years old and four were 17 years old), caregivers were invited to sit in during the informed consent; none of them advised their daughters not to take part in the interview and agreed to leave the session following the provision of informed consent. Each participant received 50 Birr ($2.50) as financial compensation. The interview lasted around two to three hours. The study was approved by Vivo International and Norwegian Church

Table 2 Self-reported age at circumcision, location, immediate complications and lifetime physical complaints due to the FGM groups

	FGM I		FGM II/III		
	$n = 60$		$n = 87$		Statistics
Age at circ. ($M \pm SD$ [CI])	3.1 ± 4.3	[2.0, 4.2]	7.6 ± 2.7	[7.0, 8.1]	$t_{(89.53)} = -7.10$***
Immediate complications (< 14 days after FGM; %, n)					
Severe pain	50%	(11)[1]	84%	(70)[2]	$Chi^2_{(1)} = 11.63$***
Excessive bleeding	5%	(1)[1]	23%	(19)[3]	$Chi^2_{(1)} = 3.72$
Infections/fever	0%	(0)[1]	36%	(30)[2]	
Lifetime chronic physical complaints due to FGM (%, n)					
Pelvic pain	10%	(6)	60%	(52)	$Chi^2_{(1)} = 36.82$***
Urination problems	10%	(6)	37%	(32)	$Chi^2_{(1)} = 13.29$***
Menstruation problem	11%	(7)	67%	(58)	$Chi^2_{(1)} = 43.55$***

*$p \leq .05$, **$p \leq .01$, ***$p \leq .001$; [1]$n = 22$, [2]$n = 83$, [3]$n = 84$

Aid (NCA). These are both international non-governmental organizations with long-standing experience in Ethiopia as well as in the Somali Region.

A team of four clinical psychologists (post-doctoral and doctoral, as well as two trained and supervised psychology master-level students) conducted the interviews with the help of English and Amhara and/or Somali-speaking interpreters in all interviews. The latter were trained in a two-day workshop introducing the applied concepts and were advised to translate literally in order to minimize the potential bias or confusion involved with personal interpretation.

Measures

Sociodemographic information was obtained from each participant by administering a semi-structured questionnaire asking for age, ethnicity, educational background in years and domestic status as well as the participant's physical health over the previous month (cough, cold/flu, shivering, fever, malaria, headache, pain, diarrhea, vomiting, scabies/skin rash, positive HIV/AIDS test, other physical pain).

To assess details on the individual's experience with FGM, we constructed a 45-item checklist (*yes/no*). In the first part, general questions regarding, for example, age at circumcision, previous knowledge regarding the tradition and location were asked. Then, with the help of anatomical sketches of the female genitalia, we asked details about the subject's own FGM, her emotional experiences during the procedure, as well as subsequent complications (short- and long-term). Finally, we asked questions regarding current attitudes on FGM. All items were evaluated separately.

Further traumatic experiences were assessed using the Checklist of Childhood Familial Violence (CFV) [29] and the event checklist part of the Posttraumatic Stress Diagnostic Scale (PDS) [30]. The 36-item CFV assesses childhood traumatic experiences at a physical, verbal-emotional, sexual and witnessed level. We added two items to assess intimate partner violence (*"Have you been beaten by your husband?"* and *"Have you been beaten by the family of your husband?"*). The PDS event checklist contains 12 potentially traumatic event types (e.g., torture, sexual abuse, accident). For both checklists, the sum of all items approved comprised the final scores.

Participant diagnostic status and PTSD symptom severity were assessed using the PTSD Symptom Scale - Interview (PSS-I) [31]. The PSS-I assesses the 17 DSM-IV [32] symptom criteria for PTSD. We assessed the symptom occurrence during the previous month (instead of over the past 2 weeks as specified by the questionnaire manual) to check the diagnostic status and to match the time period of cortisol analysis. Each item was rated on a four-point scale ranging from 0 (*not at all/only once*) to 3 (*five or more times per week/almost always*). PTSD severity was calculated by summing all of the symptom scores (possible scores range from 0 to 51). Internal consistency was excellent in this study (Cronbach's $\alpha = .95$).

To assess the syndrome of trauma-related dissociation, we applied the Shutdown Dissociation Scale (ShuD) [33]. This 13-item questionnaire assesses sensory deafferentation (e.g., transitory deafness or blindness), reduced nociception/analgesia, numbness, transitory paralysis, loss of speech/suppressed vocalization, pseudo-neurological symptoms, (pre-)syncopes and out-of-body experiences on a four-point scale (0 – *not at all* to 3 – *several times a week*). All items were added to a total score ranging from 0 to 39. Good psychometric properties were also found in the study by Schalinski et al. ([34]; Cronbach's $\alpha = .75$). In this study, Cronbach's α was .84.

The Hopkins Symptom Checklist-25 (HSCL-25) [35] was used to determine the severity of depression (15 items) and anxiety (10 items). Referring to the last 2 weeks, the subject rated each item on a four-point scale from 1 (*not at all*) to 4 (*extremely*). A separate sum score was computed for the two syndromes ranging from 15 to 60 for depression, and 10 to 40 for anxiety. The HSCL has shown good psychometric properties in previous studies [36–39]. In this study, Cronbach's α was .92 for the depression scale and .86 for the anxiety scale.

Furthermore, we applied the Mini-International Neuropsychiatric Interview (M.I.N.I., 5.0.0, January 1st, 2002) [40] to assess the diagnostic status of major depression (*A. major* depression episode), suicidal ideation (B. suicidality), drug abuse (K. non-alcohol psychoactive substance use disorder) and psychotic disorders (L. psychotic disorder). The M.I.N.I. only takes a short amount of time to administer, and has shown satisfactory concordance with the Structured Clinical Interview for DSM-IV-TR Axis I Disorders – Patient Edition (SCID-P), the Composite International Diagnostic Interview (CIDI) and with expert diagnosis [40].

Cortisol sampling

In accordance with the laboratory protocol of Stalder et al. [41] and Kirschbaum et al. [16], hair samples were cut from the posterior vertex. We used 1 cm of the segments closest to the scalp for cortisol extraction. Considering the hair growth rate of Africans (0.74 cm/month) [42], the hair segment length of 1 cm roughly signifies 1 month of growth – the time span assessed by the PSS-I. For cortisol determination, 5–10 mg of whole, nonpulverised hair was incubated in 1800 ml methanol for 18 h at 45 °C. Following extraction, cortisol levels were determined using a commercially available immunoassay with chemiluminescence detection (CLIA, IBL-Hamburg, Germany). The intra- and inter-assay coefficients of variation of this assay are below 8% [16]. The mean cortisol level was $M = 30.2$ ($SD = 16.2$, *range* 8.5–92.8), and thus comparable to other African samples [19]. Outlying values (≥ 3 *SD* above mean) were found for two women. In the presented analysis, we excluded the outliers and log-transformed HCC values (positive skewness). A total of 60 (35.9%) women refused to give hair samples because of religious or traditional objections; excluding four cases with missing data in CFV ($n = 1$), FGM ($n = 1$) and age ($n = 2$), the neuroendocrinological analyses include a total of 103 women (sociodemographic characteristics did not differ significantly between these subsamples).

Data analysis

All missing values were excluded from the analysis (see Table 1). Furthermore, we excluded women who reported having not remembered specific details during their circumcision in the descriptive analysis of the procedure; this was the case for women who reported having been circumcised at an age below 3 years as well as for one woman with FGM I and one and two women with FGM II/III (depending on the item). The descriptive data are presented as frequencies (%), means (*M*) and standard deviations (*SD*). Group differences were analyzed using independent sample *t*-tests and univariate analysis of variance (ANOVA) for continuous variables; post-hoc group differences are indicated by the reported confidence intervals in the tables. Heteroscedasticity was found in certain variables (PTSD, shutdown dissociation, depression, anxiety). Because an *F*-test performed on data with heteroscedasticity would tend to be less conservative, we computed the *Welch* statistic instead. Chi^2 tests were used for categorical variables. *Fisher's Exact* test was applied in cases of cell frequencies less than five. All statistical tests are two-tailed. Pearson's correlation coefficient was computed as measures of associations for two continuous variables.

As the group of FGM II/III presented with a higher trauma load, we conducted a stepwise linear regression model to investigate the impact of FGM on the association of lifetime traumatic events and PTSD severity. In the first step, we entered FGM to predict PTSD symptom severity; here, FGM was dummy coded with FGM I as baseline (due to low sample size and heterogeneous characteristics, the noFGM cannot be interpreted as a baseline control group). In the second step, the number of lifetime traumatic events types was entered in addition to FGM, and in the third step, the interaction term of the two predictors was entered. To address potential problems caused by heteroscedasticity, we used bootstrapping (second step); all confidence intervals of the models' standardized estimates were very close to the bootstrapped confidence intervals, suggesting that the model could be regarded as robust to heteroscedasticity. Cohen's f^2 effect size was computed, with $f^2 < .05$ constituting a small, $f^2 > .15$ a moderate, and $f^2 > .35$ a large effect [43].

For statistical analysis of the hair cortisol data, we first used random forest regression [44] with conditional inference trees (hereafter "conditional inference random forests" or RF-CI) [45] to identify the best predictors of the HCC. Here, we included all variables that would theoretically induce stress (lifetime traumatic events, childhood domestic violence, husband domestic violence, FGM, age at circumcision, PTSD, anxiety, depression, shutdown dissociation, time since the last traumatic event, physical health, HIV/AIDS, age, education). Second, to assess the predictive significance and the direction of associations of these predictors in a parametric model, we conducted a simple linear regression with the most important predictors. The number of predictors (*k*) was set according to the rule of thumb recommended in Tabachnick and Fidel [46] to test a full regression model ($50 + 8\,k$) and to interpret individual predictors (104-k).

RF-CI is a non-parametric machine learning technique. Unlike the classical random forest [44], the RF-CI does not display a bias towards predictors with many categories in the variable selection process [47]. Following the principles of ensemble methods, a certain number of trees (ntree) are aggregated to compose the random forest. Each tree is built using binary splits of the previously subsampled data (subsampling rate = 63.2%) [27, 48]. The splitting variable is chosen according to the strength of the association between the covariates and the outcome [27, 45] from a set of randomly preselected predictors (*p*, mtry, *p*/3) [49]. Next, the importance of each predictor variable is ranked based on the ensemble of trees (conditional variable importance, *cvi*) [47]. To visualize the results, we built single trees from the whole data set. These are, however, less robust (e.g., biased by outliers) and should not be interpreted without considering the results of the whole ensemble. The PDS event checklist includes a dichotomous item for familial violence and FGM. These events were excluded in the PDS sum score (lifetime traumatic events) applied in the RF-CI computation, as the FGM checklist and the CFV assess these variables more precisely. All cases with missing values in one of the predictor variables were excluded. The analysis was conducted using SPSS 21 and R (version 3.4.1). The implementation we used to compute the RF-CI was cforest [50] from the R package party [51] with unbiased variable selection [45, 50].

Results

Table 1 illustrates lifetime exposure to violence and mental health problems divided for women without FGM and women who endured FGM I, or FGM II/III, respectively. No group differences were found for childhood familial violence ($p > .05$), but for the number of lifetime traumatic events: women who endured FGM II/III also presented with a higher trauma exposure ($p < .05$).

Accordingly, in the group of FGM II/III, more women fulfilled the criteria of PTSD (FGM II/III: $n = 16$, 18%; FGM I: $n = 0$; noFGM: $n = 1$, 6%). While 11 (12%) women in the FGM II/III group fulfilled the diagnostic criteria of major depression, none of the other groups presented the required severity of symptoms. Furthermore, group comparisons revealed that PTSD and trauma-related symptoms such as shutdown dissociation, depression and anxiety were elevated in women who underwent FGM II/III (group comparisons were significant at 95% levels). Only a few women (< 5%) were diagnosed with substance dependence and/or abuse and/or psychotic disorders; for these, no group differences were found.

FGM, trauma exposure, and posttraumatic stress

Investigating the contribution of FGM to the association of the number of traumatic events and PTSD severity, we conducted a stepwise linear regression model; the results are presented in Table 3. In the first step, FGM significantly predicted PTSD severity, with elevated symptoms in the FGM II/III group ($p < .001$). In the second step, both FGM ($p < .01$) and the number of lifetime traumatic events ($p < .001$) predicted PTSD severity, and the model comparisons indicated a significant improvement in step two ($F_{(1,161)} = 75.3$, $p < .001$). In the third step, in addition to the predictors FGM and the number of lifetime traumatic events the interaction term of the two variables was inserted; the latter became the only significant predictor. The analysis explained 43.7% of variance and model comparisons indicated a better fit than the former ($F_{(2,159)} = 11.6$, $p < .001$). The last step demonstrates that, with having endured FGM II/III, the negative effects of non-FGM-related traumatic stressors are increased, and these women are more susceptible to developing PTSD. Concordantly, Fig. 1 illustrates the interaction of FGM with other lifetime traumatic events and PTSD severity as well as shutdown dissociation.

Table 3 Stepwise linear regression analysis predicting the PTSD symptom severity by FGM (dummy coded with FGM I at baseline; step 1), FGM and the number of lifetime traumatic events (step 2) and the latter variables and their interaction term

	beta (SE)	*β*	*t*
Step 1 ($F_{(2,162)} = 7.3$, $p < .001$, adjusted R2 = .07, $f^2 = .09$)			
(Intercept)	0.83 (1.34)	.09	0.42
FGM: type II/III vs. I	4.83 (1.34)	.54	3.60***
FGM: noFGM vs. type I	0.33 (2.15)	.03	0.15
Step 2 ($F_{(3,161)} = 32.2$, $p < .001$, adjusted $R^2 = .36$, $f^2 = .60$)			
(Intercept)	−2.78 (0.96)	−.32	−3.00**
FGM: type II/III vs. I	3.58 (1.12)	.40	3.19**
FGM: noFGM vs. type I	1.81 (1.79)	.20	1.01
LTE	2.68 (0.31)	.69	8.68***
Step 3 ($F_{(5,159)} = 26.5$, $p < .001$, adjusted $R^2 = .44$, $f^2 = .83$)			
(Intercept)	0.18 (1.12)	.02	0.16
FGM: type II/III vs. I	−1.21 (1.45)	−.13	−0.83
FGM: noFGM vs. type I	−0.50 (2.12)	−.05	−0.23
LTE	0.47 (0.56)	.12	0.85
Interaction: FGM type II/III vs. I and LTE	3.15 (0.66)	.81	4.76***
Interaction: FGM: noFGM vs. type I and LTE	1.30 (1.38)	.34	0.95

Unstandardized beta coefficients (*beta*) with standard error (*SE*), uncorrected standardized regression coefficients (*β*), and *t*-values (*t*) with *$p \leq .05$, **$p \leq .01$ and ***$p \leq .001$ are reported

FGM female genital mutilation, *LTE* lifetime traumatic events

Cortisol

To identify the most important predictors of the cortisol level, we used RF-CI. Then, we tested the variables in a simple linear regression model.

Predictor identification

The *cvi* was ranked as follows: years of education ($cvi = 26$), childhood familial violence ($cvi = 4$), lifetime traumatic events ($cvi = 3$), and FGM ($cvi = 1$) and the age at circumcision of < 1 year ($cvi = 1$). The *cvis* were below 0.5 for the other variables (symptom severity of PTSD, anxiety, major depression diagnosis, shutdown dissociation, and drug abuse, khat consumption, psychosis, the time since the traumatic event, physical health, intimate partner violence, and specific FGM ages beside < 1 years of age).

Linear regression

On the basis of the variable ranks (*cvi*), the linear regression model included the years of education, family violence during childhood, lifetime traumatic events, FGM (dummy coded with FGM I as a baseline) and whether FGM was endured during the first year of age (yes/no). The model explained 17% of variance with a large effect ($F_{(6,96)} = 4.5$, $p < 0.001$, $f^2 = .28$). More years of education was associated with lower HCC ($\beta = -.08$, $p < 0.01$). Regarding the FGM variables, the more invasive forms of FGM was linked with higher HCC ($\beta = .12$, $p < 0.01$). Interestingly, women who reported having been circumcision during the first year of life also presented with higher cortisol levels ($\beta = 0.16$, $p < 0.001$; see Fig. 2). Lifetime exposure to traumatic events as well as childhood familial violence did not reach significance. The results are summarized in Table 4. Figure 1 presents a single tree partitioning the sample of women who endured FGM according to FGM types and whether the circumcision was endured within the first year of life (only FGM I, none of the women in the group FGM II/III reported to be circumcised during the first year of life).

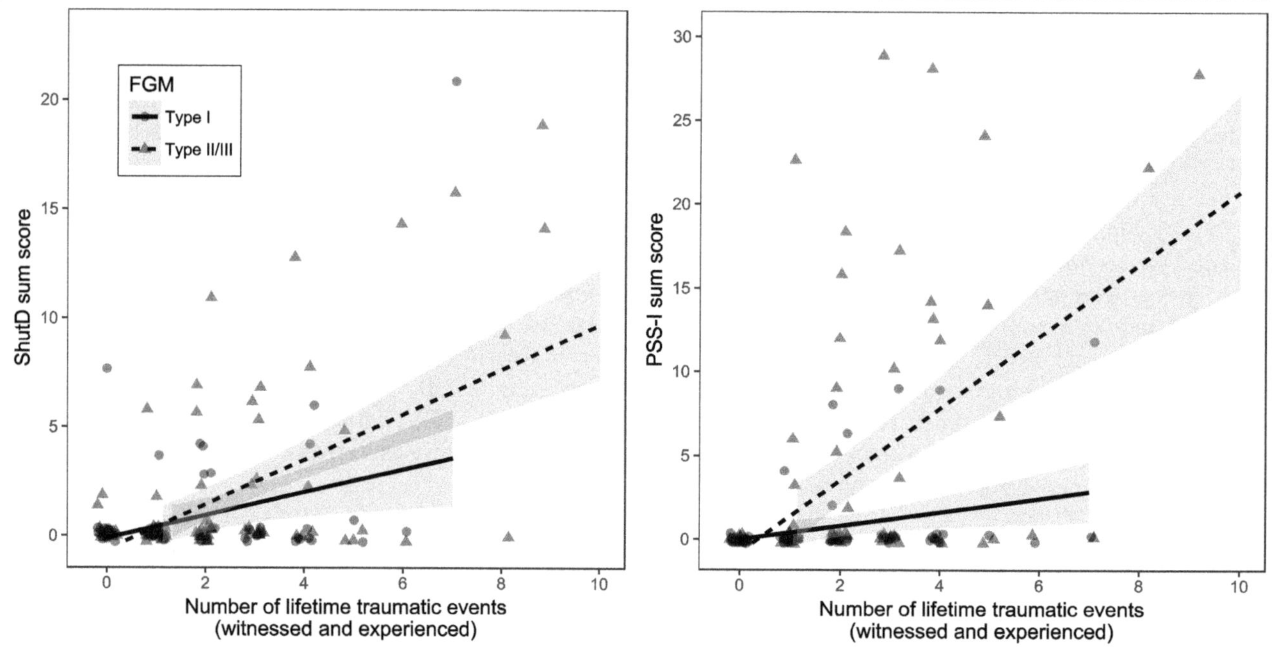

Fig. 1 The least square fitted conditional mean (smoothed with 95% CI) of the PSS-I and ShuD total score interacting with the number of lifetime traumatic events according to FGM I versus II/III. *Note:* FGM = female genital mutilation, PSS-I = Posttraumatic Stress Scale – Interview, ShuD = Shutdown Dissociation Scale, More severe forms of FGM are connected with higher levels of PTSD and, to a lesser extent, shutdown dissociation phenomena

Discussion

In this article, we aimed to investigate FGM and its psychopathological sequelae as well as neuroendocrinological associations measured by means of the HCC in an urban sample of women living in Jijiga, the capital of the Ethiopian Somali region. Group differences showed that PTSD and trauma-related symptoms such as shutdown dissociation, depression and anxiety were more severe in the subgroup of FGM II/III. The stepwise linear regression indicated an acceleration of PTSD symptom development with the accumulation of other traumatic experiences, especially for individuals with more severe forms of FGM. Using RF-CI, we found alterations in the HCC according to FGM-related variables as well as to

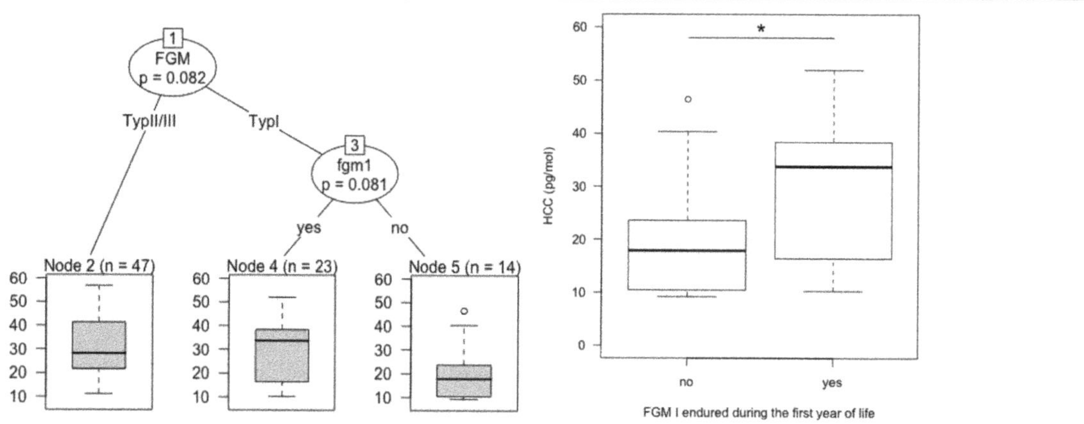

Fig. 2 Displays a single tree partitioning the sample according to FGM types and whether the circumcision was endured within the first year of life (only FGM I). Women who endured more invasive forms of FGM, but also women who endured the procedure within their first year of life, present with higher HCC. HCC comparison within the group FGM I revealed significantly higher levels for women who were circumcised in their first year of life ($t_{(29.18)} = -2.18$, $p = 0.038$)

Table 4 Linear regression analysis predicting hair cortisol levels by education, lifetime traumatic events, childhood familial violence, FGM (dummy coded with FGM I at baseline) and FGM endured during the first year of age

	HCC (mg/mol)		
	beta (SE)	*β*	*t*
(Intercept)	2.97 (0.15)	.89	19.26***
Education	−0.03 (0.01)	−.08	−2.73**
LTE	−0.02 (0.03)	−.01	−0.59
CFV	0.02 (0.01)	.04	1.94
FGM: type II/III vs. I	0.41 (0.14)	.12	2.90**
FGM: no FGM vs. type I	0.32 (0.17)	.10	1.86
FGM < 1 year of age	0.52 (0.15)	.16	3.43***

Unstandardized beta coefficients (*beta*) with standard error (*SE*), uncorrected standardized regression coefficients (*β*), and *t*-values (*t*) with $*p \leq .05$, $**p \leq .01$ and $***p \leq .001$ are displayed. $F_{(6,96)} = 4.51$, $p < 0.001$, $f^2 = .28$, multiple $R^2 = .22$, adjusted $R^2 = .17$
HCC hair cortisol concentration, *CFV* childhood family violence, *LTE* lifetime traumatic events

the years of education and childhood familial violence. More invasive forms of FGM as well as enduring FGM within the first year of life was linked to higher levels of cortisol.

FGM

In line with former studies, almost all women (92%, FGM age ≥ 3 years) reported having experienced intense fear and/or helplessness during their circumcision. Investigating this separately for the FGM groups revealed that, irrespective of the actual FGM type, the procedure applies not only in its objective characteristics to the A-criteria of PTSD as defined in the DSM-5 (severe injury, threat to life, sexual violence), but also involves intense subjective reactions of fear and helplessness.

Regarding the psychopathological sequelae of FGM, we identified women who endured FGM II/III as being particularly vulnerable to developing mental health problems. The results demonstrated that women who underwent FGM II/III suffered more often from (sub)clinical symptoms of PTSD and also reported more trauma-related complications such as shutdown dissociation, depression and anxiety than women who endured FGM I. The stepwise regression analysis revealed an interaction effect of FGM II/III and the number of lifetime traumatic events, indicating that more severe forms of FGM increase the vulnerability to PTSD, such that additional traumatic stressors exert more devastating effects [8]. This aligns with previous findings [5, 10, 11]. Notably, there is a substantial number of women who seem to be resilient (see Fig. 1a); they have a high trauma load, but do not report trauma-related symptoms. Potential resilience factors, such as an increase in social integrity, remain to be explored.

FGM and hair cortisol

In addition to the psychological variables, we measured long-term neuroendocrinological alterations by means of the HCC to explore potential adaptions of HPA axis activity in conjunction with FGM and other stress-related variables. Therefore, we statistically defined the most influential predictors (using RF-CI) and computed a parametric linear regression model, determining the direction of the associations and providing a significance test for each predictor. The results indicate long-term changes of cortisol levels in association with FGM. As implicated by the HCC as biological marker for stress, women who endured more severe forms of FGM presented with higher levels of hair cortisol. We interpret this result as evidence for the upregulation of the HPA axis activity as a consequence to the traumatic nature of the procedure itself in combination with the continuous cycle of infibulation, defibulation and re-infibulation and other physical consequences. These factors may render women who endured FGM II/III more vulnerable to the adverse effect of traumatic events at the psychological side (see Fig. 1). Furthermore, women who endured the procedure during their first year of age (in our study exclusively FGM type I) showed more pronounced levels of cortisol. This result is in line with previous research on FGM and early life stress. For example, Taddio et al. [52] found an enhanced stress reaction (facial expression, length of time screaming) at vaccination for babies that had been circumcised four to 6 months prior. Scholars agree that neonates, as well as babies in the preverbal phase, are able to respond with the full range of emotional, cognitive and physiological peritraumatic reactions (e.g. palpitation, muscle tension, tachycardia/bradycardia, vasoconstriction/vasodilatation, numbing) [53], and although they are unable to verbalize their experience of the event, the neuronal paths are generated and will be consolidated in the case of further traumatization [54]. The particular relevance of the prenatal period and the early years in life have repeatedly been demonstrated to play a critical role in the (epigenetic) programming of the HPA axis [15, 55] and other negative health outcomes [56].

This study demonstrates that even 20 years after the declaration of FGM as a human rights violation by the UN (A/RES/48/104, Article 2(b)), the practice remains widespread—even in urban regions. The findings show that the awareness of effects of FGM has to go beyond direct somatic complaints and encompass psychopathological risks as well. The provision of adequate health care which particularly addresses the consequences of traumatization is key to overcoming the manifold effects of FGM. Here, evidence-based, culturally sensitive psychotherapeutic tools have been developed to succumb these forms of traumatization, such as Narrative Exposure Therapy [57, 58]. Trauma-specific interventions should complement medical and more holistic approaches, as suggested by Mulongo et al. [59]. Cultural aspects have to be considered for all forms and regions of intervention [60].

Hair cortisol and other variables

Notably, we did not find a positive relation between other stress-related variables and HCC after controlling for the level of education and FGM-related variables. For instance, Schalinski et al. [21] found higher HCC in a sample of 42 traumatized refugees as well as Simmons et al. [61] who recently published a study with 70 children (mean age 9.5 years). In contrast, Hinkelman et al. [62] found lower HCC in individuals with a history of childhood familial violence in a sample of depressed patients and healthy participants ($N = 84$). Also Kalmakis et al. [63] reported a negative relation in healthy college students ($N = 55$), and Steudte-Schmiedgen et al. [24] in military personnel. Additionally, we did not find an association with age [64] or the number traumatic events [19–21] or major life events [22], respectively. Steudte-Schmiedgen et al. [51] found a negative correlation of HCC with the number of traumatic events and frequency of traumatization. Moreover, contradictory results were previously reported for PTSD (e.g. [19, 23, 65]), which was one of the negligible predictors ($cvi < 0.5$) in the current analyses. Similarly, inconsistent previous results were found for depression [62, 66], which was again irrelevant in the regression analysis of our study. In order to explain associations between HPA axis regulation, cortisol secretion, HCC, and clinical constructs, more research is needed. A better understanding of traumatization during specific windows of opportunity and its effect on the regulation of stress may allow to generate algorithms which eventually could validate subjective psychological reports with biological measures such as HCC.

Limitations

The lack of a comparable uncircumcised and/or non-traumatized control group constitutes a major limitation in the analysis. Moreover, in regard to the group of FGM I, where the procedure is often not remembered due to the young age at circumcision (≤ 3 years), women had to be excluded from the analysis. Furthermore, the study is correlational in nature, and thus, factors associated with the type of FGM and factors beyond the ritual itself may additionally be responsible for the observed mental health conditions. Also, the reports are retrospective and may therefore be biased, as most of the cross-sectional psychological studies. Despite the anatomical sketches, the FGM type was identified based on self-reported information and may thus not be reliable for all women; medical examinations were not feasible within the present study. Finally, the sample is not representative and generalizations may not necessarily hold up; in particular, we assume that there is a selective exclusion of women with high avoidance symptoms and other concerns regarding FGM, mental health, or research in general. To our knowledge, this is the first study associating FGM with neuroendocrinological outcomes, therefore a replication study especially including HCC would be of particular interest.

Conclusion

All forms of FGM may have negative health outcomes. Women who endured extensive forms of FGM present with a higher risk of developing mental disorders. They report more severe symptoms of PTSD and trauma-related problems, including shutdown dissociation, depression and anxiety. These findings are corroborated by heightened levels of cortisol in this group. Furthermore, women who endured FGM I during their first year of life showed higher concentration of cortisol, despite the lack of more obvious mental health implications. Evidence-based trauma interventions have been developed (e.g. [57]), and in the next step must be scaled up along with integral treatment approaches to mitigate the negative consequences of FGM.

Abbreviations

CFV: Childhood familial violence; FGM: Female genital mutilation; HCC: Hair cortisol concentrations; HSCL: Hopkins Symptom Checklist; LTE: Lifetime traumatic events; M.I.N.I.: Mini-International Neuropsychiatric Interview; PSS-I: Posttraumatic Stress Symptom Scale – Interview; PTSD: Posttraumatic stress disorder; ShuD: Shutdown Dissociation Scale

Acknowledgements

Our immense gratitude is owed to all of the participants who openly disclosed their intimate, often painful and shame-prone experiences. We are grateful to our translators from Jijiga as well as co-workers from NCA, EGLDAM, the Women's Affairs office and vivo international.

Funding

Deutsche Forschungsgesellschaft (DFG).

Authors' contributions

All of the authors contributed to the development of the study and the study design. Prof. Dr. TE wrote the grant applications for the grants that funded this work. Dr. MRL and Dipl. Psych. AK performed interviewer training and collected the data. AK performed data analysis and interpretation under the supervision of TE and MRL. AK had full access to all the data in the study and takes responsibility for the integrity of the data and the accuracy of the data analysis. AK drafted the paper, and TE and MRL provided critical revisions. All of the authors approved the final version of the paper for submission.

Competing interests

The authors declare that they have no competing interests.

References

1. WHO: Female Genital Mutilation. 2012. http://www.who.int/mediacentre/factsheets/fs241/en/.
2. UNICEF. Female Genital Mutilation/Cutting: A global concern. New York: UNICEF; 2016.
3. Banks E, Meirik O, Farley T, Akande O, Bathija H, Ali M. Female genital mutilation and obstetric outcome: WHO collaborative prospective study in six African countries. Lancet. 2006;367(9525):1835–41.
4. Dirie W, Miller C. Desert flower: The extraordinary journey of a desert nomad. New York: William Morrow; 1998.
5. Behrendt A, Moritz S. Posttraumatic stress disorder and memory problems after female genital mutilation. Am J Psychiatry. 2005;162(5):1000–2.
6. Tol WA, Stavrou V, Greene MC, Mergenthaler C, van Ommeren MA. Sexual and gender-based violence in areas of armed conflict: a systematic review of mental health and psychosocial support interventions. Confl Heal. 2013;7(1):16.
7. Wilker S, Pfeiffer A, Kolassa S, Koslowski D, Elbert T, Kolassa IT. How to quantify exposure to traumatic stress? Reliability and predictive validity of measures for cumulative trauma exposure in a post-conflict population. Eur J Psychotraumatol. 2015;6(1):28306.
8. Kolassa I-T, Elbert T. Structural and functional neurolpasticity in relation to traumatic stress. Curr Dir Psychol Sci. 2007;16(6):321–5.
9. Kessler RC, Sonnega A, Bromet E, Hughes M, Nelson CB. Posttraumatic stress disorder in the national comorbidity survey. Arch Gen Psychiatry. 1995;52(12):1048–60.
10. Pa M. The psychological impact of female genital mutilation/cutting (FGM/C) on girls/women's mental health: a narrative literature review. J Reprod Infant Psychol. 2014;32(5):469–85.
11. Knipscheer J, Vloeberghs E, van der Kwaak A, van den Muijsenbergh M. Mental health problems associated with female genital mutilation. BJPsych Bulletin. 2015;39(6):273 LP–277.
12. Meewisse ML, Reitsma JB, de Vries GJ, Gersons BP, Olff M. Cortisol and post-traumatic stress disorder in adults: systematic review and meta-analysis. Br J Psychiatry. 2007;191:387–92.
13. Steudte-Schmiedgen S, Kirschbaum C, Alexander N, Stalder T. An integrative model linking traumatization, cortisol dysregulation and posttraumatic stress disorder: insight from recent hair cortisol findings. Neurosci Biobehav Rev. 2016;69:124–35.
14. McEwen BS. Stress, adaptation, and disease: Allostasis and allostatic load. Annals of the New York academy of sciences. 1998:840(1):33–44.
15. Murgatroyd C, Spengler D. Epigenetic programming of the HPA axis: early life decides. Stress. 2011;14(6):581–9.
16. Kirschbaum C, Tietze A, Skoluda N, Dettenborn L. Hair as a retrospective calendar of cortisol production-increased cortisol incorporation into hair in the third trimester of pregnancy. Psychoneuroendocrinology. 2009;34(1):32–7.
17. Webb E, Thomson S, Nelson A, White C, Koren G, Rieder M, Van Uum S. Assessing individual systemic stress through cortisol analysis of archaeological hair. J Archaeol Sci. 2010;37:807–12.
18. Elevated content of cortisol in hair of patients with severe chronic pain: a novel biomarker for stress. Stress (Amsterdam, Netherlands). 2008;11(6):483–8.
19. Steudte S, Kolassa IT, Stalder T, Pfeiffer A, Kirschbaum C, Elbert T. Increased cortisol concentrations in hair of severely traumatized Ugandan individuals with PTSD. Psychoneuroendocrinology. 2011;36(8):1193–200.
20. Schreier HMC, Enlow MB, Ritz T, Coull BA, Gennings C, Wright RO, Wright RJ. Lifetime exposure to traumatic and other stressful life events and hair cortisol in a multi-racial/ethnic sample of pregnant women. Stress (Amsterdam, Netherlands). 2016;19(1):45–52.
21. Schalinski I, Elbert T, Steudte-Schmiedgen S, Kirschbaum C. The cortisol paradox of trauma-related disorders: lower phasic responses but higher tonic levels of cortisol are associated with sexual abuse in childhood. PLoS One. 2015;10(8):e0136921.
22. Karlen J, Ludvidsson J, Frostell A, Theodorsson E, Faresjo T. Cortisol in hair measured in young adults - a biomarker of major life stressors? BMC Clin Pathol. 2011;11(1):12.
23. Steudte S, Kirschbaum C, Gao W, Alexander N, Schnfeld S, Hoyer J, Stalder T. Hair cortisol as a biomarker of traumatization in healthy individuals and posttraumatic stress disorder patients. Biol Psychiatry. 2013;74(9):639–46.
24. Steudte-Schmiedgen S, Stalder T, Schönfeld S, Wittchen H-U, Trautmann S, Alexander N, Miller R, Kirschbaum C. Hair cortisol concentrations and cortisol stress reactivity predict PTSD symptom increase after trauma exposure during military deployment. Psychoneuroendocrinology. 2015;59:123–33.
25. Hinkelmann K, Muhtz C, Dettenborn L, Agorastos A, Wingenfeld K, Spitzer C, Otte C. Association between childhood trauma and low hair cortisol in depressed patients and healthy control subjects. Biological psychiatry. 2013;74(9):e15–e17.
26. Central Statistical Agency: Ethiopian Demographic and health survey 2005: CSA; 2005.
27. Strobl C, Malley J, Tutz G. An introduction to recursive partitioning: rationale, application and characteristics of classification and regression trees, bagging and random forests. Psychol Methods. 2009;14(4):323–48.
28. Central Statistical Agency. Ethiopian Demographic and health survey. Addis Ababa: CSA; 2005.
29. Catani C, Jacob N, Schauer E, Kohila M, Neuner F. Family violence, war, and natural disasters: a study of the effect of extreme stress on children's mental health in Sri Lanka. BMC psychiatry. 2008;8:33.
30. Foa EB, Riggs DS, Dancu CV, Rothbaum B. Reliability and validity of a brief intrument for assessing post-traumatic stress disorder. J Trauma Stress. 1993;6:459–73.
31. Foa EB, Tolin DF. Comparison of the PTSD symptom scale-interview version and the clinician-administered PTSD scale. J Trauma Stress. 2000;13(2):181–91.
32. American Psychiatric Association. Diagnostic and statistical manual of mental disorders (4th ed., Text Revision). Washington, DC: Author; 2000.
33. Schalinski I, Schauer M, Elbert T. The shutdown dissociation scale (shut-D). Eur J Psychotraumatol. 2015;6(1):25652.
34. Schalinski I, Elbert T, Schauer M. Female dissociative responding to extreme sexual violence in a chronic crisis setting: the case of eastern Congo. J Trauma Stress. 2011;24(2):235–8.
35. Derogatis LR, Lipman RS, Rickels K, Uhlenhuth EH, Covi L. The Hopkins symptom checklist (HSCL): a self-report symptom inventory. Behav Sci. 1974;19(1):1–15.
36. Hesbacher PT, Rickels K, Morris RJ, Newman H, Rosenfeld H. Psychiatric illness in family practice. J Clin Psychiatry. 1980;41(1):6–10.
37. Mollica RF, Wyshak G, de Marneffe D, Khuon F, Lavelle J. Indochinese versions of the Hopkins symptom Checklist-25: a screening instrument for the psychiatric care of refugees. Am J Psychiatr. 1987;144(4):497–500.
38. Kleijn WC, Hovens JE, Rodenburg JJ. Posttraumatic stress symptoms in refugees: assessments with the\Harvard trauma questionnaire\and the Hopkins symptom Checklist-25 in different languages. Psychol Rep. 2001;88(2):527–32.
39. Lee B, Kaaya SF, Mbwambo JK, Smith-Fawzi MC, Leshabari MT. Detecting depressive disorder with the Hopkins symptom Checklist-25 in Tanzania. Int J Soc Psychiatry. 2008;54(1):7–20.
40. Sheehan DV, Lecrubier Y, Sheehan KH, Amorim P, Janavs J, Weiller E, Hergueta T, Baker R, Dunbar GC. The mini-international neuropsychiatric interview (M.I.N.I.): the development and validation of a structured diagnostic psychiatric interview for DSM-IV and ICD-10. J Clin Psychiatry. 1998;59(Suppl 2):22–33.
41. Stalder T, Steudte S, Miller R, Skoluda N, Dettenborn L, Kirschbaum C. Intraindividual stability of hair cortisol concentrations. Psychoneuroendocrinology. 2012;37(5):602–10.
42. Loussouarn G. African hair growth parameters. Br J Dermatol. 2001;145(2):294–7.
43. Cohen J. A power primer. Psychol Bull. 1992;112(1):155.
44. Breiman L. Random forests. Mach Learn. 2001;45(1):1–35.
45. Hothorn T, Hornik K, Zeileis A. Unbiased recursive partitioning: a conditional inference framework. J Comput Graph Stat. 2006;15(3):651–74.
46. Tabachnick BG, Fidell LS: Using multivariate statistics, 5th Editio edn: Pearson Edication Inc; 2007.
47. Strobl C, Boulesteix A-L, Kneib T, Augustin T, Zeileis A. Conditional variable importance for random forests. BMC bioinformatics. 2008;9:307.
48. Strobl C. Statistical issues in machine learning: Towards reliable split selection and variable importance measures; 2008. p. 1–179.
49. Grmping U. Variable importance assessment in regression: linear regression versus random Forest. Am Stat. 2009;63(4):308–19.
50. Hothorn T, Bhlmann P, Dudoit S, Molinaro A, van der Laan MJ. Survival ensembles. Biostatistics (Oxford, England). 2006;7(3):355–73.
51. Strobl C, Hothorn T, Zeileis A. Party on! A new, conditional variable-importance measure for random Foerest available in the party package. R Journal. 2009;1(2):14–7.
52. Taddio A, Katz J, Ilersich AL, Koren G. Effect of neonatal circumcision on pain response during subsequent routine vaccination. Lancet. 1997;349(9052):599–603.
53. Schauer M, Elbert T. Dissociation following traumatic stress: etiology and treatment. J Psychol. 2011;218:109–27.

54. Geansbauer TJ. Representation of trauma in infancy: clinical and theoretical implications for the understanding of early memory. Infant Mental Health Journal. 2002;23(3):259–77.
55. Glover V, O'connor T, O'Donnell K. Prenatal stress and the programming of the HPA axis. Neurosci Biobehav Rev. 2010;35(1):17–22.
56. Maniam J, Antoniadis C, Morris MJ. Early-life stress, HPA axis adaptation, and mechanisms contributing to later health outcomes. Front Endocrinol. 2014;5. https://doi.org/10.3389/fendo.2014.00073.
57. Schauer M, Neuner F, Elbert T. Narrative exposure therapy (NET): a short-term intervention for traumatic stress disorders. 2nd ed. Cambridge/Göttingen: Hogrefe & Huber Publishers; 2011.
58. Elbert T, Schauer M, Neuner F. Narrative exposure therapy (NET): Reorganizing memories of traumatic stress, fear, and violence. In Evidence Based Treatments for Trauma-Related Psychological Disorders. Cham: Springer. 2015. pp. 229–53.
59. Mulongo P, McAndrew S, Hollins Martin C. Crossing borders: discussing the evidence relating to the mental health needs of women exposed to female genital mutilation. Int J Ment Health Nurs. 2014;23(4):296–305.
60. Kizilhan JI. Psychologie der Migration. In: Machleidt W, Heinz A, editors. Praxis der interkulturellen Psychiatrie und Psychotherapie. edn. München: Urban & Fischer; 2011.
61. Simmons JG, Badcock PB, Whittle SL, Byrne ML, Mundy L, Patton GC, Olsson CA, Allen NB. The lifetime experience of traumatic events is associated with hair cortisol concentrations in community-based children. Psychoneuroendocrinology. 2016;63:276–81.
62. Hinkelmann K, Muhtz C, Dettenborn L, Agorastos A, Wingenfeld K, Spitzer C, Gao W, Kirschbaum C, Wiedemann K, Otte C. Association between childhood trauma and low hair cortisol in depressed patients and healthy control subjects. Biol Psychiatry. 2013;74(9):e15–7.
63. Kalmakis KA, Meyer JS, Chiodo L, Leung K. Adverse childhood experiences and chronic hypothalamic–pituitary–adrenal activity. Stress. 2015;18(4):446–50.
64. Feller S, Vigl M, Bergmann MM, Boeing H, Kirschbaum C, Stalder T. Predictors of hair cortisol concentrations in older adults. Psychoneuroendocrinology. 2014;39:132–40.
65. Luo H, Hu X, Liu X, Ma X, Guo W, Qiu C, Wang Y, Wang Q, Zhang X, Zhang W, et al. Hair cortisol level as a biomarker for altered hypothalamic-pituitary-adrenal activity in female adolescents with posttraumatic stress disorder after the 2008\Wenchuan\earthquake. Biol Psychiatry. 2012;72(1):65–9.
66. Dowlati Y, Herrmann N, Swardfager W, Thomson S, Oh PI, Van US, Koren G, Lanctot KL. Relationship between hair cortisol concentrations and depressive symptoms in patients with coronary artery disease. NeuropsychiatrDisTreat. 2010;6(1178–2021 (Electronic):393–400.

12

The effect of positive psychology interventions on well-being and distress in clinical samples with psychiatric or somatic disorders

Farid Chakhssi[1,2*], Jannis T. Kraiss[2], Marion Sommers-Spijkerman[2] and Ernst T. Bohlmeijer[2]

Abstract

Background: Although positive psychology interventions (PPIs) show beneficial effects on mental health in non-clinical populations, the current literature is inconclusive regarding its effectiveness in clinical settings. We aimed to examine the effects of PPIs on well-being (primary outcome), depression, anxiety, and stress (secondary outcomes) in clinical samples with psychiatric or somatic disorders.

Methods: A systematic review and meta-analysis was conducted following PRISMA guidelines. PsycINFO, PubMed, and Scopus were searched for controlled studies of PPIs in clinical samples between Jan 1, 1998 and May 31, 2017. Methodological quality of each study was rated. We used Hedges' adjusted g to calculate effect sizes and pooled results using random-effect models.

Results: Thirty studies were included, representing 1864 patients with clinical disorders. At post-intervention, PPIs showed significant, small effect sizes for well-being (Hedges' $g = 0.24$) and depression ($g = 0.23$) compared to control conditions when omitting outliers. Significant moderate improvements were observed for anxiety ($g = 0.36$). Effect sizes for stress were not significant. Follow-up effects (8–12 weeks), when available, yielded similar effect sizes. Quality of the studies was low to moderate.

Conclusion: These findings indicate that PPIs, wherein the focus is on eliciting positive feelings, cognitions or behaviors, not only have the potential to improve well-being, but can also reduce distress in populations with clinical disorders. Given the growing interest for PPIs in clinical settings, more high quality research is warranted as to determine the effectiveness of PPIs in clinical samples.

Keywords: Well-being, Distress, Positive psychology, Chronic illness, Meta-analysis, Interventions

* Correspondence: f.chakhssi@utwente.nl
[1]Scelta, GGNet, Apeldoorn, The Netherlands
[2]Centre for eHealth and Well-being Research, Department of Psychology, Health, and Technology, University of Twente, PO Box 217, 7500 AE Enschede, The Netherlands

Background

Positive psychology is a relatively new field that focuses on enhancing well-being and optimal functioning rather than ameliorating symptoms, and complements rather than replaces traditional psychology [1]. Common themes in positive psychology include savoring, gratitude, kindness, promoting positive relationships, and pursuing hope and meaning [2].

Now that it has been repeatedly shown that well-being and psychopathology are two moderately correlated yet independent constructs of mental health [3–6], well-being receives growing attention in clinical research and practice. Even after successful treatment of psychopathology, low levels of well-being may persist in individuals, which, in turn, form a substantial risk factor for psychological distress [7]. In the light of a substantial body of evidence demonstrating that high levels of well-being buffer against psychological symptomatology, including relapse or recurrence of symptoms, besides enhancing quality of life and longevity [5, 7–14], we anticipate that clinical samples could greatly benefit from positive psychological interventions (PPIs) which explicitly aim to enhance well-being, that is, positive feelings, cognitions or behaviors [15].

Although PPIs have been mostly examined in non-clinical samples [16], some preliminary evidence exist for their efficacy in clinical samples [16, 17]. Independent lines of research have shown that PPIs improved well-being and decreased psychological distress in mildly depressed individuals [18], in patients with mood and depressive disorders [19, 20], in patients with psychotic disorders [21] and improving quality of life and well-being in breast cancer patients [22]. Thus, PPIs may have the potential to be of value to clinical samples but their effectiveness in these samples is not well established.

To date, two meta-analyses have been published that examined the effectiveness of PPIs in predominantly non-clinical samples. First, Sin and Lyubomirsky [17] included 49 controlled studies with 4235 individuals examining the effectiveness of PPIs on well-being and depression. They found that PPIs were significantly more effective than comparators (i.e. active control or treatment as usual) for enhancing well-being ($r = .29$) and decreasing depression ($r = .31$). Second, to address several methodological issues in Sin and Lyubomirsky's meta-analysis [17] such as lack of methodological quality assessment of the included studies, Bolier and colleagues [16] re-examined the literature. Using more stringent methodological and inclusion criteria, they systematically collected and synthesized the findings of 39 randomized controlled studies with 6139 individuals. Small but significant effects of PPIs on subjective well-being, psychological well-being and depression were found, with Cohen's d effect sizes of 0.34, 0.20 and 0.23, respectively.

However, these previously published meta-analyses are inconclusive regarding the effectiveness of PPIs in improving well-being and alleviating psychological distress in clinical samples. Although both meta-analyses included a number of studies with clinical samples, 12 out of 49 studies [17] and 4 out of 39 studies [16], respectively, these were limited to psychiatric samples with depressive or anxiety symptoms. To our knowledge, no attempt has been made to systematically examine the effects of PPIs in samples with somatic disorders who may benefit from improvements in well-being [23].

Since there is growing interest in the application of PPIs targeting clinical samples, the aim of the study was to add to the existing literature on the effectiveness of PPIs in primarily non-clinical samples [16, 17] through meta-analytically testing the effects of PPIs on well-being and distress across a broad range of clinical samples with psychiatric and somatic disorders.

Methods

This study was prepared and conducted according to the preferred reporting items for systematic reviews and meta-analyses (PRISMA) guidelines [24] and registered on April 29, 2016 in PROSPERO (#CRD42016037451), an international prospective register for systematic reviews.

Search strategy

The electronic databases PsycINFO, PubMed, and Scopus were searched from 1998 (the start of the positive psychology movement) to March 31, 2016, and an update of the search was conducted on May 31, 2017. For each database, text word search terms, medical subject headings (PubMed) or thesaurus terms (PsycINFO) were used relating to 'well-being' and 'positive psychology', in combination with terms related to 'interventions', 'disorders and illness' and 'outcome' (see Additional file 1 for more detailed information on the search terms). Studies cited in the previously published meta-analytic reviews [16, 17, 22] were cross-checked. Additionally, three clinical trial registers (www.clinicaltrialsregister.eu, www.clinicaltrials.gov, www.isrctn.com) were searched on August 31, 2016, to detect trials with unpublished results available.

Selection of studies

Potentially eligible studies were screened on title in the first phase, on abstract in the second phase, and on full paper in the third phase. Studies were included in the meta-analysis if they: 1) examined the effects of an intervention developed in line with the theoretical tradition of positive psychology cfm. Sin and Lyubomirsky (2009), that is, a psychological intervention (i.e. training, exercise, therapy) aimed at raising positive feelings, cognitions or behaviors; 2) included adult participants (18 years or older) with clinical psychiatric or somatic disorders [according to the International Classification of Diseases and Related Health Problems; [25]; 3) used an outcome measure of social, emotional or psychological well-being; 4) used a control condition; and 5) provided an effect size or sufficient information to calculate an effect size. Studies were excluded if they: 1) were not published in an English language peer-reviewed journal; 2) examined physical exercises aimed at improving well-being; or 3) used an intervention that is primarily based on reminiscence, mindfulness and/or meditation. With regard to the third exclusion criterion, extensive meta-analyses have already been published for these types of interventions [26–30]. Published abstracts and/or study protocols were also excluded.

The first (FC) and second author (JTK) independently conducted the screening of titles. The interrater reliability was high (kappa = 0.84; $n = 1000$). Disagreements between raters during the screening of abstracts and full texts were discussed until consensus was reached. Any remaining ambiguity was resolved with the third (MSS) and fourth author (ETB).

Data extraction

Data were collected on: 1) population characteristics, including age, gender, disorder, and sample size (per condition); 2) intervention characteristics, including type of PPI, delivery mode, number of sessions, duration in weeks, retention rate, and guidance (i.e. with or without therapist); 3) methodological characteristics, including study design, type of control group, assessment points (i.e. pre, post and/or follow up), and outcome measures. Eight authors were contacted because information regarding study characteristics or to calculate effect sizes was lacking, of whom six provided additional data on request.

Quality assessment

All studies were rated on methodological quality using criteria based on the Cochrane Collaboration's tool for assessing risk of bias [31] and the Jadad scale [32]. This rating consists of seven items that are rated as 0 ("absent") or 1 ("present"), resulting in a maximum quality score of 7 points. Studies were identified as "good" when all seven criteria were met, "fair" when five or six criteria were met, and "poor" when four or less criteria were met [33]. The included items cover: 1) random sequence generation and allocation concealment (i.e. sufficient description of the method used to generate and conceal the allocation sequence); 2) blinding of outcome assessments (i.e. outcome assessments are either administered online or by an independent person who is not involved in the study), 3) reporting incomplete outcome data (i.e. dropout analysis is conducted or reasons for drop-out are reported), 4) using intention-to-treat analysis, 5) group similarity at baseline regarding prognostic factors (e.g. demographics) or adjustments were made to correct for baseline imbalance, 6) adequate sample size/power analysis (i.e. an adequate power analysis was conducted or the study included 50 or more persons in the analysis), and 7) reliability of the diagnostic assessment (i.e. assessment was conducted by a professional and not based on self-report or screening or there were no diagnostic assessments). The first (FC) and second author (JTK) independently conducted the quality assessment, whereby disagreements were discussed until consensus was reached.

Primary and secondary outcomes

The primary outcome was the mean well-being score at the end of the intervention, assessed with validated measures of social, emotional, and/or psychological well-being. In the absence of well-being measures, measures, constructs related to well-being such as hope, happiness, life satisfaction, personal growth, optimism or positive affect were included if available. If more than one measure for well-being was used, we used the most validated measure, to ensure each study had one primary outcome for the analysis. Secondary outcomes included depression, anxiety and stress.

Statistical analysis

For each study, means and standard deviations were extracted, where possible based on the intention-to-treat method; otherwise, the reported means and standard deviations for the patients that completed the interventions were used. Effect sizes were calculated in three steps. First, standardized pre-post effect sizes were calculated per condition (i.e. PPI or control condition) by subtracting the average pre-intervention score from the average post-intervention score and subsequently dividing this score by the pooled standard deviation. Second, the difference in effect size (Δd) between PPI condition and control condition was computed. Third, Δd was adjusted for small sample bias, indicated as Hedges' g. Where possible, pre-to-follow-up effect sizes were calculated in a similar manner, thereby only using studies with a follow-up period between 8 and 12 weeks.

Using Comprehensive Meta-Analysis version 2.2.064, separate meta-analyses were performed for 1) well-being, 2) depression, 3) anxiety, and 4) stress in which data were pooled using the random-effects model accounting for diversity across studies (e.g. in terms of populations, types of PPIs and outcome measures). Effect sizes of 0.56 to 1.2 can be considered large, effect sizes of 0.33 to 0.55 moderate, and effect sizes of 0 to 0.32 small [34].

Heterogeneity of effect sizes was examined using Q and I^2 statistics. The Q-test assesses whether the observed effect sizes are significantly more different from one another than would be expected based on chance alone. A significant Q-statistic indicates heterogeneity. The I^2 statistic captures the percentage of the total variance across the included studies attributable to heterogeneity. A value of zero indicates true homogeneity, while values of 25, 50, and 75% indicate low, moderate, and high levels of heterogeneity, respectively [35].

Publication bias was assessed using funnel plots, Egger's Test, Duval and Tweedie's trim-and-fill procedure, and fail-safe N. First, a funnel plot was created by plotting the overall mean effect size against study size. Whereas a symmetric distribution of studies around the effect size indicates the absence of publication bias, a higher concentration of studies on one side of the effect size than on the other indicates publication bias [36]. Second, Egger's test [37] was used to examine the symmetric distribution of studies around the effect size with a quantitative test statistic (considered significant funnel plot asymmetry if $p < 0.05$). Third, Duval and Tweedie's [38] trim-and-fill procedure was applied. This procedure imputes the effect sizes of missing studies and produces an adjusted effect size accounting for these missing studies. Adjusted values were only reported for pooled effect sizes when these were statistically significant. Finally, a fail-safe N, a test of funnel plot asymmetry, was calculated for each analysis. The fail-safe N indicates the number of unpublished non-significant studies that would be required to lower the overall effect size below significance [37]. The findings were considered robust if the fail-safe $N \geq 5n + 10$, where n is the number of comparisons [39].

Pre-specified exploratory subgroup analyses were performed to examine differences in effect sizes based on: 1) population type: psychiatric vs somatic disorders; 2) intervention type: individual vs. group format, with vs. without therapist guidance; and 3) duration of the intervention: short (≤ 8 weeks) vs long (> 8 weeks). Mixed effects analysis was used to tests for differences between subgroups. Additional ad hoc analyses were performed to explore differences in effect sizes based on: 1) type of PPI: PPI therapy programs (e.g. meaning-centered group approach, well-being therapy) vs single PPIs (e.g. three good things/signature strengths); and 2) control group: no intervention (i.e. did not receive any intervention at all)/waitlist (i.e. did receive the intervention after the experimental group) vs. active/treatment-as-usual. Finally, meta-regression analysis was performed to investigate if effect sizes were moderated by study quality.

Results

Selection of studies

A total of 10,886 studies were produced in the electronic database searches. After the exclusion of duplicates (n = 1578) and the removal of studies at the title screening phase (n = 9069), 239 abstracts were reviewed (Fig. 1). Of the 101 articles identified for full text review, 30 controlled studies were included. The 30 studies comprised 33 comparisons for well-being, 26 comparisons for depression, 14 comparisons for anxiety and 6 comparisons for stress [40–69]. Fourteen studies were conducted in the United States, three each in Iran, Canada, and Spain, two each in the United Kingdom and Italy, and one each in Australia, Germany, and Taiwan. The characteristics of the included studies are presented in Table 1.

Population characteristics

The included studies comprised 1864 adult participants, 960 in the PPI conditions and 904 in the control conditions. The mean age of the participants at pre-intervention was 47.8 years (SD = 11.5, range 26.4–68.9), and more than half were women (61.5%). In 16 studies, clinical samples with somatic disorders were included, with cancer being the most prevalent disorder (8 out of 16 studies). Other somatic disorders included cardiac diseases (n = 4), HIV (n = 1), brain injuries (n = 1), diabetes (n = 1) and chronic pain (n = 1). The remaining 14 studies included samples with psychiatric disorders, with depressive disorder as the most prevalent disorder (7 out of 13 studies), followed by anxiety disorders (n = 2), severe emotion dysregulation (n = 1), psychotic disorders (n = 1), post-traumatic stress syndrome (n = 1), and various mental health problems (n = 2).

Intervention, comparison and outcome characteristics

In 20 studies, PPIs were compared to treatment as usual or an active control condition, such as supportive psychotherapy [44], cognitive behavioral therapy [47], dialectical behavior therapy [69] or mood monitoring [57]. Ten studies compared PPIs to a no intervention/waitlist condition. The names of the PPIs as provided by the authors of the studies are also displayed in Table 1. All interventions were explicitly aimed at raising positive feelings, cognitions or behaviors. The 24 studies used empirically validated PPIs (see [2, 18]) or programs that have incorporated PPIs such as positive psychotherapy [67] or well-being therapy [51]. In 24 studies, therapist guidance was part of the PPI. The intervention duration varied

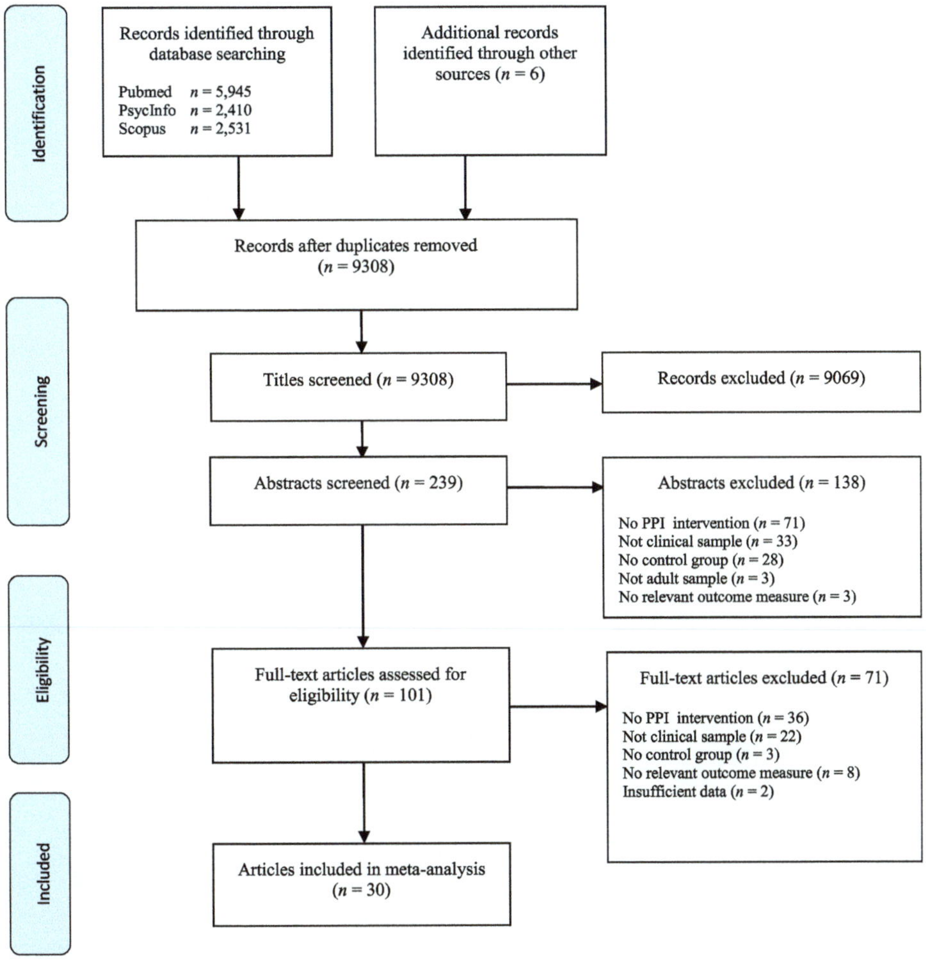

Fig. 1 Flowchart of the study selection process

from 3 days to 16 weeks. The mean retention rate, based on dropouts at post-intervention, was 81.4% (available for 26 studies). For the PPI conditions, the mean retention rate was 81.0% and for the control conditions 81.8%. For the 12 studies that included follow-up measurements, the average follow-up time was 12.9 weeks after post-intervention.

Quality of studies

The quality scores of the studies are displayed in Table 2. If a criterion was not reported in the paper, it was labeled "unclear", and the criterion was rated as not met. All studies were either of medium quality ($n = 12$) or of low quality ($n = 18$). None of the included studies met all quality criteria. The use of intention-to-treat analyses was the most poorly rated, with only 11 studies meeting this criterion.

Meta-analyses

Table 3 summarizes findings from the meta-analyses per outcome, i.e. well-being, depression, anxiety, and stress. The meta-analyses were run separately for all studies at post-intervention with the outliers included, with the outliers excluded and with the low quality omitted. The meta-analyses at follow-up were run including outliers and low quality studies. The effect sizes of the individual studies at post-intervention are plotted in Figs. 2, 3, 4 and 5.

Post-intervention effects on well-being

For well-being (33 comparisons), a significant, small effect was observed ($g = 0.28$, 95% CI: 0.07 to 0.48, $p = 0.008$) at post-intervention. The level of heterogeneity was high ($I^2 = 78.20$). Four outliers were detected [41, 46, 52, 61]. After omitting these studies from the analysis, we found a similar effect, with $g = 0.24$ (95% CI: 0.13 to 0.35, $p < 0.001$), and heterogeneity reduced substantially ($I^2 = 20.29$). When studies scored as low quality were excluded from the analysis (including outliers), again a small significant effect size was observed ($g = 0.19$, 95% CI: 0.02 to 0.37, $p = 0.030$), with a moderate level of heterogeneity ($I^2 = 40.88$).

Table 1 Characteristics of studies included in the systematic review and meta-analysis

First author (Year)	Disorder	% female	Mean age (SD)	PPI name (*n*)	Format (guidance)	Duration in days or weeks (n sessions)	Control group (*n*)	Retention rate post-treatment		Follow-up (in weeks)	Outcome measure			
								PPI	Control		WB	DEP	ANX	S
Andrewes (2014) [40]	Brain injury	10%	42.2 (8.5)	Three good things in life / Signature strengths (4)	Individual (Yes)	2w (1–2)	CBT (5)	80%	100%	10	AHI			
Asgharipoor (2012) [41]	Major Depressive Disorder	72%	26.4 (5.9)	Positive psychotherapy (9)	Group (Yes)	12w (12)	CBT (5)	100%	100%	–	EWBS	BDI-II		SUDS
Breitbart (2010) [43]	Advanced cancer	51%	60.1 (11.8)	Meaning-centered group psychotherapy (49)	Group (Yes)	8w (8)	Supportive Psychotherapy (41)	71.4%	48.8%	8	FACIT-SP	HADS-D	HADS-A	
Breitbart (2012) [42]	Advanced cancer	61%	54.4 (11.6)	Meaning-centered group psychotherapy (64)	Individual (Yes)	7w (7)	Massage (56)	64.1%	66.1%	8	FACIT-SP	HADS-D	HADS-A	
Breitbart (2015) [44]	Advanced cancer	70%	58.2 (11.0)	Meaning-centered group psychotherapy (132)	Group (Yes)	8w (8)	Supportive Psychotherapy (121)	52.3%	47.9%	8	FACIT-SP	BDI-II	HADS-A	
Celano (2016) [55]	Major Depressive Disorder	69%	44 (16.6)	Positive Psychology Intervention (32)	Individual (Yes)	6w (6)	Cognition Focused Intervention (33)	90.6%	87.8%	6	PA	QIDS-SR		
Cerezo (2014) [46]	Breast cancer	100%	50 (9.7)	Positive Psychology Intervention (87)	Group (Yes)	14w (14)	Waitlist (88)	86.1%	83%	–	SWLS			
Chaves (2017) [47]	Depression/ Dysthymia	100%	51.7 (10.4)	Positive Psychology Intervention (47)	Group (Yes)	10w (10)	CBT (49)	72.4%	79.6%	–	SWLS	BDI-II	BAI	
Cohn (2014) [48]	Type 2 diabetes	51%	54 (U)	DAHLIA: Developing Affective HeaLth to Improve Adherence (29)	Individual (No)	5w (0)	Emotion reporting (20)	86.2%	85%	–	PA	CES-D		PSS
Coote (2012) [49]	Depression	71%	52.5 (13.4)	Goal-setting and Planning (26)	Individual (No)	5w (0)	Waitlist (29)	92.3%	62.1%	5	PA	CES-D		
Elham (2015) [50]	Cardiovascular diseases	41%	68.9 (8.3)	Need-based spiritual/ religious interventions (33)	Individual (Yes)	3 days (3)	No treatment (33)	100%	100%	–	SWBS		STAI	
Fava (1998) [51]	Affective disorders	55%	28.4 (6.6)	Well-being therapy (10)	Group (Yes)	16w (8)	CBT (10)	100%	100%	–	PWB	CID-D	SQ-A	
Fava (2005) [52]	Generalized anxiety disorder	65%	41.9 (11.9)	Well-being therapy (10)	Group (Yes)	16w (8)	CBT (10)	80%	80%	52	PWB	CID-D	CID-A	
Henry (2010) [53]	Stage III or IV ovarian cancer	100%	55 (9.7)	The Meaning-Making intervention (12)	Individual (Yes)	8w (3)	TAU (12)	80%	92.3%	12	FACIT-SP	HADS-D	HADS-A	
Hsiao (2012) [54]	Breast cancer	100%				8w (8)		69.2%	95.4%	32	MLQ	BDI-II		

Table 1 Characteristics of studies included in the systematic review and meta-analysis *(Continued)*

First author (Year)	Disorder	% female	Mean age (SD)	PPI name (*n*)	Format (guidance)	Duration in days or weeks (n sessions)	Control group (*n*)	Retention rate post-treatment		Follow-up (in weeks)	Outcome measure			
								PPI	Control		WB	DEP	ANX	S
			46.2 (8.6)	Body-mind-spirit (BMS) group therapy (26)	Group (Yes)		One psycho-educational session (22)							
Huffman (2016) [55]	Coronary syndrome	40%	62.8 (11.5)	Positive Psychology Interventions (23)	Individual (Yes)	8w (8)	TAU (25)	87%	88%	–	PA	HADS-D	HADS-A	
Kent (2011) [56]	Posttraumatic Stress Disorder	33%	54 (8.34)	Resilience-Oriented Treatment (20)	Group (Yes)	12w (12)	Waitlist (19)	95%	89.5%	–	PWB	BDI-II	STAI	PDS
Kerr (2015) (Group 1 gratitude)	Various mental problems	75%	43 (11.1)	Gratitude Interventions (16)	Individual (No)	2w (14)	Mood monitoring (15)	?	?	–	MLQ	DASS-D	DASS-A	DASS-S
Kerr (2015) (Group 2 Kindness)	Various mental problems	75%	43 (11.1)	Kindness Interventions (16)	Individual (No)	2w (14)	Mood monitoring (15)	?	?	–	MLQ	DASS-D	DASS-A	DASS-S
Krentzman (2015) [58]	Alcohol use disorder	48%	46.3 (10.9)	Web-based gratitude exercise (11)	Individual (No)	2w (14)	Placebo (11)	?	?	8	PA			
Lee (2006) [59]	Breast or colorectal cancer	81%	56.7 (10)	Meaning-making intervention (35)	Individual (Yes)	4.5w (4)	No treatment (39)	85.4%	95.1%	–	LOT-R			
Lcuro (2016) [60]	Colorectal cancer	34%	(U)	Enhancing Positive Emotions Procedure (31)	Group (Yes)	6w (4)	No treatment (21)	77.4%	95.2%	4	PA			
Mann (2001) [61]	HIV patients	100%	38.5 (8.2)	Future Writing and Optimism (21)	Individual (No)	4w (8)	No treatment (23)	95.2%	87%	–	LOT-R			
Muller (2016) [62]	Physical disability and chronic pain	70%	59.4 (11.8)	Computer-based positive psychology intervention (51)	Individual (No)	8w (0)	Writing exercises (45)	76.5%	74.5%	10	PWI	HADS-D		
Nikrahan (2016) [63] (group 1)	Heart diseases	24%	56.6 (8.7)	Fordyce's positive CBT (15)	Group (Yes)	6w (6)	Waitlist (14)	66.7%	85.7%	–	SWLS	BDI-II		
Nikrahan (2016) [63] (group 2)	Heart diseases	24%	56.6 (8.7)	Lyubomirsky's the how of happiness (13)	Group (Yes)	6w (6)	Waitlist (14)	92.3%	85.7%	–	SWLS	BDI-II		
Nikrahan (2016) [63] (group 3)	Heart diseases	24%	56.6 (8.7)	Seligman's authentic Happiness (13)	Group (Yes)	6w (6)	Waitlist (14)	76.9%	85.7%	–	SWLS	BDI-II		
Pietrowsky (2012) [64]	Depression	53%	38.9 (8.6)	Positive Psychology Interventions (9)	Group (Yes)	4w (3)	TAU (8)	77.8%	75%	–	SWLS	BDI-II		
Sanjuan (2016) [65]	Cardiac diseases	18%	54.4 (9.1)	Program to improve Well-being (57)	Group (Yes)	6w (24)	Relaxation (51)	87.7%	84.3%	–	PA	SCL90-D		
Schrank (2016) [66]	Psychosis	40%	42.5 (11.3)	Positive psychotherapy (47)	Group (Yes)	11w (11)	TAU (47)	91.5%	87.2%	–	WEMWBS	SDHS		

Table 1 Characteristics of studies included in the systematic review and meta-analysis *(Continued)*

First author (Year)	Disorder	% female	Mean age (SD)	PPI name (*n*)	Format (guidance)	Duration in days or weeks (n sessions)	Control group (*n*)	Retention rate post-treatment		Follow-up (in weeks)	Outcome measure			
								PPI	Control		WB	DEP	ANX	S
Seligman (2006) [67] (study 2)	Depression	76%	(U)	Positive psychotherapy (11)	Individual (Yes)	12w (14)	TAU (9)	84.6%	60%	–	SWLS	ZSRS		
Taylor (2017) [68]	Depression / Anxiety	62.5%	29.4 (12.1)	Positive Activity Intervention (16)	Individual (Yes)	10w (10)	Waitlist (12)	100%	92.3%	–	SWLS	BDI-II	STAI	
Uliaszek (2016) [69]	Severe emotion dysregulation	78%	22.2 (5.0)	Positive Psychotherapy	Group (Yes)	12w (12)	DBT	55.6%	85.2%	–	PPTI	SCL-90-D	SCL-R-A	DTS

Note. AHI Authentic Happiness Index, *ANX* Anxiety, *BAI* Beck Anxiety Inventory, *BDI-II* Beck Depression Inventory-II, *CES-D* Center for Epidemiologic Studies Depression Scale, *CID-A* Clinical Interview for Depression - Anxiety subscale, *CID-D* Clinical Interview for Depression - Depression subscale, *EWBS* Emotional Well-Being Scale, *DBT* Dialectical Behaviour Therapy, *DEP* Depression, *DTS* Distress Tolerance Scale, *FACIT-SP* Functional Assessment of Chronic Illness Therapy - Spiritual Well-being Scale, *HADS* Hospital Anxiety and Depression Scale, *HADS-A* Hospital Anxiety and Depression Scale – Anxiety Scale, *HADS-D* Hospital Anxiety and Depression Scale - Depression Scale, *HS* The Hope Scale, *LOT-R* Life Orientation Test – Revised, *MLQ* The Meaning in Life Questionnaire, *PA* The Positive and Negative Affect Scale - Positive Affect Scale, *PDS* Posttraumatic Stress Diagnostic Scale, *PPI* Positive Psychological Intervention, *PPTI* Positive Psychotherapy Inventory, *PSS* Perceived Stress Scale, *PWB* The Ryff Scales of Psychological Well-Being, *PWBS* Psychological Well-Being Scale, *PWI* Personal Well-being Index, *QIDS-SR* Quick Inventory of Depressive Symptomatology, Self-Report, *S* Stress, *SCL-90-A* Symptom Checklist 90 – Anxiety subscale, *SCL-90-D* Symptom Checklist 90 - Depression subscale, *STAI* Spielberger State – Trait Anxiety Inventory, *SQ-A* Symptom Questionnaire - Anxiety subscale, *SUDS* Subjective Units of Distress Scale, *SWB* Subjective Well-Being, *SWBS* Spiritual Well-Being Scale, *SWLS* Satisfaction with Life Scale, *TAU* Treatment-as-Usual, *U* Unknown, *WB* Well-being, *WEMMWB* Warwick-Edinburgh Mental Well-Being Scale

Table 2 Methodological quality of studies included in the meta-analysis

First author (year)	1. Adequate allocation sequence generation and allocation concealment	2. Blinding of main outcome assessments	3. Description of withdrawals/ drop-outs	4. Intention-to-treat analysis is performed or there are no drop-outs	5. The sample size is based on an adequate power analysis.	6. The groups are similar on prognostic indicators at baseline (and this was explicitly assessed) or adjustments were made to correct for baseline imbalance (using appropriate covariates).	7. Diagnostic assessment was conducted by a professional, or there were no diagnostic assessments necessary for the recruitment	Score
Andrewes (2014) [40]	Yes	No	Yes	No	No	Yes	Yes	4
Asgharipoor (2012) [41]	Unclear	No	Unclear	Unclear	No	Yes	Yes	2
Breitbart (2010) [43]	Unclear	Unclear	Yes	No	Yes	Yes	Yes	4
Breitbart (2012) [42]	Yes	Unclear	Yes	No	Yes	Yes	Yes	5
Breitbart (2015) [44]	Unclear	Unclear	Yes	No	Yes	Yes	Yes	4
Celano (2016) [55]	Yes	Yes	No	Yes	Yes	Yes	Yes	6
Cerezo (2014) [46]	Yes	Unclear	No	No	Yes	Yes	Yes	4
Chaves (2017) [47]	Unclear	Yes	Yes	Yes	Yes	Yes	Yes	6
Cohn (2014) [48]	Yes	Yes	No	No	Yes	Yes	Unclear	4
Coote (2012) [49]	Unclear	Yes	No	No	Yes	Yes	No	3
Elham (2015) [50]	No	No	Yes	Yes	Yes	Yes	Yes	5
Fava (1998) [51]	Unclear	Yes	Yes	Yes	No	Unclear	Yes	4
Fava (2005) [52]	Unclear	Yes	No	No	No	Unclear	Yes	2
Henry (2010) [53]	Yes	Yes	Yes	No	No	Yes	Yes	5
Hsiao (2012) [54]	Yes	Unclear	Yes	No	No	Yes	Yes	4
Huffman (2016) [55]	No	No	Yes	No	No	Yes	Yes	3
Kent (2011) [56]	Unclear	Unclear	Yes	Yes	No	Yes	Yes	4
Kerr (2015)	Unclear	Unclear	Yes	Yes	No	Yes	Yes	4
Krentzman(2015) [58]	Unclear	Yes	No	No	No	Yes	Yes	3
Lee (2006) [59]	Yes	Yes	Yes	No	Yes	Yes	Yes	6
Louro (2016) [60]	No	No	Yes	No	No	Yes	Yes	3
Mann (2001) [61]	Unclear	No	No	No	No	Yes	Yes	2
Muller (2016) [62]	Yes	Yes	Yes	No	Yes	Yes	Yes	6
Nikrahan (2016) [63]	Unclear	Unclear	Yes	Yes	Yes	Yes	Yes	5
Pietrowsky (2012) [64]	Unclear	No	No	Yes	No	Yes	Yes	3
Sanjuan 2016 [65]	Yes	Unclear	Yes	No	Yes	Yes	Yes	5
Schrank (2016) [66]	Yes	No	Yes	Yes	Yes	Yes	Yes	6
Seligman (2006) [67] (study 2)	Unclear	Yes	Yes	No	No	Yes	Yes	4
Taylor (2017) [68]	Yes	Unclear	Yes	Yes	No	Yes	Yes	5
Uliaszek (2016) [69]	Yes	No	No	Yes	Yes	Yes	Yes	5

Table 3 Between-group effects

Outcome measures	N_{comp}	Hedges' *g*	95% CI	*Z*	Heterogeneity Q-value	I^2	Fail-safe *N*
All studies post-intervention (including outliers)							
Well-being	33	0.28	0.07–0.48	2.66**	146.81***	78.20	271
Depression	26	0.27	0.09–0.45	2.97**	66.40***	62.34	132
Anxiety	14	0.47	0.23–0.71	3.78***	36.83***	64.71	135
Stress	6	0.00	-0.62–0.62	0.00	25.35***	80.28	0
All studies post-intervention (excluding outliers)[a]							
Well-being	29	0.24	0.13–0.35	4.16***	35.13	20.29	137
Depression	21	0.23	0.11–0.34	3.74***	22.26	10.16	66
Anxiety	13	0.36	0.20–0.53	4.24***	16.96	29.26	81
Stress	5	0.27	−0.19–0.73	1.16	11.02	63.69	0
Medium or high quality studies post-intervention							
Well-being	14	0.19	0.02–0.37	2.17*	21.99	40.88	17
Depression	12	0.07	-0.19–0.32	0.53	32.43	66.08	0
Anxiety	6	0.22	−0.05–0.49	1.57	8.39	40.39	1
Stress	1	−0.32	− 0.85–0.21	−1.19	0.00	0.00	–
Studies with 8–12 week follow up (including outliers)							
Well-being	7	0.41	0.08–0.74	2.46*	19.24**	68.82	28
Depression	5	0.21	0.05–0.37	2.53*	2.55	0.00	4
Anxiety	4	0.35	0.12–0.59	2.91**	4.45	32.54	10
Stress	–	–	–	–	–	–	–

Note. N_{comp}, number of comparisons, *CI* confidence interval. **p* < 0.05. ** *p* < 0.01. *** *p* < 0.001. [a] The effect size for well-being ($g = 0.24$) corresponds with a standardized mean difference Cohen's $d = 0.24$ and unweighted mean $r = 0.12$; the effect size for depression ($g = 0.23$) corresponds with $d = 0.23$ and $r = 0.11$; the effect size for anxiety (g = 0.36) corresponds with $d = 0.37$ and $r = 0.18$; the effect size for stress ($g = 0.27$) corresponds with $d = 0.28$ and $r = 0.14$

Post-intervention effects on depression

Based on 26 comparisons, we found a significant, small effect of PPIs on depression, with $g = 0.27$ (95% CI: 0.09 to 0.45, $p = 0.003$) at post-intervention. The level of heterogeneity was moderate ($I^2 = 62.34$). Five outliers were detected [45, 51, 56, 68, 69]. After removal of the outliers, a small effect size was observed ($g = 0.23$, 95% CI: 0.11 to 0.34, $p < 0.001$). The level of heterogeneity was low ($I^2 = 10.16$). After removal of low quality studies, the effect size for depression was not significant with $g = 0.07$ (95% CI: -0.19 to 0.32, $p = 0.598$), and heterogeneity was moderate ($I^2 = 66.08$).

Post-intervention effects on anxiety

For anxiety (14 comparisons), a significant, moderate effect was found ($g = 0.47$, 95% CI: 0.23 to 0.71, $p <$ 0.001) at post-intervention. Heterogeneity was moderate ($I^2 = 62.34$), and one outlier was detected [52]. After removal of the outlier, the effect size dropped to $g = 0.36$ (95% CI: 0.20 to 0.53, $p < 0.001$), but still remained in the moderate range, and the level of heterogeneity was low ($I^2 = 10.16$). After removal of low quality studies from the analysis, the effect size for anxiety was small and not significant ($g = 0.22$, 95% CI: -0.05 to 0.49, $p = 0.233$), with moderate heterogeneity ($I^2 = 40.39$).

Post-intervention effects on stress

The overall mean effect size for 5 comparisons on stress was not significant ($g = 0.00$; 95% CI: -0.62 to 0.62, $p = 0.999$) at post-intervention. After the removal of one outlier [41], the effect size increased to the small range ($g = 0.27$; 95% CI: -0.19 to 0.73, $I^2 = 43.89$) but remained non-significant ($p = .247$). Only 1 study that included stress as an outcome had a medium quality rating (see Table 1).

Effects at follow-up

At follow-up, a significant, moderate effect was observed for well-being ($g = 0.41$, 95% CI: 0.08 to 0.74, $p = 0.014$), a significant, small effect for depression ($g = 0.21$, 95% CI: 0.05 to 0.37, $p = 0.011$), and a significant, moderate effect for anxiety ($g = 0.35$, 95% CI: 0.12 to 0.59, $p = 0.004$). There were no follow-up assessments conducted between 8 to 12 weeks with stress as outcome.

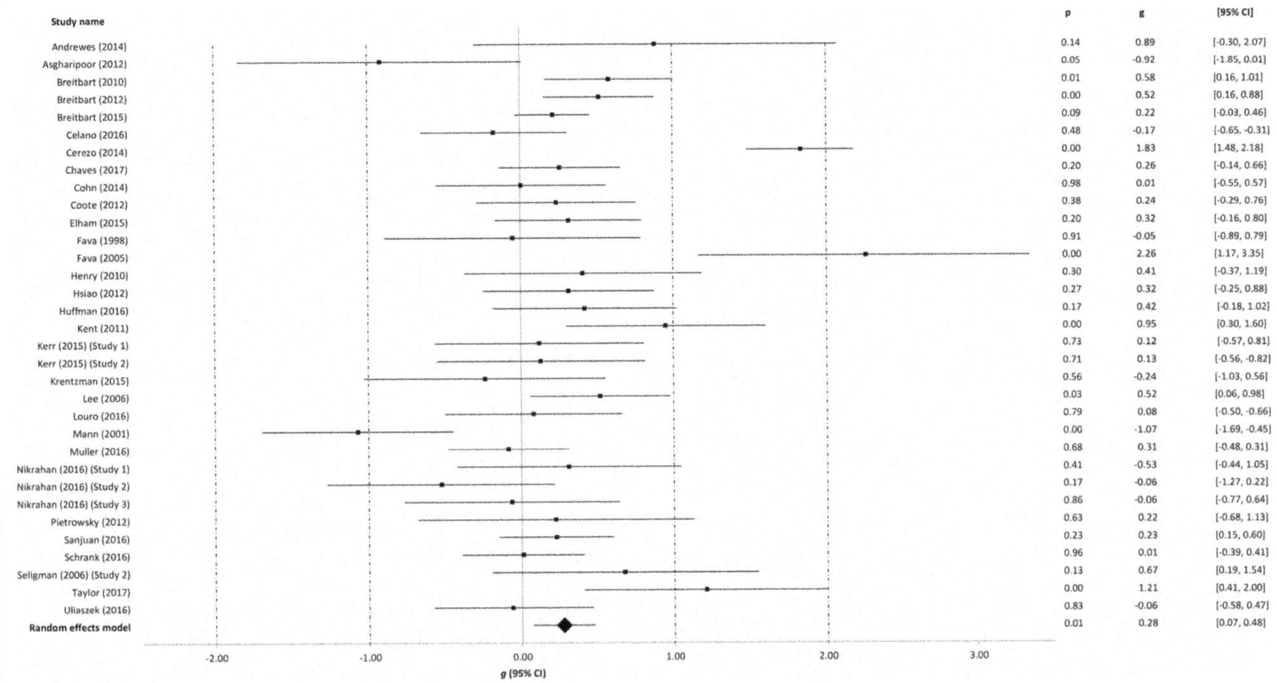

Fig. 2 Post-intervention effects of positive psychology interventions on well-being. The square boxes show Hedges' g effect size in each study, and the line the 95% confidence interval. The diamond reflects the pooled effect size and the line the width of the 95% confidence interval

Subgroup analyses

Exploratory subgroup analyses are presented in Table 4. For well-being ($Q = 6.412$, $df = 1$, $p = 0.011$) a significantly higher effect size was found for PPIs with therapist guidance ($g = 0.39$) than for PPIs without therapist guidance ($g = -0.12$). For stress, PPIs were found significantly more effective in studies using a no intervention/waitlist control condition ($g = 1.12$ vs $g = -0.21$; $Q = 8.283$, $df = 1$, $p = 0.004$) than in studies using an active or treatment-as-usual control condition. Effect sizes did not significantly vary based on population type (i.e. psychiatric vs somatic disorders), intervention format (i.e. individual vs group), intervention duration (i.e. shorter vs longer than 8 weeks) and/or type of PPI (i.e. PPI therapy programs vs single PPIs). For depression and anxiety, no significant differences between subgroups were found.

Meta-regression analysis

Using meta-regression analysis, we found no evidence that effect sizes for well-being and stress were moderated by study quality. The study quality had a significant negative influence on the effect size for depression and anxiety, with lower study quality scores resulting in lower effect sizes for depression (slope: -0.17, $Z = -3.23$, $p = 0.001$) and anxiety (slope: -0.28, $Z = -3.25$, $p = 0.001$).

Publication bias

First, inspection of the funnel plots showed that only for stress the funnel plot was skewed in favor of studies with a positive outcome at post-intervention. Second, Egger's test statistic showed no significant funnel plot asymmetry for all analyses (all p-values > .05). Third, after adjusting for potential publication bias with Duval and Tweedie's trim-and-fill procedure, the effect sizes for well-being and stress remained the same. However, for depression, four studies were trimmed and the adjusted effect size was $g = 0.15$ (95% CI: 0.05 to 0.25). Also for anxiety, four studies were trimmed and the adjusted effect size was $g = 0.27$ (95% CI: 0.14 to 0.39). Finally, the fail-safe N indicated that the findings for well-being and anxiety were robust, whereas the fail-safe numbers for depression (132) and stress (0) were lower than required (140 and 35, respectively). After omitting outliers, the findings for anxiety remained robust. The fail-safe N for well-being (137), depression (66) and stress (0) were lower than required (respectively 155, 115 and 35). At follow-up, the fail-safe N for well-being (28), depression (4) and anxiety (10) were lower than required (respectively 45, 35, and 30).

Discussion

To our knowledge, this is the first meta-analysis examining the effects of PPIs on well-being and distress in clinical samples with psychiatric and somatic disorders. When

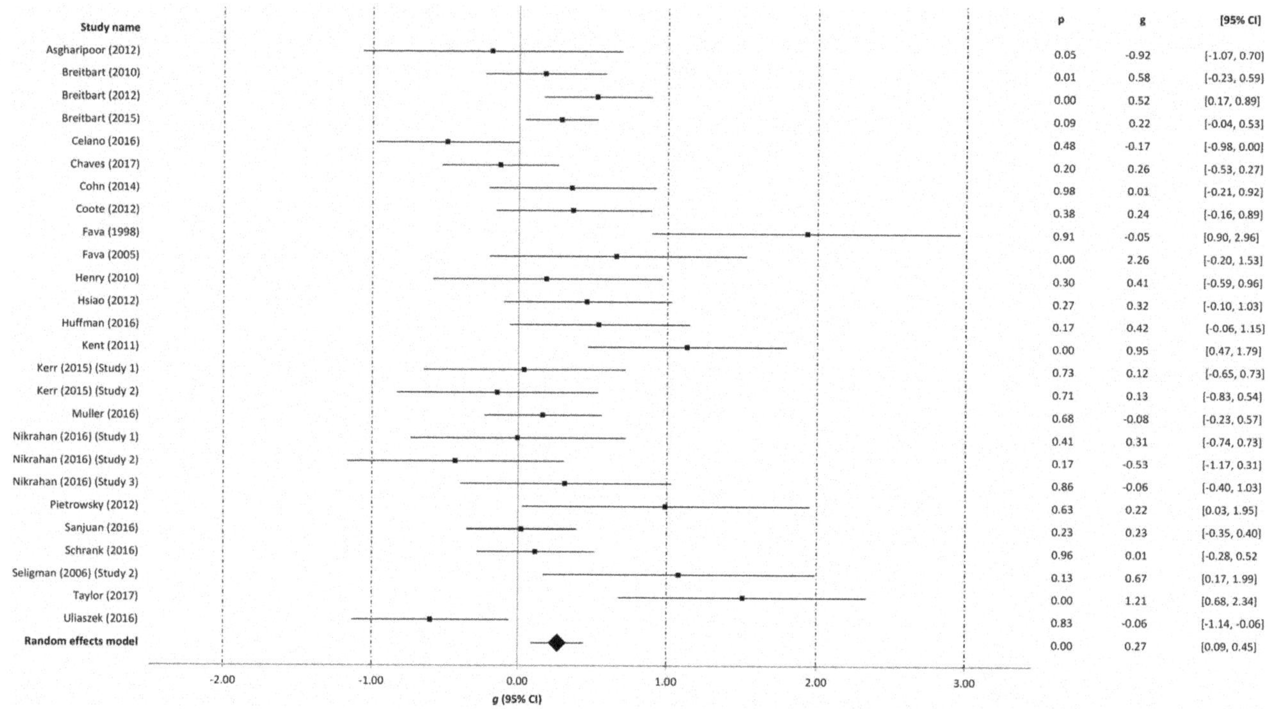

Fig. 3 Post-intervention effects of positive psychology interventions on depression. The square boxes show Hedges' g effect size in each study, and the line the 95% confidence interval. The diamond reflects the pooled effect size and the line the width of the 95% confidence interval

excluding outliers, our analyses suggest that PPIs have a small but significant effect on well-being compared to control conditions. At follow-up, a significant moderate effect size of PPIs on well-being was observed. For the secondary outcomes, a small but significant effect size was found for depression at post-intervention and follow-up and moderate significant effect sizes for anxiety at post-intervention and follow-up. Effect sizes for stress were not significant. These findings suggest that PPIs not only have the potential to improve well-being, but can also reduce distress in populations with clinical disorders.

The effect sizes at post-intervention and follow-up for well-being and distress were comparable with those found in Bolier et al's meta-analysis of controlled PPIs studies in predominantly non-clinical samples [16], but were lower than those in the earlier meta-analysis of Sin and Lyubomirsky [17]. However, in the meta-analysis conducted by Sin and Lyubomirsky [17] less stringent inclusion criteria were used and other interventions such as mindfulness and life-review were included that are commonly not regarded as PPIs [2, 16]. Nonetheless, our findings show promise for PPIs in samples with psychiatric and somatic disorders, and suggest that PPIs, wherein the focus is on eliciting positive feelings, cognitions or behaviors, may also be relevant for clinical populations.

In the field of psychology, especially clinical psychology, the focus lies primarily on examining distress-reducing treatment approaches. As PPIs explicitly aim to improve well-being, the findings of the current study are important because well-being is often impaired in individuals with clinical disorders [23] and low levels of well-being form a substantial risk for relapse or recurrence of symptoms [5, 7]. More importantly, recent studies suggest that well-being and psychological distress are two separate constructs, and that the treatment of symptoms does not necessarily result in improved well-being (e.g., [6, 14]). In the light of these findings, we encourage researchers to further establish the effectiveness of well-being enhancing approaches including PPIs.

Explorative subgroup analyses suggest that guided PPIs are more effective in improving well-being compared to unguided PPIs, such as self-help. Similar findings were found in earlier meta-analytic reviews [16, 17] regarding PPIs in predominantly nonclinical samples, where larger effect sizes were found in therapist-guided interventions (compared with unguided self-help), when the interventions were offered to people with mental health problems. This is also in line with findings regarding supported versus unsupported conventional psychological treatments, such as cognitive behavioral therapy (e.g., [70, 71]) where significant larger effect sizes are observed for supported psychological treatments. Therapist guidance may potentially improve outcomes of PPIs on well-being in samples with psychiatric and/or somatic disorders. However, based on the explorative nature of the subgroup analyses, these

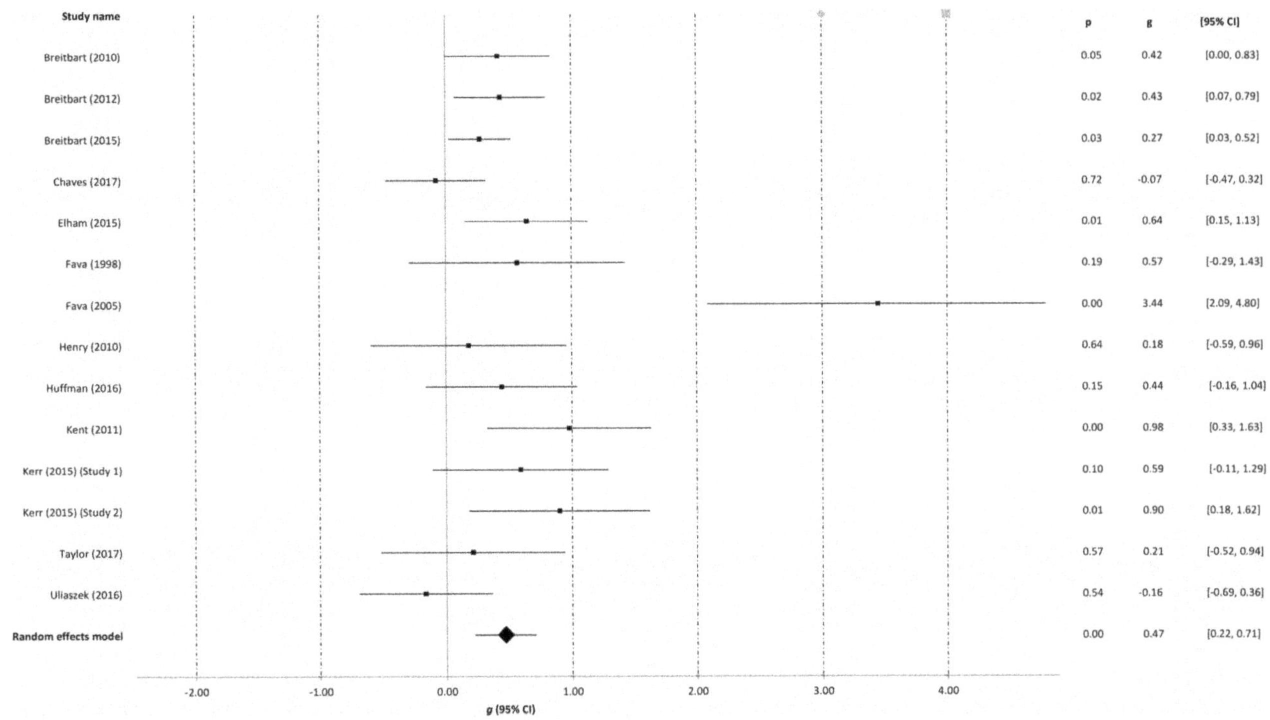

Fig. 4 Post-intervention effects of positive psychology interventions on anxiety. The square boxes show Hedges' g effect size in each study, and the line the 95% confidence interval. The diamond reflects the pooled effect size and the width of the 95% confidence interval

findings should be treated with caution and future research should examine the effect of therapist guidance compared to self-help in controlled studies.

No other significant pre-specified moderators of outcome were observed. There was no significant effect of disorder type (i.e. psychiatric vs somatic disorders) and intervention format (i.e. individual vs group). Although, the moderating effect of intervention duration was not significant, the results showed that PPIs with a shorter duration than 8 weeks did not have a significant effect on well-being whereas PPIs with a longer duration had a significant effect on well-being. This finding is in line with earlier meta-analytic reviews [4, 5] and suggests that PPIs are more effective when offered during a longer period of time (more than 8 weeks). In the additional moderator analyses, no significant differences in effect sizes were found for empirically validated PPIs vs other PPIs. For stress, a significantly higher effect size was found for PPIs that had no intervention/waitlist as control condition than for PPIs that had an active control condition or treatment-as-usual as control condition. However, the sample sizes were relatively small in the exploratory subgroup analyses, which limits the interpretation of the differences between groups, and the results should therefore be considered with caution.

The current systematic review and meta-analysis highlights the need to improve the research methodology and reporting within the field of PPIs. The quality of the included studies was low to medium. Although the quality of the studies may have been underestimated since we rated a criterion as not met if it was not reported in the paper, it seems that the methodological quality of studies in this field could be considerably improved if authors routinely report on sequence generation, allocation concealment and blinding of assessors. Furthermore, only one third of the included studies reported using the intention-to-treat principle to analyze the results and almost half of the included studies did not report using a power analysis to determine the sample size. Inadequate statistical power and not adhering to the intention-to-treat principle introduces bias into the results of individual studies, and distorts the results from meta-analyses [72]. This was reflected in the meta-regression analysis which indicated that the effects of PPIs on depression and anxiety were moderated by the methodological quality of the studies, with a lower study quality resulting in smaller effect sizes. Therefore, we recommend researchers conducting studies on PPIs in clinical samples to comply with the quality criteria when designing studies, in order to perform more high quality research to accurately determine the effectiveness of PPIs in clinical samples with psychiatric and somatic

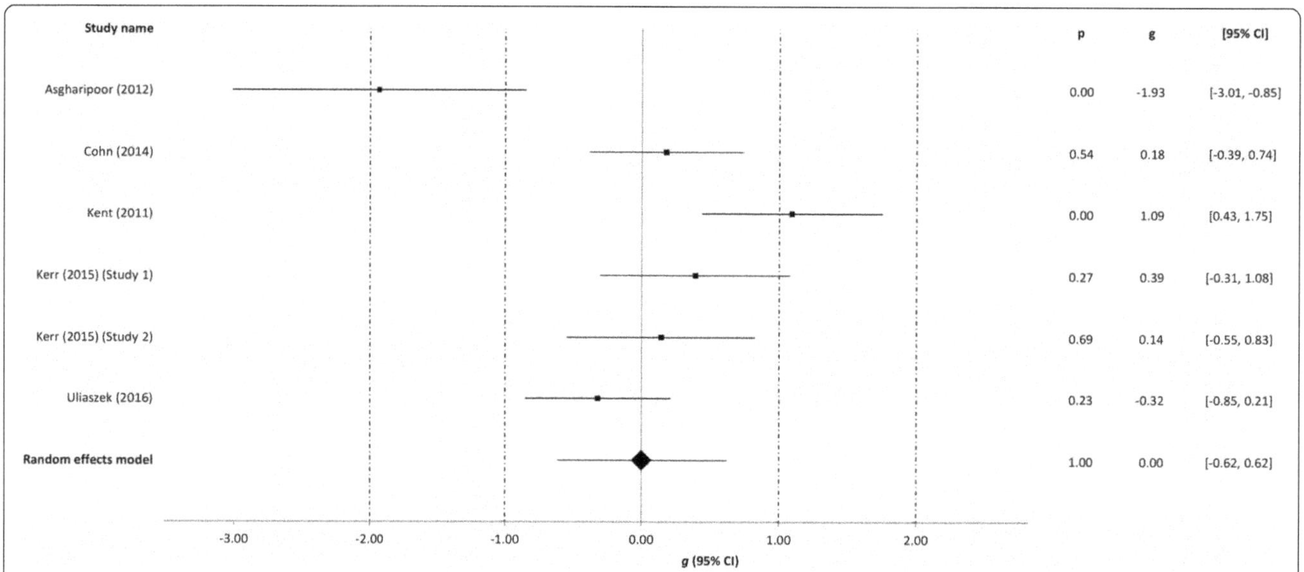

Fig. 5 Post-intervention effects of positive psychology interventions on stress. The square boxes show Hedges' g effect size in each study, and the line the 95% confidence interval. The diamond reflects the pooled effect size and the width of the 95% confidence interval

disorders. Moreover, the number of studies including post-treatment follow-up measures is relatively low (12 out of 30). We encourage researchers in the field to include follow-up measurements as to determine whether possible favorable effects of PPIs can be sustained in the long run.

Our systematic review and meta-analysis focused on controlled studies of PPIs in clinical samples. We identified a number of studies in different clinical disorders, age groups and settings. Drawing upon these findings in one place has generated the first evidence-based overview of the effectiveness of PPIs in clinical populations. However, several limitations should be noted. One important limitation is that well-being was not always the primary outcome in the included studies. Also, different definitions of well-being were used across the included studies. Incorporating validated measures of well-being, preferably ones that encompass emotional, psychological, and social dimensions of well-being [73], in future studies of PPIs is recommended. Second, the effects of the PPIs may also have been overestimated due to publication bias. Although the results of this meta-analysis point at significant but small effects of PPIs, after adjustment for publication bias, caution is needed. Third, our conclusions are based on the overall effect after the exclusion of outliers, including studies of low quality. When considering only studies of at least medium quality, the effects of PPIs are substantially lower but the sample size of the studies also decreases substantially. Since this is the first study meta-analyzing the effects of PPIs in clinical samples, we based our conclusions on the analyses (i.e. after excluding outliers) with the largest sample size to present a more comprehensive representation of the field. Fourth, we observed a broad range of PPIs in our meta-analysis that varied in delivery mode and intensity. Future research should examine which clinical populations may benefit from PPIs, in terms of type, delivery mode and intensity, and whether there are differential mediators of outcome. Still, this is one of the first meta-analyses in this field providing an overview of PPIs in clinical samples.

Conclusions

In conclusion, this systematic review and meta-analysis provides evidence that PPIs are effective in improving well-being as well as in alleviating common psychological symptoms, including depression and anxiety, in clinical samples with psychiatric and somatic disorders. At present, the most promising PPIs seem to be those that are guided. Given the growing interest for PPIs in clinical settings [15, 16], it is timely and important to further establish the potential of PPIs in the context of clinical populations using large-scale and methodologically sound trials.

Abbreviations

AHI: Authentic happiness index; ANX: Anxiety; BAI: Beck anxiety inventory; BDI-II: Beck depression inventory-II; CES-D: Center for epidemiologic studies depression scale; CI: Confidence interval; CID-A: Clinical interview for depression - anxiety subscale; CID-D: Clinical interview for depression -

Table 4 Subgroup analyses (including outliers)

Outcome measure	Criterion	Subgroup	N_{comp}	Hedges' *g*	95% CI	I^2	*Z*
Well-being	Duration	<= 8 weeks	22	0.15	0.00–0.30	42.23	1.95
		> 8 weeks	11	0.59	0.06–1.11	88.74	2.19*
	Format	Group	17	0.33	0.01–0.66	84.87	2.01*
		Individual	16	0.20	−0.03–0.43	58.89	1.74
	Guidance	Therapist	26	0.39	0.16–0.62	78.63	3.30***
		Without therapist	7	−0.12	−0.43–0.20	49.96	−0.73
	Disorder	Psychiatric	15	0.26	−0.02–0.53	62.56	1.83
		Somatic	18	0.28	−0.01–0.57	83.99	1.91
Depression	Duration	<= 8 weeks	16	0.18	0.03–0.33	27.56	2.38*
		> 8 weeks	10	0.54	0.08–0.99	80.02	2.31*
	Format	Group	15	0.23	−0.01–0.47	64.37	1.91
		Individual	11	0.33	0.04–0.61	61.60	2.26*
	Guidance	Therapist	21	0.31	0.09–0.52	68.95	2.74**
		Without therapist	5	0.19	−0.05–0.43	0.00	1.55
	Disorder	Psychiatric	14	0.37	0.01–0.73	76.94	2.03*
		Somatic	12	0.26	0.13–0.39	0.00	3.86***
Anxiety	Duration	<= 8 weeks	7	0.41	0.25–0.57	0.00	5.02***
		> 8 weeks	7	0.59	0.03–1.16	81.11	2.05*
	Format	Group	7	0.52	0.08–0.96	81.15	2.31**
		Individual	7	0.49	0.28–0.70	0.00	4.53***
	Guidance	Therapist	12	0.43	0.17–0.70	67.87	3.21**
		Without therapist	2	0.74	0.24–1.24	0.00	2.89**
	Disorder	Psychiatric	8	0.65	0.12–1.18	79.75	2.41**
		Somatic	6	0.38	0.21–0.54	0.00	4.56***
Stress	Duration	<= 8 weeks	3	0.23	−0.14–0.59	0.00	1.20
		> 8 weeks	3	−0.33	−1.77–1.11	91.69	−0.45
	Format	Group	3	−0.33	−1.77–1.11	91.69	−0.45
		Individual	3	0.23	−0.14–0.59	0.00	1.20
	Guidance	Therapist	3	−0.33	−1.77–1.11	91.69	−0.45
		Without therapist	3	0.23	−0.14–0.59	0.00	1.20
	Disorder	Psychiatric	5	−0.06	−0.84–0.73	84.16	−0.14
		Somatic	1	0.18	−0.39–0.74	0.00	0.61

Note. N_{comp}, number of comparisons; *CI* confidence interval. *$p < 0.05$. ** $p < 0.01$. *** $p < 0.001$

depression subscale; DBT: Dialectical behaviour therapy; DEP: Depression; DTS: Distress tolerance scale; EWBS: Emotional well-being scale; FACIT-SP: Functional assessment of chronic illness therapy - spiritual well-being scale; HADS: Hospital anxiety and depression scale; HADS-A: Hospital anxiety and depression scale – anxiety scale; HADS-D: Hospital anxiety and depression scale - depression scale; HS: The hope scale; LOT-R: Life orientation test – revised; MLQ: The meaning in life questionnaire; N_{comp}: Number of comparisons; PA: The positive and negative affect scale - positive affect scale; PDS: Posttraumatic stress diagnostic scale; PPI: Positive psychological intervention; PPTI: Positive psychotherapy inventory; PRISMA: Preferred reporting items for systematic reviews and meta-analyses; PSS: Perceived stress scale; PWB: The Ryff scales of psychological well-being; PWBS: Psychological Well-Being Scale; PWI: Personal well-being index; QIDS-SR: Quick inventory of depressive symptomatology, self-report; S: Stress; SCL-90-A: Symptom checklist 90 – anxiety subscale; SCL-90-D: Symptom checklist 90 - depression subscale; SQ-A: Symptom questionnaire - anxiety subscale; STAI: Spielberger state – trait anxiety inventory; SUDS: Subjective units of distress scale; SWB: Subjective well-being; SWBS: Spiritual well-being scale; SWLS: Satisfaction with Life Scale; TAU: Treatment-as-usual; U: Unknown; WB: Well-being; WEMMWB: Warwick-Edinburgh mental well-being scale

Acknowledgements

We thank Peter Noort for his support by providing his expertise for developing the search strategy.

Authors' contributions

FC, JTK, MSS and ETB designed the study. JTK conducted the literature searches. Selection of studies and data extraction: FC and JTK. Disagreements were resolved by discussion or arbitration by MSS and ETB. Statistical analysis: FC, MSS and ETB. FC drafted the manuscript. FC, JTK, MSS and ETB critically revised the manuscript and approved the final version.

Competing interests

The authors declare that they have no competing interests.

References

1. Duckworth AL, Steen TA, Seligman ME. Positive psychology in clinical practice. Annu Rev Clin Psychol. 2005;1:629–51.
2. Schueller SM, Parks AC. The science of self-help. Eur Psychol. 2014;19(2):145–55.
3. Huppert FA, Whittington JE. Evidence for the independence of positive and negative well-being: implications for quality of life assessment. Br J Health Psychol. 2003;8(Pt 1):107–22.
4. Keyes CL. Mental illness and/or mental health? Investigating axioms of the complete state model of health. J Consult Clin Psychol. 2005;73(3):539–48.
5. Lamers S, Westerhof GJ, Glas CA, Bohlmeijer ET. The bidirectional relation between positive mental health and psychopathology in a longitudinal representative panel study. J Posit Psychol. 2015;10(6):553–60.
6. Westerhof GJ, Keyes CL. Mental illness and mental health: the two continua model across the lifespan. J Adult Dev. 2010;17(2):110–9.
7. Wood AM, Joseph S. The absence of positive psychological (eudemonic) well-being as a risk factor for depression: a ten year cohort study. J Affect Disord. 2010;122(3):213–7.
8. Chida Y, Steptoe A. Positive psychological well-being and mortality: a quantitative review of prospective observational studies. Psychosom Med. 2008;70(7):741–56.
9. Diener E, Ryan K. Subjective well-being: a general overview. South African Journal of Psychology. 2009;39(4):391–406.
10. Howell RT, Kern ML, Lyubomirsky S. Health benefits: meta-analytically determining the impact of well-being on objective health outcomes. Health Psychol Rev. 2007;1(1):83–136.
11. Keyes CL, Dhingra SS, Simoes EJ. Change in level of positive mental health as a predictor of future risk of mental illness. Am J Public Health. 2010; 100(12):2366–71.
12. Lamers SM, Bolier L, Westerhof GJ, Smit F, Bohlmeijer ET. The impact of emotional well-being on long-term recovery and survival in physical illness: a meta-analysis. J Behav Med. 2012;35(5):538–47.
13. Ryff CD. Psychological well-being revisited: advances in the science and practice of eudaimonia. Psychother Psychosom. 2014;83(1):10–28.
14. Trompetter H, Lamers S, Westerhof G, Fledderus M, Bohlmeijer E. Both positive mental health and psychopathology should be monitored in psychotherapy: confirmation for the dual-factor model in acceptance and commitment therapy. Behav Res Ther. 2017;91:58–63.
15. Wood AM, Tarrier N. Positive clinical psychology: a new vision and strategy for integrated research and practice. Clin Psychol Rev. 2010;30(7):819–29.
16. Bolier L, Haverman M, Westerhof GJ, Riper H, Smit F, Bohlmeijer E. Positive psychology interventions: a meta-analysis of randomized controlled studies. BMC Public Health. 2013;13(1):119.
17. Sin NL, Lyubomirsky S. Enhancing well-being and alleviating depressive symptoms with positive psychology interventions: a practice-friendly meta-analysis. J Clin Psychol. 2009;65(5):467–87.
18. Seligman ME, Steen TA, Park N, Peterson C. Positive psychology progress: empirical validation of interventions. Am Psychol. 2005;60(5):410–21.
19. Fava GA, Ruini C. Development and characteristics of a well-being enhancing psychotherapeutic strategy: well-being therapy. J Behav Ther Exp Psychiatry. 2003;34(1):45–63.
20. Rashid T. Positive psychotherapy: a strength-based approach. J Posit Psychol. 2015;10(1):25–40.
21. Meyer PS, Johnson DP, Parks A, Iwanski C, Penn DL. Positive living: a pilot study of group positive psychotherapy for people with schizophrenia. J Posit Psychol. 2012;7(3):239–48.
22. Casellas-Grau A, Font A, Vives J. Positive psychology interventions in breast cancer. A systematic review. Psychooncology. 2014;23(1):9–19.
23. de Ridder D, Geenen R, Kuijer R, van Middendorp H. Psychological adjustment to chronic disease. Lancet. 2008;372(9634):246–55.
24. Moher D, Liberati A, Tetzlaff J, Altman DG. Preferred reporting items for systematic reviews and meta-analyses: the PRISMA statement. Ann Intern Med. 2009;151(4):264–9.
25. World Health Organization. International statistical classification of diseases and health related problems, 10th revision. Geneva: WHO; 1992.
26. Bohlmeijer E, Prenger R, Taal E, Cuijpers P. The effects of mindfulness-based stress reduction therapy on mental health of adults with a chronic medical disease: a meta-analysis. J Psychosom Res. 2010;68(6):539–44.
27. Bohlmeijer E, Roemer M, Cuijpers P, Smit F. The effects of reminiscence on psychological well-being in older adults: a meta-analysis. Aging Ment Health. 2007;11(3):291–300.
28. Gotink RA, Chu P, Busschbach JJ, Benson H, Fricchione GL, Hunink MG. Standardised mindfulness-based interventions in healthcare: an overview of systematic reviews and meta-analyses of RCTs. PLoS One. 2015;10(4):e0124344.
29. Khoury B, Lecomte T, Fortin G, Masse M, Therien P, Bouchard V, Chapleau MA, Paquin K, Hofmann SG. Mindfulness-based therapy: a comprehensive meta-analysis. Clin Psychol Rev. 2013;33(6):763–71.
30. Strauss C, Cavanagh K, Oliver A, Pettman D. Mindfulness-based interventions for people diagnosed with a current episode of an anxiety or depressive disorder: a meta-analysis of randomised controlled trials. PLoS One. 2014;9(4):e96110.
31. Higgins JP, Altman DG, Gøtzsche PC, Jüni P, Moher D, Oxman AD, Savović J, Schulz KF, Weeks L, Sterne JA. The Cochrane Collaboration's tool for assessing risk of bias in randomised trials. BMJ. 2011;343:d5928.
32. Jadad AR, Moore RA, Carroll D, Jenkinson C, Reynolds DJM, Gavaghan DJ, McQuay HJ. Assessing the quality of reports of randomized clinical trials: is blinding necessary? Control Clin Trials. 1996;17(1):1–12.
33. Spijkerman MPJ, Pots WTM, Bohlmeijer ET. Effectiveness of online mindfulness-based interventions in improving mental health: a review and meta-analysis of randomised controlled trials. Clin Psychol Rev. 2016;45:102–14.
34. Lipsey MW, Wilson DB. The efficacy of psychological, educational, and behavioral treatment. Confirmation from meta-analysis. Am Psychol. 1993; 48(12):1181–209.
35. Higgins JP, Thompson SG. Quantifying heterogeneity in a meta-analysis. Stat Med. 2002;21(11):1539–58.
36. Sterne JA, Egger M, Moher D. Addressing reporting biases. Cochrane handbook for systematic reviews of interventions; 2008. p. 297–333.
37. Egger M, Smith GD, Schneider M, Minder C. Bias in meta-analysis detected by a simple, graphical test. BMJ. 1997;315(7109):629–34.
38. Duval S, Tweedie R. Trim and fill: a simple funnel-plot–based method of testing and adjusting for publication bias in meta-analysis. Biometrics. 2000;56(2):455–63.
39. Rosenberg MS. The file-drawer problem revisited: a general weighted method for calculating fail-safe numbers in meta-analysis. Evolution. 2005;59(2):464–8.
40. Andrewes HE, Walker V, O'Neill B. Exploring the use of positive psychology interventions in brain injury survivors with challenging behaviour. Brain Inj. 2014;28(7):965–71.
41. Asgharipoor N, Asgharnejad FA, Arshadi H, Sahebi A. A comparative study on the effectiveness of positive psychotherapy and group cognitive-behavioral therapy for the patients suffering from major depressive disorder. Iran J Psychiatry Behav Sci. 2012;6(2):33–41.
42. Breitbart W, Poppito S, Rosenfeld B, Vickers AJ, Li Y, Abbey J, Olden M, Pessin H, Lichtenthal W, Sjoberg D, et al. Pilot randomized controlled trial of individual meaning-centered psychotherapy for patients with advanced cancer. J Clin Oncol. 2012;30(12):1304–9.
43. Breitbart W, Rosenfeld B, Gibson C, Pessin H, Poppito S, Nelson C, Tomarken A, Timm AK, Berg A, Jacobson C, et al. Meaning-centered group psychotherapy for patients with advanced cancer: a pilot randomized controlled trial. Psychooncology. 2010;19(1):21–8.
44. Breitbart W, Rosenfeld B, Pessin H, Applebaum A, Kulikowski J, Lichtenthal WG. Meaning-centered group psychotherapy: an effective intervention for improving psychological well-being in patients with advanced cancer. J Clin Oncol. 2015;33(7):749–54.
45. Celano C, Beale E, Mastromauro C, Stewart J, Millstein R, Auerbach R, Bedoya C, Huffman J. Psychological interventions to reduce suicidality in high-risk patients with major depression: a randomized controlled trial. Psychol Med. 2017;47(5):810–21.
46. Cerezo MV, Ortiz-Tallo M, Cardenal V, De La Torre-Luque A. Positive psychology group intervention for breast cancer patients: a randomised trial. Psychol Rep. 2014;115(1):44–64.
47. Chaves C, Lopez-Gomez I, Hervas G, Vazquez C. A comparative study on the efficacy of a positive psychology intervention and a cognitive behavioral therapy for clinical depression. Cognit Ther Res. 2017;41(3):417–33.
48. Cohn MA, Pietrucha ME, Saslow LR, Hult JR, Moskowitz JT. An online positive affect skills intervention reduces depression in adults with type 2 diabetes. J Posit Psychol. 2014;9(6):523–34.
49. Coote HM, MacLeod AK. A self-help, positive goal-focused intervention to increase well-being in people with depression. Clin Psychol Psychother. 2012;19(4):305–15.

50. Elham H, Hazrati M, Momennasab M, Sareh K. The effect of need-based spiritual/religious intervention on spiritual well-being and anxiety of elderly people. Holist Nurs Pract. 2015;29(3):136–43.
51. Fava GA, Rafanelli C, Cazzaro M, Conti S, Grandi S. Well-being therapy. A novel psychotherapeutic approach for residual symptoms of affective disorders. Psychol Med. 1998;28(2):475–80.
52. Fava GA, Ruini C, Rafanelli C, Finos L, Salmaso L, Mangelli L, Sirigatti S. Well-being therapy of generalized anxiety disorder. Psychother Psychosom. 2005;74(1):26–30.
53. Henry M, Cohen SR, Lee V, Sauthier P, Provencher D, Drouin P, Gauthier P, Gotlieb W, Lau S, Drummond N, et al. The meaning-making intervention (MMi) appears to increase meaning in life in advanced ovarian cancer: a randomized controlled pilot study. Psychooncology. 2010;19(12):1340–7.
54. Hsiao FH, Jow GM, Kuo WH, Chang KJ, Liu YF, Ho RT, Ng SM, Chan CL, Lai YM, Chen YT. The effects of psychotherapy on psychological well-being and diurnal cortisol patterns in breast cancer survivors. Psychother Psychosom. 2012;81(3):173–82.
55. Huffman JC, Millstein RA, Mastromauro CA, Moore SV, Celano CM, Bedoya CA, Suarez L, Boehm JK, Januzzi JL. A positive psychology intervention for patients with an acute coronary syndrome: treatment development and proof-of-concept trial. J Happiness Stud. 2016;17(5):1985–2006.
56. Kent M, Davis MC, Stark SL, Stewart LA. A resilience-oriented treatment for posttraumatic stress disorder: results of a preliminary randomized clinical trial. J Trauma Stress. 2011;24(5):591–5.
57. Kerr SL, O'Donovan A, Pepping CA. Can gratitude and kindness interventions enhance well-being in a clinical sample? J Happiness Stud. 2015;16(1):17–36.
58. Krentzman AR, Mannella KA, Hassett AL, Barnett NP, Cranford JA, Brower KJ, Higgins MM, Meyer PS. Feasibility, acceptability, and impact of a web-based gratitude exercise among individuals in outpatient treatment for alcohol use disorder. J Posit Psychol. 2015;10(6):477–88.
59. Lee V, Robin Cohen S, Edgar L, Laizner AM, Gagnon AJ. Meaning-making intervention during breast or colorectal cancer treatment improves self-esteem, optimism, and self-efficacy. Soc Sci Med. 2006;62(12):3133–45.
60. Louro AC, Fernández-Castro J, Blasco T. Effects of a positive emotion-based adjuvant psychological therapy in colorectal cancer patients: a pilot study. Psicooncología. 2016;13(1):113.
61. Mann T. Effects of future writing and optimism on health behaviors in HIV-infected women. Ann Behav Med. 2001;23(1):26–33.
62. Muller R, Gertz KJ, Molton IR, Terrill AL, Bombardier CH, Ehde DM, Jensen MP. Effects of a tailored positive psychology intervention on well-being and pain in individuals with chronic pain and a physical disability: a feasibility trial. Clin J Pain. 2016;32(1):32–44.
63. Nikrahan GR, Suarez L, Asgari K, Beach SR, Celano CM, Kalantari M, Abedi MR, Etesampour A, Abbas R, Huffman JC. Positive psychology interventions for patients with heart disease: a preliminary randomized trial. Psychosomatics. 2016;57(4):348–58.
64. Pietrowsky R, Mikutta J. Effects of positive psychology interventions in depressive patients—a randomized control study. Psychology. 2012;03(12):1067–73.
65. Sanjuan P, Montalbetti T, Perez-Garcia AM, Bermudez J, Arranz H, Castro A. A randomised trial of a positive intervention to promote well-being in cardiac patients. Appl Psychol Health Well Being. 2016;8(1):64–84.
66. Schrank B, Brownell T, Jakaite Z, Larkin C, Pesola F, Riches S, Tylee A, Slade M. Evaluation of a positive psychotherapy group intervention for people with psychosis: pilot randomised controlled trial. Epidemiol Psychiatr Sci. 2016;25(3):235–46.
67. Seligman ME, Rashid T, Parks AC. Positive psychotherapy. Am Psychol. 2006; 61(8):774–88.
68. Taylor CT, Lyubomirsky S, Stein MB. Upregulating the positive affect system in anxiety and depression: outcomes of a positive activity intervention. Depress Anxiety. 2017;34(3):267–80.
69. Uliaszek AA, Rashid T, Williams GE, Gulamani T. Group therapy for university students: a randomized control trial of dialectical behavior therapy and positive psychotherapy. Behav Res Ther. 2016;77:78–85.
70. Andersson G, Cuijpers P. Internet-based and other computerized psychological treatments for adult depression: a meta-analysis. Cogn Behav Ther. 2009;38(4):196–205.
71. Richards D, Richardson T. Computer-based psychological treatments for depression: a systematic review and meta-analysis. Clin Psychol Rev. 2012;32(4):329–42.
72. Juni P, Altman DG, Egger M. Systematic reviews in health care: assessing the quality of controlled clinical trials. BMJ. 2001;323(7303):42–6.

13

Factors associated with health service utilisation for common mental disorders

Tessa Roberts[1,2*], Georgina Miguel Esponda[1], Dzmitry Krupchanka[3,4], Rahul Shidhaye[5,6], Vikram Patel[7] and Sujit Rathod[1]

Abstract

Background: There is a large treatment gap for common mental disorders (CMD), with wide variation by world region. This review identifies factors associated with formal health service utilisation for CMD in the general adult population, and compares evidence from high-income countries (HIC) with that from low-and-middle-income countries (LMIC).

Methods: We searched MEDLINE, PsycINFO, EMBASE and Scopus in May 2016. Eligibility criteria were: published in English, in peer-reviewed journals; using population-based samples; employing standardised CMD measures; measuring use of formal health services for mental health reasons by people with CMD; testing the association between this outcome and any other factor(s). Risk of bias was assessed using the adapted Mixed Methods Appraisal Tool. We synthesised the results using "best fit framework synthesis", with reference to the Andersen socio-behavioural model.

Results: Fifty two studies met inclusion criteria. 46 (88%) were from HIC.
Predisposing factors: There was evidence linking increased likelihood of service use with female gender; Caucasian ethnicity; higher education levels; and being unmarried; although this was not consistent across all studies.
Need factors: There was consistent evidence of an association between service utilisation and self-evaluated health status; duration of symptoms; disability; comorbidity; and panic symptoms. Associations with symptom severity were frequently but less consistently reported.
Enabling factors: The evidence did not support an association with income or rural residence. Inconsistent evidence was found for associations between unemployment or having health insurance and use of services.
There was a lack of research from LMIC and on contextual level factors.

Conclusion: In HIC, failure to seek treatment for CMD is associated with less disabling symptoms and lack of perceived need for healthcare, consistent with suggestions that "treatment gap" statistics over-estimate unmet need for care as perceived by the target population. Economic factors and urban/rural residence appear to have little effect on treatment-seeking rates. Strategies to address potential healthcare inequities for men, ethnic minorities, the young and the elderly in HIC require further evaluation. The generalisability of these findings beyond HIC is limited. Future research should examine factors associated with health service utilisation for CMD in LMIC, and the effect of health systems and neighbourhood factors.

Keywords: Common mental disorders, Depression, Anxiety, Treatment seeking, Health service utilisation, Andersen behavioural model, Systematic review, Healthcare access, Barriers to care

* Correspondence: tessa.roberts@lshtm.ac.uk; tessa.roberts@kcl.ac.uk
[1]Centre for Global Mental Health, Department of Population Health, Faculty of Epidemiology and Population Health, London School of Hygiene and Tropical Medicine, Keppel Street, London WC1E 7HT, UK
[2]Health Service and Population Research Department, Institute of Psychiatry, Psychology and Neuroscience, King's College London, London, UK
Full list of author information is available at the end of the article

Background

Common mental disorders (CMD) comprise depressive disorders and anxiety disorders, according to the World Health Organisation's definition [1], and are a leading cause of disability worldwide [2, 3]. Depressive disorders include major depressive disorder and dysthymia, while anxiety disorders include generalised anxiety disorder (GAD), panic disorder, phobias, social anxiety disorder, obsessive-compulsive disorder (OCD) and post-traumatic stress disorder (PTSD). More than 300 million people were estimated to suffer from depression in 2015 (4.4% of the global population), with almost as many affected by anxiety disorders, although there is substantial comorbidity between the two [1].

Despite evidence of effective treatments for CMD [4], there is a large "treatment gap" for CMD globally, with only 42–44% of those affected worldwide seeking treatment for these symptoms from any medical or professional service provider, including specialists and non-specialists, in the public or private sectors [5]. This proportion has been shown to be much lower in low- and middle-income countries, with estimates of as little as 5% seeking treatment, even when traditional providers are also included [6–8].

Within the Global Mental Health literature, these statistics have been used to call for the scaling up of mental health services in order to reduce the treatment gap [9–14], on the assumption that meeting clinical criteria for CMD indicates – or acts as a proxy for – a need for treatment.

Access to health services has been conceptualised as the "fit between the patient and the health care system" [15]. Donabedian (1973) defines access as "a group of factors that intervene between capacity to provide services and actual provision or consumption of services" [16]. Identifying those factors that are associated with seeking treatment for CMD can help us to better understand the reasons for the treatment gap, and inform service planning to expand access to care.

The Andersen behavioural model of health service utilisation [17] provides a useful framework to inform analyses of factors that influence health service utilisation. The Andersen model is a sociological model of health service utilisation that has been extensively applied [18, 19]. This model proposes that the use of health services is affected by:

(a) one's *predisposition* to seek help from health services when needed (a product of socio-demographic characteristics, attitudes and beliefs);
(b) one's *need* for care (both objective measures and subjective perceptions of one's health needs); and
(c) the structural or *enabling* factors that facilitate or impede service utilisation (such as financial situation, health insurance and social support).

In later iterations of the model it was recognised that these predisposing, enabling and need factors can operate at both the individual level and the contextual level [20, 21].

A substantial body of evidence exists on the factors that influence health service utilization for health conditions such as HIV treatment and maternal health care [22–24], and more recently, depression [25]. However, the latter review included treatment-seeking by adolescents and by specific sub-groups of the population, and as such its results may not be generablisable to the general adult population. Furthermore, since depressive and anxiety disorders are closely related and frequently co-occur [26, 27], with many individuals experiencing mixed anxiety-depression disorders [28], we believe that it is more appropriate when studying non-clinical populations to consider the larger construct of CMD rather than separating these disorders, as has been argued elsewhere [29–31]. To date, there has been no comprehensive review of the factors associated with health service utilisation for symptoms of CMDs in the general adult population.

The aim of this review is to investigate factors associated with the use of health services for CMD symptoms, in observational, population-based studies.

Specific objectives are:

(1) To identify factors associated with health service utilisation for CMD among adults in the general population, and to assess the quality and consistency of evidence supporting an association between each factor and health service utilisation for CMD.
(2) To evaluate the evidence for these associations from high-income countries (HIC) compared to that from low- or middle-income countries (LMIC).

Methods

The protocol for this study was registered with PROSPERO (registration number 42016046551) [32].

Results are presented according to PRISMA (Preferred Reporting Items for Systematic Reviews and Meta-Analyses) guidelines (see Additional file 1).

Information sources and search strategy

We searched four databases; MEDLINE, PsycINFO, EMBASE and Scopus. We combined two key concepts (CMD and health service utilisation) using keywords and subject headings in the respective databases. Results were retrieved on 5th May 2016. The search strategy can be found in the Additional file 2. We supplemented the database search by hand searching and reference searches. We only included articles published in English.

Eligibility criteria

Since the population of interest is the general adult population, we included only population-based studies, defined as community-based epidemiological studies that are representative of the adult population. We excluded studies that focused only on specific sub-populations such as veterans, students, or prisoners, whose experiences may not be representative of the wider population and warrant separate reviews.

The primary outcome measure of interest was any contact with formal health services – including private, public, generalist and specialist – for mental health reasons (also referred to as "treatment-seeking") by adults aged 18 and above with CMD. Reflecting the definition of the treatment gap, we focussed specifically on use of services as a binary outcome – i.e. any versus no use – rather than volume of treatment received or quality of care.

To be eligible for inclusion, the study must have tested the association between treatment seeking and any other factors. We therefore included only quantitative studies, published in peer-reviewed journals, and excluded narrative reviews and commentaries. We included only studies in which the analyses were restricted to those individuals who either met diagnostic criteria or screened positive for CMD using a standardised instrument.

For the purposes of this article, CMD is defined as those ICD-10 (International Classification of Diseases - 10th Revision) disorders measured by the Clinical Interview Schedule - Revised [33] – often considered the gold standard for measuring CMD [34, 35] – namely, depressive disorders, generalised anxiety disorder, panic disorder, phobias, obsessive compulsive disorder, and mixed anxiety-depression disorder.

We excluded papers that measured only intentions to seek help, or perceived barriers to care, since multiple studies have found that these are not closely correlated with behaviour [36–40].

No restrictions were placed on geographic area or date of publication. Table 1 provides full details of the inclusion criteria applied.

Study selection

The first author completed title and abstract screening for all references retrieved. Subsequently two researchers (GME and DK) independently screened a random sample of 10% of the references, and inter-rater reliability was calculated at 94%. Full texts were retrieved for all studies included after the title/abstract screening. The first author screened all full texts, while the second author (GME) screened a purposive sample of 10%. At both stages, disagreements were resolved through discussion.

We assessed the quality of the relevant evidence extracted from the included studies using the Mixed-Method Appraisal Tool (MMAT) [41], which has been shown to be quick and reliable to apply [42]. Table 2 sets out the criteria used. Extracted evidence for the purposes of this review was rated as poor, fair, good or excellent if 0–1, 2, 3 or 4 of these criteria were met, respectively. These ratings are not intended to reflect the study quality in relation to its own primary aims, but only of the quality of the evidence that related to this review.

Data extraction and synthesis

The following data were extracted for all papers that were included in the full text search: study title, authors, publication date and journal; country; study design; population; CMD measure; outcome (i.e. health service utilisation) measure; and factors associated with the outcome (including null associations). An association was regarded as detected when it was associated with the outcome in the most fully-adjusted model presented, with a p-value of < 0.05. The corresponding authors were contacted for clarification in case of any ambiguities.

Due to the number of different factors investigated, and heterogeneity in the measures used, it was not feasible to attempt a meta-analysis of the effect of each factor. Instead, the "best fit" framework synthesis method [43] was used to compare the fit of the data with an existing model of factors affecting health service utilisation. This technique was originally developed for the synthesis of qualitative research, but has since been applied to reviews of quantitative and mixed methods studies [44, 45].

The first author extracted the data from each of the included papers and coded these deductively using the Andersen framework described above [17]. Any data that did not fit any of the headings in the Andersen model headings were to be coded separately under a new theme in a subsequent inductive phase.

To avoid bias in the synthesis and interpretation of results due to pre-conceived ideas about which factors are associated with treatment-seeking, we created a priori definitions with which to categorise the associations found for each factor. These definitions (summarised in Table 3) were created for the purposes of the current review, and are intended to be conservative.

No prior studies were found to guide the operationalisation of these definitions, and therefore the cut-off points chosen are necessarily arbitrary. However, we have tried to be entirely transparent in how these have been applied, and present the full findings and quality ratings in the appendices provided so the reader can examine how the evidence relates to the conclusions drawn.

Table 1 Inclusion and exclusion criteria applied

	Include	Exclude
Participants	- Population-based studies, in which participants are randomly sampled from a sampling frame that can be reasonably expected to include the majority of the adult population - Studies in which CMD is measured and analyses are restricted to those who "screen positive" for CMD.[a]	- Any studies including people aged under 18 (unless these are presented separately in analyses) - Studies with exclusion criteria that would rule out a large proportion of the adult population (e.g. over-55 s only, people of a particular minority ethnic group only, women who have recently given birth) - Studies in which participants do not live in community settings (e.g. prisoners, inpatients, residents of elderly care homes) or are defined by their occupation (e.g. doctors, police officers, students) - Studies in which all participants have used health services for mental health reasons - Studies that combine people with CMD and those with other conditions and do not report results separately in analyses - Ecological level studies in which CMD is not controlled at the individual level (i.e. it's not possible to tell whether the people using services are the same individuals who have CMD) - Studies that apply overly restrictive exclusion criteria for participants, e.g. focussed solely on individuals with a specific comorbid condition, or restricted to only specific ethnic groups
Design	- Observational - Quantitative or qualitative comparison of treatment-seekers and non-treatment-seekers - Cross-sectional or longitudinal - Articles published in peer-reviewed journals only	- Reviews/commentaries/opinion pieces - Conference abstracts/dissertations/book chapters - Case studies that lack quantitative evaluation
Outcomes	- Studies reporting on the use/non-use (as a binary variable) of formal, face-to-face health services (either specialist or non-specialist, public or private) for mental health reasons - Timeframe in which service use is measured must be clearly defined (e.g. past 12 months)	- Studies reporting on general health care use (i.e. including for reasons other than mental health problems) - Studies examining use of only one specific treatment type (e.g. antidepressant use only, counselling only) - Studies reporting on volume of treatment (i.e. number of visits to a treatment provider), adherence to treatment or quality of treatment - Studies reporting on rates of detection or referral - Studies reporting on theoretical access rather than actual use (e.g. insurance coverage, being registered with a clinic) - Studies reporting on the use of online or telephone-based services - Studies examining the use of informal care (e.g. friends/family/religious support) or complementary/alternative treatments (i.e. those provided outside of the formal health sector) - Studies reporting on willingness or intentions to use services, or recommendations for service use in case of experiencing CMD symptoms, with no measure of actual behaviour - Studies that report participation in screening as the outcome rather than active treatment-seeking or uptake of services post-screening
Correlates	- Any factors that are correlated with the outcome of interest, including (but not limited to): • demographic factors • health status (e.g. severity/disability/comorbid conditions etc.) • distance/transport to services • insurance coverage • interventions • specific symptoms • behavioural/personality factors • neighbourhood characteristics • characteristics of the healthcare provider • health systems factors • stigma/attitudes towards services	- Studies reporting on the magnitude of the treatment gap, without any correlates of treatment-seeking - Studies that report predictors of service type (e.g. generalist vs. specialist, pharmacological vs. psychological) rather than any vs. no use - Studies reporting barriers and facilitators to the use of health services, without examining the association between these barriers and actual treatment-seeking behaviour
Dates	Any year of publication	
Region	Any country or region	

[a]Defined as any of the following: depression, generalised anxiety disorder (GAD), panic disorder, phobias, obsessive compulsive disorder (OCD), or CMD not otherwise specified

Table 2 Operationalisation of quality appraisal criteria, based on the Mixed-Method Appraisal Tool (MMAT)

Criterion	Definition	Example
Appropriate sampling strategy	Population-based sample using a sampling frame that can reasonably be assumed to include the majority of the non-institutionalised adult population. (Justification of sample size was not included in this criterion since none of the included studies justified their sample size with reference to the research questions addressed in this review.)	*Meets criterion:* Simple random sample of households chosen from a government list of residential addresses, then one resident aged > = 18 randomly chosen to participate. *Doesn't meet criterion:* Males and females sampled through separate means (males at compulsory conscription, females at enrolment on the electoral register).
Sample representative of target population	Sample representative of non-institutionalised adult population, with minimal exclusion criteria applied.	*Meets criterion:* All adults eligible in urban area where study was conducted. Sample representative of urban residents with regard to major socio-demographic factors tested. *Doesn't meet criterion:* Participants excluded due to age, ethnicity, chronicity of symptoms, comorbid conditions etc.
Appropriate measures used	Validated measure of CMD (either screening tool or diagnostic instrument), timeframe for health service utilisation limited and specified.	*Meets criterion:* CIDI, AUDADIS-IV, CIS-R, SPIKE, PHQ-9, GAD-7, DIS, Burnam depression screener 12 month help-seeking from health services for MH reasons *Doesn't meet criterion:* Self-defined depression/anxiety, prior receipt of diagnosis Lifetime use of health services (due to limited accuracy of recall)
Acceptable response rate	> 60% response rate for cross-sectional studies > 60% response rate and < 30% attrition rate for longitudinal studies	*Meets criterion:* > 60% response rate across all study sites, or across all major groups compared *Doesn't meet criterion:* < 60% response rate overall, in some study sites, or for one gender

Results

Search results

Figure 1 summarises the search process. After removing duplicates, 10,331 papers were retrieved. Fifty-two papers were found to meet the criteria at the full text screening stage. Of these, eleven were cohort studies while forty-one were cross-sectional.

Thirty-two (62%) of these studies reported data from North America, nine (16%) from Europe, two (4%) from Australasia, three (6%) from Africa, one (2%) from Asia, two (4%) from Latin America and three (6%) used international data from across world regions.

Table 3 Definitions used to grade consistency of evidence when synthesising findings from included studies

Evidence level	Criteria
Good evidence of an association	≥75% of studies that investigated this factor report an association, of which ≥2 (using different datasets) are of good/excellent quality
Good evidence of no association	< 25% of studies that investigated this factor report an association, of which ≥2 (using different datasets) are of good/excellent quality
Inconsistent evidence	25–75% of studies that investigated this factor report an association, of which ≥2 (using different datasets) are of good/excellent quality
Poor quality evidence only	< 2 studies of good/excellent quality (using different datasets) investigated the association between this factor and treatment-seeking for CMD
Not examined	No studies investigated the association between this factor and treatment-seeking for CMD

The study sizes varied considerably, from 56 participants to 18,972 participants with elevated levels of CMD symptoms.

In terms of quality, evidence from one study was rated as poor, evidence from 16 was classified as fair, evidence from 20 was classified as good, and evidence from 15 studies was rated excellent. Additional file 3 presents the characteristics of the included studies.

Factors associated with health service utilisation for CMD

Table 4 shows the number of studies that investigated each of the factors in the Andersen model.

Compared to other factors, we identified the highest number of studies on the association between socio-demographic factors (classified according to the Andersen model as "predisposing" factors) and treatment-seeking for CMD. We also found a large number of studies that investigated symptom severity, symptom profile and comorbidity (termed "need" factors in the Andersen model) as correlates of treatment-seeking. Fewer of the included studies examined enabling factors such as insurance, household wealth and social support. There was a lack of published evidence on some factors implicated by the Andersen model, such as psychological factors (e.g. beliefs and attitudes, classified as "predisposing" factors) and health systems factors (e.g. the availability and accessibility of services).

Almost all of the factors identified were individual rather than contextual level factors. No factors were identified that could not be accommodated by the model.

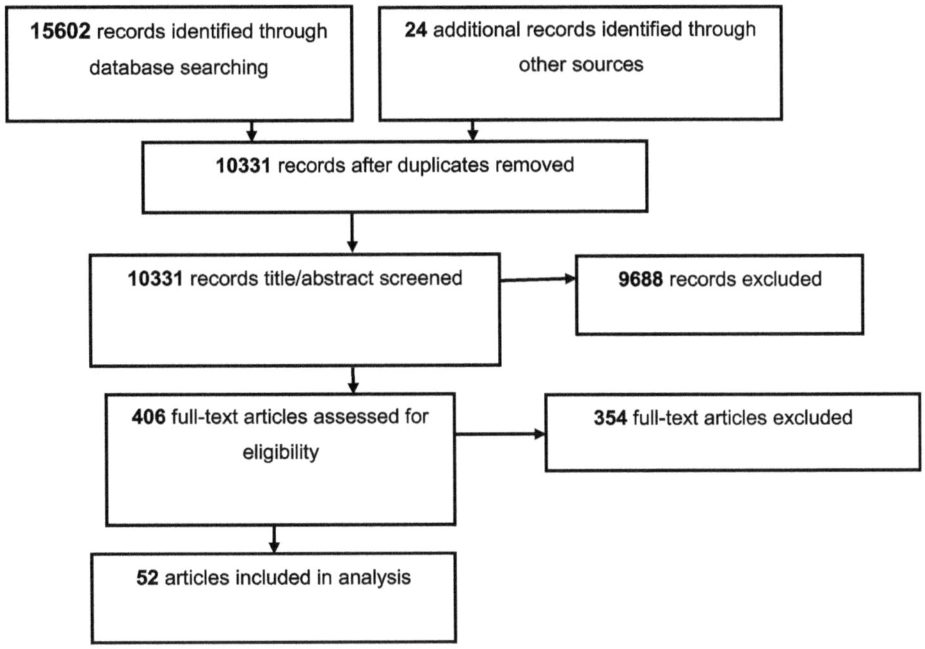

Fig. 1 PRISMA flowchart showing selection of studies

A summary of findings for each factor group is presented below. For more detailed results see the Additional file 4.

Predisposing factors

Overall synthesis of findings on predisposing factors As shown in Table 4, while several trends were identified, no predisposing factors were consistently found to be associated with seeking treatment.

Factor-by-factor synthesis of evidence from included studies *General trends across studies.*

Having sought mental health treatment previously was generally associated with increased likelihood of seeking treatment [46–48]. The relationship between age and health service utilisation for CMD was commonly found to be hill-shaped, with middle-aged respondents most likely to seek treatment [49–68]. Female gender was frequently found to be associated with increased treatment-seeking [46, 47, 49–55, 57–62, 64, 65, 67–77], as was being Caucasian, which represented the majority ethnic group in the context of most of the included studies [46, 47, 49–51, 53, 55, 57–60, 64, 68, 70, 78–87]. Several studies reported that higher education levels were associated with health service utilisation for CMD, although this was not found across all studies [46, 47, 49–51, 53, 55, 57–65, 68, 70, 76, 77]. Being married was negatively associated with treatment-seeking, though it was unclear whether this is due to greater use of services by the never married or by those who are separated or divorced group [46, 47, 49–51, 55, 57–59, 62, 64–68, 70, 73].

Findings related to other predisposing factors.

There was mixed evidence with regard to immigration status [46, 48, 68, 73, 82, 88], change in marital status [46, 47, 71], and personality factors [51, 61, 66, 74]. There was limited published evidence available on age of onset, from just three studies, but the findings generally indicated increased likelihood of seeking treatment with later onset [46, 71, 77]. There was also a lack of published evidence on the effect of stigma or other beliefs and attitudes [66, 67].

Need factors

Overall synthesis of findings on need factors Need factors were most consistently associated with the use of health services for CMD symptoms across studies, as seen in Table 4.

Factor-by-factor synthesis of evidence from included studies *Consistent findings.*

Five factors were consistently found to be associated with treatment-seeking across studies. These were self-evaluated health status or healthcare needs [50, 53, 67, 68, 70, 74, 83, 86]; duration or chronicity of symptoms [49, 66, 71]; disability or functioning [48, 51, 63, 65, 68, 73, 74, 76]; comorbid mental disorders [46, 49–52, 54, 59, 65, 66, 70, 71, 73, 76, 77, 89–91]; and panic symptoms [46, 51, 52, 71, 91].

General trends across studies.

Symptom severity was generally reported to be associated with an increased likelihood of seeking treatment [50, 51, 53, 54, 58, 59, 61, 65, 67, 71, 73, 74, 76, 78, 79, 85].

Table 4 Synthesis of associations found between factors in Andersen socio-behavioural model of health service utilisation and treatment-seeking for CMD

Type	Factor	Summary of associations found	Evidence level	No. of studies	Relationship	No. of good quality studies	No. of longitudinal studies	Total sample size	Total number of studies from each region	No. of studies from LMIC
Predisposing factors										
Demographic	Age	Hill-shaped relationship commonly reported, with highest use by middle-aged individuals and lower use by the young and the elderly	Inconsistent	25	Hill-shaped	9	3	33,779	10 N. America 1 Australasia 1 L. America	1
					Positive/Consistent with hill-shape	2	2	3162	1 Africa 1 L. America 2 Europe	2
					Mixed	0	1	1926	2 Europe	0
					Null	4	0	6501	2 Africa 2 N. America 2 Europe	2
	Age of onset	Older age of onset associated with service use in some studies	Inconsistent	3	Positive	2	1	14,640	2 N. America	0
					Other	0	1	1572	1 Europe	0
	Gender	Female gender generally associated with greater service utilisation	Inconsistent	29	Positive (women)	9	5	28,201	10 N. America 1 L. America 1 Africa 1 Europe	1
					Other/mixed	4	2	29,838	3 N. America 2 Africa 1 Europe	2
					Null	5	2	6380	1 Africa 1 Asia 2 N. America 1 Australasia 4 Europe	1
					Negative (women)	1	0	531	1 L. America	1
Social structure	Ethnicity	Caucasian ethnicity commonly associated with greater use than other ethnic groups	Inconsistent	23	Positive (white)	7	2	60,534	11 N. America 1 L. America	1
					Positive compared to some ethnicities only	2	0	17,299	3 N. America	0
					Mixed	4	1	36,558	5 N. America 1 South Africa	1
					Null	2	1	2658	2 N. America 1 Australasia	0
	Immigration status	No clear pattern found	Inconsistent	6	Negative (born abroad)	0	1	2026	1 Europe	0
					Null	2	1	15,056	2 N. America 1 Australasia	0
					Mixed	0	0	7687	2 N. America	0

Table 4 Synthesis of associations found between factors in Andersen socio-behavioural model of health service utilisation and treatment-seeking for CMD *(Continued)*

Type	Factor	Summary of associations found	Evidence level	No. of studies	Relationship	No. of good quality studies	No. of longitudinal studies	Total sample size	Total number of studies from each region	No. of studies from LMIC
	Marital Status	Being married associated with lower service use in some studies	Inconsistent	18	Negative (married)	5	2	10,367	5 N. America 1 Europe 1 Australasia	0
					Null	5	1	17,493	1 L. America 2 Africa 2 N. America 2 Europe	3
					Positive (married)	1	1	337	1 N. America	0
					Mixed	2	1	13,590	1 N. America 1 Europe	0
	Education	Higher levels of education associated with greater service use in some studies	Inconsistent	20	Positive (higher)	6	4	31,441	6 N. America 1 Europe 1 L. America 1 Africa	2
					Null	7	1	11,377	5 N. America 2 Europe 1 Australasia 1 Africa	1
					Mixed	0	1	2130	1 N. America 1 Europe	0
Personality	Conscientiousness	No clear pattern found	Poor	1	Positive	0	1	354	1 Europe	0
	Mastery	No clear pattern found	Poor	1	Mixed	0	1	903	1 Europe	0
	Neuroticism		Inconsistent	2	Positive	1	1	2005	1 Australasia	0
					Null	1	1	102	2 Europe	0
Health beliefs	Prior use of services	Prior use associated with greater use	Good	3	Positive	2	2	13,672	4 N. America	0
					Null	0	0	0	0	0
	Stigma	No clear pattern found	Poor	2	Null	0	0	102	1 Europe	0
					Mixed	1	0	56	1 Asia	1
	Mental Health Literacy	Not investigated		0	N/A	0	0	0		0
Enabling factors										
Assets	Income/ wealth	Most studies did not find any association	Good – no association	11	Null	5	0	7623	3 N. America 3 Africa 1 Europe	3
					Positive	1	0	7209	1 N. America 1 Asia	1
					Mixed	1	0	2510	2 N. America	0

Table 4 Synthesis of associations found between factors in Andersen socio-behavioural model of health service utilisation and treatment-seeking for CMD *(Continued)*

Type	Factor	Summary of associations found	Evidence level	No. of studies	Relationship	No. of good quality studies	No. of longitudinal studies	Total sample size	Total number of studies from each region	No. of studies from LMIC
	Employment	Being employed associated with lower use in some studies	Inconsistent	8	Negative (being employed)	2	2	3452	2 N. America 2 Europe	0
					Null	3	0	3059	2 Africa 1 Europe 1 Australasia	2
	Social support	Greater social support linked to use in some studies	Poor	5	Positive	0	1	661	1 Europe 1 Africa	1
					Null	1	1	1275	2 N. America 1 Europe	0
	Insurance	Having health insurance associated with use in some studies	Inconsistent	7	Positive	2	1	10,393	4 N. America	0
					Null	1	0	956	2 N. America	0
					Mixed	0	0	558	1 N. America	0
Need factors										
Perceived	Self-rated health/ perceived need for care	Better self-rated health (/lower perceive need for care) associated with lower service use	Good	8	Negative	2	2	2738	2 N. America 1 Europe	0
					Mixed or indirect	2	0	2865	3 N. America	0
					Null	0	1	491	1 N. America 1 Asia	1
Evaluated	Symptom severity	Greater severity commonly associated with service use	Inconsistent	16	Positive	5	5	23,165	7 N. America 2 Europe 1 Australasia	0
					Mixed	1	0	298	1 Europe	0
					Null	3	1	4052	2 N. America 2 Europe 1 Asia	1
	Chronicity/ duration	Longer duration associated with service use	Good	3	Positive	3	0	8603	2 N. America 1 Europe	0
	Disability	Greater impairment associated with service use	Good	8	Positive	3	1	4794	1 N. America 3 Europe 1 Australasia	0
					Mixed/ borderline	0	1	2199	2 N. America 1 Europe	0
	Comorbid conditions – total	No clear pattern found	Poor	4	Null	1	1	7565	1 N. America 1 Europe 1 L. America	1
	Non-psychiatric	No clear pattern found	Inconsistent	14	Positive	3	2	17,455	3 N. America	1

Table 4 Synthesis of associations found between factors in Andersen socio-behavioural model of health service utilisation and treatment-seeking for CMD *(Continued)*

Type	Factor	Summary of associations found	Evidence level	No. of studies	Relationship	No. of good quality studies	No. of longitudinal studies	Total sample size	Total number of studies from each region	No. of studies from LMIC
	chronic conditions								1 Europe 1 International	(combined HIC/LMIC)
					Negative	1	0	220	1 Europe	0
					Mixed	1	0	7460	1 N. America 1 Africa	1
					Null	5	1	4567	3 Europe 2 N. America 1 Australasia	0
	Psychiatric comorbidities (general)	Comorbid mental disorders (in general) associated with service use	Good	6	Positive	5	3	6295	3 N. America 2 Europe 1 Australasia	0
	Comorbid SUD	No clear pattern found	Inconsistent	8	Positive	3	1	24,189	3 N. America	0
					Negative	1	1	1,1,56	2 N. America	0
					Mixed	0	1	1572	1 Europe	0
					Null	2	1	20,445	2 N. America	0
	Comorbid mood/ anxiety disorders	Comorbid mood/anxiety disorders associated with service use	Good	6	Positive	5	4	26,714	3 N. America 2 Europe	0
					Null	1	0	102	1 Europe	0
	Other comorbid mental disorders	No clear pattern found	Inconsistent	3	Mixed	3	1	8719	3 N. America	0
	Panic symptoms	Panic symptoms associated with service use	Good	6	Positive	5	2	26,350	4 N. America 1 Australasia	0
					Negative	0	0	558	1 N. America	0
	Suicidality	No clear pattern found	Inconsistent	3	Positive	2	0	1646	1 N. America 1 Europe	0
					Null	1	1	2864	1 N. America	0
	Somatisation	No evidence of any association	Good – no	2	Null	2	1	1566	2 N. America	0
	Other CMD symptoms	No clear pattern found	Inconsistent	5	Mixed	2	1	15,941	3 N. America 2 Europe	0
	Adverse childhood events	No clear pattern found	Poor	4	Positive	0	2	1926	2 Europe	0
					Mixed	1	1	1201	2 Europe	0
Contextual factors										
Place of residence	Urban/rural residence	No evidence of any association	Good – no	7	Null	6	1	16,677	3 N. America 2 Europe 1 Australasia 1 L. America	1

Table 4 Synthesis of associations found between factors in Andersen socio-behavioural model of health service utilisation and treatment-seeking for CMD *(Continued)*

Type	Factor	Summary of associations found	Evidence level	No. of studies	Relationship	No. of good quality studies	No. of longitudinal studies	Total sample size	Total number of studies from each region	No. of studies from LMIC
	Country	No clear pattern found	Inconsistent	3	Mixed	2	0	4111	1 N. America/ Europe 1 N. America/ Australasia	0
					Null	0	0	751	1 N. America	0
	Region (within-country)	No clear pattern found	Inconsistent	3	Positive	1	1	7620	1 N. America 1 L. America	1
					Null	1	0	7153	1 N. America	0
Health service factors	Service availability (perceived)	No clear pattern found	Poor	1	Positive	0	1	435	1 N. America	0
	Service accessibility	No clear pattern found	Poor	1	Null	0	0	56	1 Asia	1
	Regular source of care	No clear pattern found	Poor	2	Mixed	1	0	436	2 N. America	0
	Organisation of services (gatekeeper)	No clear pattern found	Poor	1	Negative	1	0	1498	1 N. America	0
	Service capacity/ waiting times/ opening hours	Not investigated		0	N/A	0	0	0		0
	Resources available	Not investigated		0	N/A	0	0	0		0
	Healthcare policy	Not investigated		0	N/A	0	0	0		0
	Quality of care	Not investigated		0	N/A	0	0	0		0
Social factors	Neighbourhood norms	Not investigated		0	N/A	0	0	0		0

Findings related to other need factors.

There was mixed evidence for an association with suicidality or specific CMD symptoms [46, 47, 51, 52, 59, 63, 66, 71, 76, 77, 85, 91, 92], substance use and non-psychiatric conditions [47, 49–51, 53, 54, 57, 63, 65, 66, 68, 71, 73–75, 93–95] and adverse childhood events [61, 74, 76, 77].

Enabling factors

Overall synthesis of findings on enabling factors As indicated in Table 4, there was inconsistent evidence for an association between treatment-seeking for CMD and enabling factors.

Factor-by-factor synthesis of evidence from included studies *Consistent findings.*

The studies included here did not support an association between wealth or income and the use of health services for CMD symptoms [47, 55, 58, 60, 62, 64, 65, 67, 68, 75].

General trends across studies.

Some studies indicated a positive association between treatment-seeking and being in employment although this was not found across all studies [50, 51, 58, 62, 65, 73, 75, 76]. Having health insurance was frequently, but not consistently, reported to be correlated with health service utilisation for CMD [47, 49, 50, 53, 60, 63, 68].

Findings related to other enabling factors.

There was mixed evidence with regard to social support [50, 61, 66, 68, 75], and limited published evidence available on the effect of having a regular source of care [47, 48].

Contextual level factors

Overall synthesis of findings on contextual factors Overall, limited published evidence was found testing the association between contextual level factors and health service utilisation for CMD.

Consistent findings.

The studies included here suggest that living in a rural area is not associated with lower rates of treatment-seeking [49, 51, 54, 55, 57, 65, 76].

Findings related to other contextual factors.

Few studies compared treatment-seeking between countries or by geographic region within countries, and those that did reported inconsistent findings [49, 57, 59, 78, 96, 97]. There was a dearth of published evidence on the association between the health care environment and utilisation of services for CMD, with just one study on the effect of managed care [53], one on perceived availability of services [50], and one on perceived accessibility of services [67].

Comparison of evidence from LMIC and HIC

There was a clear discrepancy in the quantity of research identified between high-income and low-and-middle-income countries, with just six of the included studies originating from LMIC and one international study that included data from both HIC and LMIC [93]. Five of the LMIC-only studies were from middle-income countries; two from South Africa [64, 75], and one from Brazil [57], Mexico [69] and China [67]. The only study from a low-income country was from Ethiopia [62].

Evidence from three out of six LMIC studies was rated as good or excellent. On average LMIC studies were smaller than HIC studies, with a mean of 1742 participants with high CMD symptoms, compared to 3374 for HICs.

The LMIC studies identified predominantly reported on the effect of predisposing factors, such as age, gender, and education levels, and on measures of income or wealth.

There was insufficient published evidence from LMIC to compare the factors associated with treatment-seeking for CMD between HIC and LMIC.

Methodological limitations of included studies

The majority of studies used secondary datasets, which limited the choice of variables to those that are typically collected as part of multi-purpose epidemiological surveys. The frequent use of cross-sectional data also limits our ability to disentangle the direction of causation when associations are found. The majority of studies used multivariate logistic regression models for analysis. The use of hierarchical models, or structural equation modelling that explicitly recognises the potential interactions between some of these factors, may have led to differing conclusions. Although several studies cited the Andersen model to justify their choice of variables, there seems to be little agreement as to how the model should be operationalised and much heterogeneity in the measures used, making it difficult to compare the results across studies. In particular, agreement is needed on how variables indicating level of "need for care" should be measured in the context of CMD, so that is it possible to control for this consistently when investigating whether the use of health services is equitable. Finally, many of the included studies did not correct for multiple testing when investigating multiple associations simultaneously, and as such their findings should be viewed as hypothesis-generating rather than hypothesis-testing.

Discussion

Principal findings

This review furthers our understanding of the treatment gap for CMD by summarising patterns of treatment-seeking. Need factors were most consistently found to be associated with treatment-seeking for CMD symptoms. Enabling factors were not found to be consistently associated with treatment seeking for CMD. The evidence on predisposing factors was inconsistent, although there was weak evidence for an association with demographic factors, specifically age, gender, ethnicity, education level and marital status. Finally, the current results suggest that urban or rural residence is not associated with treatment-seeking.

With regard to the second objective, there was insufficient published evidence from LMIC to draw any firm conclusions about whether the factors associated with health service utilisation for CMD differ from high-income countries.

Strengths and weaknesses

This review has several strengths: It employed a broad search strategy, informed by previous reviews [22–24], since the literature on this topic spans several disciplines with varying terminology. It followed an a priori protocol, had screening verified at multiple stages by a second researcher, and employed a widely recognised theoretical framework to analyse the results. Compared to the most recent review in this area [25], we searched a larger number of databases in order to make the review as comprehensive as possible.

This review adds to previous research by considering the wider category of CMD rather than a single diagnostic category, which several researchers have argued is a more appropriate grouping for community and primary care settings [26, 28–31]. It was also deliberately more liberal in terms of its definition of CMD symptoms, since it is generally accepted that CMD symptoms are better conceptualised as a spectrum rather than a dichotomy between those who meet diagnostic criteria and those who do not [27]. Since conducting full diagnostic interviews in large population studies is often not feasible, it was hoped that this broader definition would lead to the inclusion of studies from a wider range of settings.

Other related reviews have been restricted to young adults [98] or to one country only [99]. While the results reported here are broadly consistent with the findings of these reviews, this study extends previous research by (a) comparing results across settings; (b) including only population-based studies to ensure the generalisability of findings; (c) examining a set of symptoms that typically present together in community settings, making the results a stronger basis for informing interventions at the population level; and (d) separating service utilisation by adults from that of children or adolescents, since in many countries services are delivered separately for these two groups, and decisions regarding treatment-seeking may follow different paths for minors (defined here as those aged under 18).

However, the current review nonetheless has several limitations that must be acknowledged. One is that it was not possible to assess the power of each study to detect an association, meaning that in studies where no association was found with a given factor, this cannot be interpreted with confidence to indicate a lack of association rather than a lack of statistical power. Secondly, it is possible that some studies in which this was not the primary research question may have been erroneously excluded if associations with treatment-seeking were not reported in the title or abstract of the paper. This is more likely to be the case when no associations are found, leading to potential selection bias. For reasons of feasibility, the search was restricted to studies published in English.

We were not able to present data on the amount of variance explained by the factors included in the studies reviewed, since this was not reported in the majority of these studies. Nor was it possible to discuss the confounding factors controlled for in every analysis, due to the large number of studies included. To definitively assess the causal effect of any one factor on treatment-seeking for CMD a meta-analysis of that specific association would be recommended; this was not the purpose of the current review, which set out to summarise associations, not to make causal claims.

The inclusion of multiple measures of CMD symptoms also means that these will not be exactly comparable across studies. Furthermore, when the quality of studies was assessed, we considered the measure of CMD used and the measure of treatment-seeking from the formal health sector; however, due to the number of factors investigated it was not possible to assess the appropriateness of measures used for each of these factors. Finally, as mentioned in the methods section, although the consistency of evidence for each factor was graded according to pre-defined criteria, other ways of operationalising levels of evidence are possible, which could lead to more or less conservative conclusions. Full details of all studies and the criteria applied are presented in the appendices.

Comparison with previous literature

Our findings are consistent with previous research pointing to need factors as the strongest determinants of health service utilisation for mental disorders [100–103]. This is also consistent with the finding from the World Mental Health Surveys (WMHS) – which included both LMICs and HICs and measured substance use disorders and bipolar disorder as well as CMD – that low perceived need was the most common reason cited for not seeking treatment [104].

The same associations with female gender, middle age, higher levels of education, and being unmarried were found in the WMHS [8].

The fact that the evidence included in the current study did not support an association with economic factors was surprising, given the evidence that socio-economic factors affect the type of provider contacted [63, 68, 77], the quality of care received [63], adherence [105–109] and response to treatment [110, 111]. However, a recent analysis of WMHS data by Evans-Lacko et al. (2017) found that differences in treatment rates in the WMHS by socio-economic status were predominantly accounted for by education rather than income [112].

Thus our findings on treatment-seeking for CMD are largely in keeping with the largest international study of mental disorders and service utilisation to date. The WMHS did not investigate rural/urban residence, or any of the other factors included in the Andersen model besides those listed above.

Implications

Need factors, reflecting the extent to which CMD symptoms interfere with people's lives and whether outside help is needed, appear to be central to explaining treatment-seeking behaviour. This suggests that many of those who do not seek care from formal health services for their CMD symptoms fail to do so not because of limited supply, but because of lack of demand for services.

Whether meeting criteria for a disorder is a good indication of a "need for health services" is an ongoing debate in the context of mental health care [113]. The limited demand for interventions for CMD, compared to the number of people who meet criteria for CMD, can be conceptualised as a lack of education or awareness about mental health issues, indicating a need for information, education and communication campaigns. On the other hand, it may be an indication that current diagnostic categories are overly broad, and include a large number of people who do not require formal medical care. Patel (2014) has argued that current prevalence estimates should not be regarded as the number of individuals in need of care, since a large proportion of these individuals do not require formal interventions through the health system [31]. Measures of functioning or quality of life may represent better indicators of "need for care" than meeting diagnostic criteria (it is notable that the latter concept was not investigated by any of the studies included here).

Patel's argument that increasing the supply of mental health services will not alone make a substantial impact on the treatment gap for mental disorders is supported by the current findings that; (a) lack of perceived need is a major determinant of failure to seek help from health services, and (b) that enabling factors do not appear to be a major determinant of treatment-seeking (discussed below). Many individuals with less disabling symptoms are likely to view informal support – such as social interventions in the community, or advice on self-care, listed at the bottom of the World Health Organization (WHO) Service Organization Pyramid [114] – as more appropriate for their needs. As such, encouraging these individuals to seek care through the health system may not be the best use of resources.

The lack of evidence for an association between enabling factors and health service utilisation, even in settings with weak public health systems, such as South Africa, and without universal health coverage, like the USA, was surprising. Of course, absence of evidence is not proof of a lack of association, especially given that the studies included here were not explicitly powered to detect this relationship. There is also the potential for information bias, given the sensitivity of financial topics, since most studies used self-reported data.

However, the hypothesis that economic factors do not play a major role in determining whether people with CMD initially seek care from health services is backed up by findings from Evans-Lacko et al. (2017) [112], as well as Andrews et al. (2001), who found no association at the ecological level with health spending or out-of-pocket costs [112, 115]. Furthermore, Andrade et al. (2014) found that attitudinal barriers (most commonly, wanting to handle the problem alone) were reported much more often than structural barriers (which are linked to enabling factors), with the exception of severe cases. It is possible that the inclusion in this review of individuals with milder conditions, for whom low perceived need primarily inhibits treatment-seeking, might be obscuring the real impact of enabling factors such as cost and travel distance on the sub-group with severe CMD, who are most in need of care. Future research could usefully examine the extent to which supply side factors such as the availability, affordability and accessibility of care affect service utilisation by those with the most severe needs.

If equitable access to health care is defined as equal utilisation by those with equal need for care [116], then there is some evidence pointing to the need to target underserved groups such as men, ethnic minority groups, the elderly and young adults, at least in HIC. However, the extent to which need factors such as symptom severity and disability were controlled in these analyses varied between studies, so we cannot definitively rule out the possibility that these differences can be explained by variability in need for treatment.

Attempts to address these inequities have been made in HIC through strategies such as enhancing cultural competence in mental health services [117] and targeting underserved groups through social marketing [118], with some success [119, 120]. Evaluations of these interventions typically measure adherence/attrition, patient satisfaction or attitudes towards seeking care rather than treatment-seeking behaviour, so their effectiveness in reducing mental health care inequities is still to be determined.

Regarding geographic location, some studies indicate that this may affect the type of provider chosen and the quality of care received [54, 121]. It is possible that the initial decision of whether or not to seek treatment is made independently of location of residence, but the subsequent decision of where to seek treatment, and the health system's response, is influenced by geography. This wants further investigation (see "Unanswered questions and future research", below).

Finally, although it was not the topic of this review, there was some evidence to suggest that the factors associated with health service utilisation for CMD may vary between the specialist and generalist sectors [64, 77, 87], which has been highlighted in other studies [100, 112]. This warrants further investigation as it has important implications for service planning. Thornicroft and Tansella (2013) advocate a stepped care model of mental health services, with the majority of services delivered through primary care in low-resource settings [122]. However, it remains to be investigated which balance leads to the most equitable use of services for CMD, and whether some groups are more likely to seek treatment through primary care in LMIC.

Unanswered questions and future research

This review identified three major gaps in our knowledge: Firstly, a lack of research from LMIC; secondly, a dearth of research on contextual factors, particularly health systems factors; and thirdly, an absence of studies that are explicitly powered to test associations between the factor of interest and treatment-seeking for CMD.

The first of these gaps directly relates to the second objective of this review. Although we have drawn some tentative conclusions above, the generalisability of these findings to LMIC is questionable at best, since nearly 90% of the studies identified were from high-income countries. In contrast, 85% of the world's population is expected to live in LMIC by 2030 [123], making this is an extremely important omission.

Not only was there a noticeable lack of population-based studies from LMIC, but those studies that were identified were less consistent in their findings than those from HICs. This may be in part due to the reduced statistical power of studies from areas where treatment rates are low, meaning that larger sample sizes are needed to detect an association. More research is urgently needed in LMIC – especially in those countries for which no population-based studies were identified – to determine whether the same factors are associated with treatment-seeking for CMD in non-Western settings, using large enough samples to detect an association.

Secondly, there was also a notable lack of published evidence on several contextual factors, in particular health systems factors that are likely to affect treatment-seeking. This includes the availability of services, the geographical accessibility of those services, and characteristics of services such as opening times, which are central to several models of access to health care [15, 124, 125]. This is a crucial gap, as such evidence could usefully inform service planning to expand access to care.

The extent to which distance affects treatment-seeking has particular relevance to debates around decentralisation and integration of mental health care [126]. Facility-based studies have pointed to distance and travel time as a potentially important determinant of health service utilisation [127–131], which contrasts with the lack of evidence supporting an association with urban/rural residence found in this review. However, these studies cannot disentangle geographic differences in prevalence from differences in treatment seeking behaviour. Furthermore, unless they assess the use of *all* health facilities in a given area – both public and private – it is not clear if distance affects whether affected individuals seek any care, or if it merely influences the choice of provider among those who do decide to seek treatment. This review showed that there is a lack of population-based data on the influence of geographic accessibility on the uptake of health services for CMD, with the exception of crude comparisons of rural and urban areas, for which no association was found with treatment-seeking.

Finally, none of the studies included here justified their sample size with regard to the relationship between treatment-seeking and the factors investigated. It is therefore possible that the lack of associations identified in some of the studies included here are the result of under-powered studies, rather than a genuine lack of association. To build the evidence base in this area and confirm the hypotheses generated by the current review, future studies should ensure that they have sufficient statistical power to detect an association with the factors investigated.

Conclusions

This review found that the set of factors most consistently associated with formal health service utilisation for CMD among the adult population were need factors, with inconsistent evidence of an association with predisposing factors – specifically demographic factors – and little evidence to support an association with enabling factors. Health system factors, such as the availability and accessibility of services, are under-researched in population-based studies. Research in low and middle-income countries is urgently needed to enhance our understanding of treatment-seeking for CMD in order to inform efforts to expand access to effective interventions and increase health service utilisation for CMD by those with greatest need for care.

Abbreviations

CIS-R: Clinical Interview Schedule - Revised; CMD: Common mental disorder; HIC: High-income countries; ICD-10: International Statistical Classification of Diseases and Related Health Problems - 10th Revision; LMIC: Low- and middle-income countries; MMAT: Mixed-Method Appraisal Tool; PHQ-9: Patient Health Questionnaire-9; PRISMA: Preferred Reporting Items for Systematic Reviews and Meta-Analyses; WHO: World Health Organization; WMHS: World Mental Health Surveys

Funding

There was no specific funding provided for this study. The first author is supported by a Bloomsbury Colleges PhD studentship. Bloomsbury Colleges had no role in the design or conduct of this study, or in the decision of whether or where to publish it.

Authors' contributions

TR was the lead author, and was ultimately responsible for the study design, title/abstract screening, full text screening, data extraction, synthesis of results, and the writing of the manuscript. GME provided input to the development of the inclusion and exclusion criteria, conducted title/abstract screening, conducted full text screening, assisted in developing the main table of results (Table 4), and provided comments and feedback on earlier drafts of the paper. DK also conducted title/abstract screening, and offered comments and feedback on earlier drafts of the paper. RS advised on the design of the study and the presentation of the results, and provided comments and feedback on earlier drafts of the paper. VP also advised on the study design and methodology, and offered comments and feedback on earlier drafts of the paper. Finally, SR provided extensive guidance through the process of study design, screening, data extraction, synthesis and writing, and also gave detailed comments and feedback on earlier drafts. All authors read and approved the final manuscript.

Consent for publication

Not applicable.

Competing interests

The authors declare that they have no competing interests.

Author details

[1]Centre for Global Mental Health, Department of Population Health, Faculty of Epidemiology and Population Health, London School of Hygiene and Tropical Medicine, Keppel Street, London WC1E 7HT, UK. [2]Health Service and Population Research Department, Institute of Psychiatry, Psychology and Neuroscience, King's College London, London, UK. [3]Department of Social Psychiatry, National Institute of Mental Health, Prague, Czech Republic. [4]Institute of Global Health, University of Geneva, Geneva, Switzerland. [5]Centre for Chronic Conditions and Injuries, Public Health Foundation of India, New Delhi, India. [6]Care and Public Health Research Institute, Maastricht University, Maastricht, Netherlands. [7]Department of Global Health and Social Medicine, Harvard Medical School, Boston, USA.

References

1. World Health Organization. Depression and Other Common Mental Disorders: Global Health Estimates. Geneva; 2017. Available from: http://apps.who.int/iris/bitstream/handle/10665/254610/WHOMSD?sequence=1 [Accessed 02/07/2018]
2. Ormel J, VonKorff M, Ustun TB, Pini S, Korten A, Oldehinkel T. Common mental disorders and disability across cultures: results from the WHO collaborative study on psychological problems in general health care. JAMA. 1994;272(22):1741–8.
3. Vos T, Flaxman AD, Naghavi M, Lozano R, Michaud C, Ezzati M, et al. Years lived with disability (YLDs) for 1160 sequelae of 289 diseases and injuries 1990–2010: a systematic analysis for the global burden of disease study 2010. Lancet. 2013;380(9859):2163–96.
4. Patel V, Araya R, Chatterjee S, Chisholm D, Cohen A, De Silva M, et al. Treatment and prevention of mental disorders in low-income and middle-income countries. Lancet. 2007;370(9591):991–1005.
5. Kohn R, Saxena S, Levav I, Saraceno B. The treatment gap in mental health care. Bull World Health Organ. 2004;82(11):858–66.
6. Sagar R, Pattanayak RD, Chandrasekaran R, Chaudhury PK, Deswal BS, Singh RL, et al. Twelve-month prevalence and treatment gap for common mental disorders: findings from a large-scale epidemiological survey in India. Indian J Psychiatry. 2017;59(1):46.
7. Demyttenaere K, Bruffaerts R, Posada-Villa J, Gasquet I, Kovess V, Lepine J, et al. Prevalence, severity, and unmet need for treatment of mental disorders in the World Health Organization world mental health surveys. JAMA. 2004;291(21):2581–90.
8. Wang PS, Aguilar-Gaxiola S, Alonso J, Angermeyer MC, Borges G, Bromet EJ, et al. Use of mental health services for anxiety, mood, and substance disorders in 17 countries in the WHO world mental health surveys. Lancet. 2007;370(9590):841–50.
9. Chisholm D, Flisher A, Lund C, Patel V, Saxena S, Thornicroft G, et al. Scale up services for mental disorders: a call for action. Lancet. 2007;370(9594):1241–52.
10. Patel V, Boyce N, Collins PY, Saxena S, Horton R. A renewed agenda for global mental health. Lancet (London, England). 2011;378(9801):1441.
11. Eaton J, McCay L, Semrau M, Chatterjee S, Baingana F, Araya R, et al. Scale up of services for mental health in low-income and middle-income countries. Lancet. 2011;378(9802):1592–603.
12. Lund C, Tomlinson M, De Silva M, Fekadu A, Shidhaye R, Jordans M, et al. PRIME: a programme to reduce the treatment gap for mental disorders in five low-and middle-income countries. PLoS Med. 2012;9(12):e1001359.
13. Organization WH. mhGAP: Mental Health Gap Action Programme: scaling up care for mental, neurological and substance use disorders. 2008.
14. De Silva MJ, Lee L, Fuhr DC, Rathod S, Chisholm D, Schellenberg J, et al. Estimating the coverage of mental health programmes: a systematic review. Int J Epidemiol. 2014;43(2):341–53.
15. Penchansky R, Thomas JW. The concept of access: definition and relationship to consumer satisfaction. Med Care. 1981;19:127–40.
16. Donabedian A. Aspects of medicalcare administration: specifying requirements for health care. 1973.
17. Andersen RM. A Behavioral Model of Families' Use of Health Services. Chicago, IL: Center for Health Administration Studies, University of Chicago. 1968. Research Series no. 25.
18. Babitsch B, Gohl D, von Lengerke T. Re-revisiting Andersen's behavioral model of health services use: a systematic review of studies from 1998–2011. GMS Psycho-Social-Medicine. 2012;9:Doc11.
19. Andersen RM. Revisiting the behavioral model and access to medical care: does it matter? J Health Soc Behav. 1995;36:1–10.
20. Andersen RM, Davidson PL, Baumeister SE. Improving access to care. Changing the US health care system: Key issues in health services policy and management; 2013. p. 33–69.
21. Phillips KA, Morrison KR, Andersen R, Aday LA. Understanding the context of healthcare utilization: assessing environmental and provider-related variables in the behavioral model of utilization. Health Serv Res. 1998;33(3 Pt 1):571.
22. Çalışkan Z, Kılıç D, Öztürk S, Atılgan E. Equity in maternal health care service utilization: a systematic review for developing countries. Int J Public Health. 2015;60(7):815–25.
23. Brennan A, Morley D, O'Leary AC, Bergin CJ, Horgan M. Determinants of HIV outpatient service utilization: a systematic review. AIDS Behav. 2015;19(1):104–19.
24. Say L, Raine R. A systematic review of inequalities in the use of maternal health care in developing countries: examining the scale of the problem and the importance of context. Bull World Health Organ. 2007;85(10):812–9.
25. Magaard JL, Seeralan T, Schulz H, Brütt AL. Factors associated with help-seeking behaviour among individuals with major depression: a systematic review. PLoS One. 2017;12(5):e0176730.
26. Goldberg DP, Huxley P. Common mental disorders: a bio-social model:

Tavistock/Routledge; 1992.
27. Goldberg D. Plato versus Aristotle: categorical and dimensional models for common mental disorders. Compr Psychiatry. 2000;41(2):8–13.
28. Das-Munshi J, Goldberg D, Bebbington PE, Bhugra DK, Brugha TS, Dewey ME, et al. Public health significance of mixed anxiety and depression: beyond current classification. Br J Psychiatry. 2008;192(3):171–7.
29. Jacob K, Prince M, Goldberg D. Confirmatory factor analysis of common mental disorders. Diagnostic Issues in Depression and Generalized Anxiety Disorder: Refining the Research Agenda for DSM-V. 2010.
30. Jacob K, Patel V. Classification of mental disorders: a global mental health perspective. Lancet. 2014;383(9926):1433–5.
31. Patel V. Rethinking mental health care: bridging the credibility gap. Intervention. 2014;12:15–20.
32. Roberts T, Rathod, S., Patel, V., Shidhaye, R. Review protocol: factors associated with health service utilisation for symptoms of common mental disorders PROSPERO international prospective register of systematic reviews: University of York: Centre for Reviews and Dissemination; 2016 [updated 07 July 20170e7 July 2017]. Available from: https://www.crd.york.ac.uk/PROSPERO/display_record.asp?ID=CRD42016046551.
33. Lewis G, Pelosi AJ, Araya R, Dunn G. Measuring psychiatric disorder in the community: a standardized assessment for use by lay interviewers. Psychol Med. 1992;22(02):465–86.
34. Patel V, Araya R, Chowdhary N, King M, Kirkwood B, Nayak S, et al. Detecting common mental disorders in primary care in India: a comparison of five screening questionnaires. Psychol Med. 2008;38(2):221–8.
35. Stansfeld S, Clark C, Bebbington P, King M, Jenkins R, Hinchliffe S. Common mental disorders. Mental health and wellbeing in England: Adult Psychiatric Morbidity Survey. 2014.
36. Franz A. Predictors of help-seeking behavior in emerging adults. 2012.
37. Pescosolido BA, Olafsdottir S. The Cultural Turn in Sociology: Can It Help Us Resolve an Age-Old Problem in Understanding Decision Making for Health Care? Sociological Forum 2010 Dec (Vol. 25, No. 4, pp. 655-676). Oxford: Blackwell Publishing Ltd.
38. Armitage CJ, Norman P, Alganem S, Conner M. Expectations are more predictive of behavior than behavioral intentions: evidence from two prospective studies. Ann Behav Med. 2015;49(2):239–46.
39. Chin WY, Chan KT, Lam CL, Lam T, Wan EY. Help-seeking intentions and subsequent 12-month mental health service use in Chinese primary care patients with depressive symptoms. BMJ Open. 2015;5(1): e006730.
40. Stefl ME, Prosperi DC. Barriers to mental health service utilization. Community Ment Health J. 1985;21(3):167–78.
41. Pluye P, Gagnon M-P, Griffiths F, Johnson-Lafleur J. A scoring system for appraising mixed methods research, and concomitantly appraising qualitative, quantitative and mixed methods primary studies in mixed studies reviews. Int J Nurs Stud. 2009;46(4):529–46.
42. Pace R, Pluye P, Bartlett G, Macaulay AC, Salsberg J, Jagosh J, et al. Testing the reliability and efficiency of the pilot mixed methods appraisal tool (MMAT) for systematic mixed studies review. Int J Nurs Stud. 2012;49(1):47–53.
43. Carroll C, Booth A, Leaviss J, Rick J. "Best fit" framework synthesis: refining the method. BMC Med Res Methodol. 2013;13(1):37.
44. Teo CH, Ng CJ, Booth A, White A. Barriers and facilitators to health screening in men: a systematic review. Soc Sci Med. 2016;165:168–76.
45. Coxon K, Chisholm A, Malouf R, Rowe R, Hollowell J. What influences birth place preferences, choices and decision-making amongst healthy women with straightforward pregnancies in the UK? A qualitative evidence synthesis using a 'best fit'framework approach. BMC Pregnancy Childbirth. 2017;17(1):103.
46. Iza M, Olfson M, Vermes D, Hoffer M, Wang S, Blanco C. Probability and predictors of first treatment contact for anxiety disorders in the United States: analysis of data from the National Epidemiologic Survey on alcohol and related conditions (NESARC). J Clin Psychiatry. 2013;74(11):1093–100.
47. Bucholz KK, Robins LN. Who talks to a doctor about existing depressive illness? J Affect Disord. 1987;12(3):241–50.
48. Gwynn RC, McQuistion HL, McVeigh KH, Garg RK, Frieden TR, Thorpe LE. Prevalence, diagnosis, and treatment of depression and generalized anxiety disorder in a diverse urban community. Psychiatr Serv. 2008;59(6):641–7.
49. Carragher N, Adamson G, Bunting B, McCann S. Treatment-seeking behaviours for depression in the general population: results from the National Epidemiologic Survey on alcohol and related conditions. J Affect Disord. 2010;121(1):59–67.
50. Fortney J, Rost K, Zhang M. A joint choice model of the decision to seek depression treatment and choice of provider sector. Med Care. 1998;36(3):307–20.
51. Issakidis C, Andrews G. Service utilisation for anxiety in an Australian community sample. Soc Psychiatry Psychiatr Epidemiol. 2002;37(4):153–63.
52. Mackenzie CS, Reynolds K, Cairney J, Streiner DL, Sareen J. Disorder-specific mental health service use for mood and anxiety disorders: associations with age, sex, and psychiatric comorbidity. Depress Anxiety. 2012;29(3):234–42.
53. Ojeda VD, McGuire TG. Gender and racial/ethnic differences in use of outpatient mental health and substance use services by depressed adults. Psychiatry Q. 2006;77(3):211–22.
54. Rost K, Zhang M, Fortney J, Smith J, Smith GR Jr. Rural-urban differences in depression treatment and suicidality. Med Care. 1998;36(7):1098–107.
55. Roy-Byrne PP, Joesch JM, Wang PS, Kessler RC. Low socioeconomic status and mental health care use among respondents with anxiety and depression in the NCS-R. Psychiatr Serv. 2009;60(9):1190–7.
56. Starkes JM, Poulin CC, Kisely SR. Unmet need for the treatment of depression in Atlantic Canada. Can J Psychiatry. 2005;50(10):580–90.
57. Lopes CS, Hellwig N, Silva GA E, Menezes PR. Inequities in access to depression treatment: results of the Brazilian National Health Survey–PNS. Int J Equity Health. 2016;15(1):154.
58. Olfson M, Klerman G. Depressive symptoms and mental health service utilization in a community sample. Soc Psychiatry Psychiatr Epidemiol. 1992;27(4):161–7.
59. Chartrand H, Robinson J, Bolton JM. A longitudinal population-based study exploring treatment utilization and suicidal ideation and behavior in major depressive disorder. J Affect Disord. 2012;141(2):237–45.
60. González HM, Vega WA, Williams DR, Tarraf W, West BT, Neighbors HW. Depression care in the United States: too little for too few. Arch Gen Psychiatry. 2010;67(1):37–46.
61. Schomerus G, Appel K, Meffert PJ, Luppa M, Andersen RM, Grabe HJ, et al. Personality-related factors as predictors of help-seeking for depression: a population-based study applying the behavioral model of health services use. Soc Psychiatry Psychiatr Epidemiol. 2013;48(11):1809–17.
62. Hailemariam S, Tessema F, Asefa M, Tadesse H, Tenkolu G. The prevalence of depression and associated factors in Ethiopia: findings from the National Health Survey. Int J Ment Heal Syst. 2012;6(1):23.
63. Wang PS, Berglund P, Kessler RC. Recent care of common mental disorders in the United States. J Gen Intern Med. 2000;15(5):284–92.
64. Seedat S, Williams DR, Herman AA, Moomal H, Williams SL, Jackson PB, et al. Mental health service use among South Africans for mood, anxiety and substance use disorders. S Afr Med J. 2009;99(5):346–52.
65. Gabilondo A, Rojas-Farreras S, Rodráguez A, Ferníndez A, Pinto-Meza A, Vilagut G, et al. Use of primary and specialized mental health care for a major depressive episode in Spain by ESEMeD respondents. Psychiatr Serv. 2011;62(2):152–61.
66. Boerema AM, Kleiboer A, Beekman AT, van Zoonen K, Dijkshoorn H, Cuijpers P. Determinants of help-seeking behavior in depression: a cross-sectional study. BMC Psychiatry. 2016;16(1):78.
67. Chen J. Seeking help for psychological distress in urban China. J Comm Psychology. 2012;40(3):319–41.
68. Vasiliadis H-M, Lesage A, Adair C, Wang PS, Kessler RC. Do Canada and the United States differ in prevalence of depression and utilization of services? Psychiatr Serv. 2007;58(1):63–71.
69. Rafful C, Medina-Mora ME, Borges G, Benjet C, Orozco R. Depression, gender, and the treatment gap in Mexico. J Affect Disord. 2012;138(1):165–9.
70. Burnett-Zeigler I, Zivin K, Islam K, Ilgen MA. Longitudinal predictors of first time depression treatment utilization among adults with depressive disorders. Soc Psychiatry Psychiatr Epidemiol. 2012;47(10): 1617–25.
71. Galbaud du Fort G, Newman S, Boothroyd L, Bland R. Treatment seeking for depression: role of depressive symptoms and comorbid psychiatric diagnoses. J Affect Disord. 1999;52(1):31–40.
72. Vesga-López O, Schneier F, Wang S, Heimberg R, Liu S-M, Hasin DS, et al. Gender differences in generalized anxiety disorder: results from the National Epidemiologic Survey on alcohol and related conditions (NESARC). J Clin Psychiatry. 2008;69(10):1606.
73. Wallerblad A, Möller J, Forsell Y. Care-seeking pattern among persons with depression and anxiety: a population-based study in Sweden. Int J Family Med. 2012;2012:895425.

74. Angst J, Gamma A, Clarke D, Ajdacic-Gross V, Rössler W, Regier D. Subjective distress predicts treatment seeking for depression, bipolar, anxiety, panic, neurasthenia and insomnia severity spectra. Acta Psychiatr Scand. 2010;122(6):488–98.
75. Andersson LM, Schierenbeck I, Strumpher J, Krantz G, Topper K, Backman G, et al. Help-seeking behaviour, barriers to care and experiences of care among persons with depression in eastern cape, South Africa. J Affect Disord. 2013;151(2):439–48.
76. Hamalainen J, Isometsa E, Sihvo S, Pirkola S, Kiviruusu O. Use of health services for major depressive and anxiety disorders in Finland. Depress Anxiety. 2008;25(1):27–37.
77. ten Have M, de Graaf R, Vollebergh W, Beekman A. What depressive symptoms are associated with the use of care services?: results from the Netherlands mental health survey and incidence study (NEMESIS). J Affect Disord. 2004;80(2):239–48.
78. Mojtabai R, Olfson M. Treatment seeking for depression in Canada and the United States. Psychiatr Serv. 2006;57(5):631–9.
79. Sussman LK, Robins LN, Earls F. Treatment-seeking for depression by black and white Americans. Soc Sci Med. 1987;24(3):187–96.
80. Alegría M, Chatterji P, Wells K, Cao Z, Chen CN, Takeuchi D, et al. Disparity in depression treatment among racial and ethnic minority populations in the United States. Psychiatr Serv. 2008;59(11):1264–72.
81. Keyes KM, Hatzenbuehler ML, Alberti P, Narrow WE, Grant BF, Hasin DS. Service utilization differences for Axis I psychiatric and substance use disorders between white and black adults. Psychiatr Serv. 2008;59(8):893–901.
82. Bauldry S, Szaflarski M. Immigrant-based disparities in mental health care utilization. Socius. 2017;3:2378023116685718.
83. Ault-Brutus AA. Changes in racial-ethnic disparities in use and adequacy of mental health care in the United States, 1990–2003. Psychiatr Serv. 2012; 63(6):531–40.
84. Lee SY, Martins SS, Keyes KM, Lee HB. Mental health service use by persons of Asian ancestry with DSM-IV mental disorders in the United States. Psychiatr Serv. 2011;62(10):1180–6.
85. Lee SY, Xue Q-l, Spira AP, Lee HB. Racial and ethnic differences in depressive subtypes and access to mental health care in the United States. J Affect Disord. 2014;155:130–7.
86. Ault-Brutus A, Alegria M. Racial/ethnic differences in perceived need for mental health care and disparities in use of care among those with perceived need in 1990–1992 and 2001–2003. Ethn Health. 2016;23(2): 142-57.
87. Hankerson SH, Fenton MC, Geier TJ, Keyes KM, Weissman MM, Hasin DS. Racial differences in symptoms, comorbidity, and treatment for major depressive disorder among black and white adults. J Natl Med Assoc. 2011; 103(7):576–84.
88. Pirkis J, Burgess P, Meadows G, Dunt D. Access to Australian mental health care by people from non-English-speaking backgrounds. Aust N Z J Psychiatry. 2001;35(2):174–82.
89. Chen L-Y, Crum RM, Martins SS, Kaufmann CN, Strain EC, Mojtabai R. Service use and barriers to mental health care among adults with major depression and comorbid substance dependence. Psychiatr Serv. 2013;64(9):863–70.
90. Robinson JA, Sareen J, Cox BJ, Bolton JM. Correlates of self-medication for anxiety disorders: results from the National Epidemiolgic Survey on alcohol and related conditions. J Nerv Ment Dis. 2009;3(12):873–8.
91. Bucholz KK, Dinwiddie SH. Influence of nondepressive psychiatric symptoms on whether patients tell a doctor about depression. Am J Psychiatry. 1989; 146(5):640.
92. Vigod SN, Levitt AJ. Seasonal severity of depressive symptoms as a predictor of health service use in a community-based sample. J Psychiatr Res. 2011; 45(5):612–8.
93. Nakash O, Levav I, Aguilar-Gaxiola S, Alonso J, Andrade LH, Angermeyer MC, et al. Comorbidity of common mental disorders with cancer and their treatment gap: findings from the world mental health surveys. Psycho-Oncology. 2014;23:40–51.
94. Demyttenaere K, Bonnewyn A, Bruffaerts R, Brugha T, De Graaf R, Alonso J. Comorbid painful physical symptoms and depression: prevalence, work loss, and help seeking. J Affect Disord. 2006;92(2):185–93.
95. Demyttenaere K, Bonnewyn A, Bruffaerts R, De Graaf R, Haro JM, Alonso J. Comorbid painful physical symptoms and anxiety: prevalence, work loss and help-seeking. J Affect Disord. 2008;109(3):264–72.
96. Tempier R, Meadows GN, Vasiliadis H-M, Mosier KE, Lesage A, Stiller A, et al. Mental disorders and mental health care in Canada and Australia: comparative epidemiological findings. Soc Psychiatry Psychiatr Epidemiol. 2009;44(1):63–72.
97. Tempier R, Vasiliadis H-M, Gilbert F, Demyttenaere K, Bruffaerts R, Lépine J-P, et al. Comparing mental health of francophones in Canada, France, and Belgium: 12-month and lifetime rates of mental health service use (part 2). Can J Psychiatry. 2010;55(5):295–304.
98. Li W, Dorstyn DS, Denson LA. Predictors of mental health service use by young adults: a systematic review. Psychiatr Serv. 2016;67(9):946–56.
99. Twomey CD, Baldwin DS, Hopfe M, Cieza A. A systematic review of the predictors of health service utilisation by adults with mental disorders in the UK. BMJ Open. 2015;5(7):e007575.
100. Leaf PJ, Bruce ML, Tischler GL, Freeman DH Jr, Weissman MM, Myers JK. Factors affecting the utilization of specialty and general medical mental health services. Med Care. 1988;26:9–26.
101. Padgett D, Struening EL, Andrews H. Factors affecting the use of medical, mental health, alcohol, and drug treatment services by homeless adults. Med Care. 1990;28:805–21.
102. Parslow RA, Jorm AF. Who uses mental health services in Australia? An analysis of data from the National Survey of mental health and wellbeing. Aust N Z J Psychiatry. 2000;34:997–1008.
103. Graham A, Hasking P, Brooker J, Clarke D, Meadows G. Mental health service use among those with depression: an exploration using Andersen's behavioral model of health service use. J Affect Disord. 2017;208:170–6.
104. Andrade LH, Alonso J, Mneimneh Z, Wells J, Al-Hamzawi A, Borges G, et al. Barriers to mental health treatment: results from the WHO world mental health surveys. Psychol Med. 2014;44(06):1303–17.
105. Olfson M, Marcus SC, Tedeschi M, Wan GJ. Continuity of antidepressant treatment for adults with depression in the United States. Am J Psychiatr. 2006;163(1):101–8.
106. Baekeland F, Lundwall L. Dropping out of treatment: a critical review. Psychol Bull. 1975;82(5):738.
107. Garfield SL. Research on client variables in psychotherapy. 1994.
108. Barrett MS, Chua W-J, Crits-Christoph P, Gibbons MB, Thompson D. Early withdrawal from mental health treatment: Implications for psychotherapy practice. Psychotherapy: Theory, Research, Practice, Training. 2008;45(2):247.
109. Wierzbicki M, Pekarik G. A meta-analysis of psychotherapy dropout. Professional Psychology: Research and Practice. 1993;24(2):190.
110. Cohen A, Gilman SE, Houck PR, Szanto K, Reynolds CF. Socioeconomic status and anxiety as predictors of antidepressant treatment response and suicidal ideation in older adults. Soc Psychiatry Psychiatr Epidemiol. 2009;44(4):272.
111. Jain FA, Hunter AM, Brooks JO, Leuchter AF. Predictive socioeconomic and clinical profiles of antidepressant response and remission. Depress Anxiety. 2013;30(7):624–30.
112. Evans-Lacko S, Aguilar-Gaxiola S, Al-Hamzawi A, Alonso J, Benjet C, Bruffaerts R, Chiu WT, Florescu S, de Girolamo G, Gureje O, Haro JM. Socio-economic variations in the mental health treatment gap for people with anxiety, mood, and substance use disorders: results from the WHO World Mental Health (WMH) surveys. Psychol Med. 2018;48(9):1560-71.
113. Mechanic D. Is the prevalence of mental disorders a good measure of the need for services? Health Aff. 2003;22(5):8–20.
114. Funk M, Saraceno B, Drew N, Lund C, Grigg M. Mental health policy and plans: promoting an optimal mix of services in developing countries. Int J Ment Health. 2004;33(2):4–16.
115. Andrews G, Issakidis C, Carter G. Shortfall in mental health service utilisation. Br J Psychiatry. 2001;179(5):417–25.
116. Oliver A, Mossialos E. Equity of access to health care: outlining the foundations for action. J Epidemiol Community Health. 2004;58(8):655–8.
117. Hernandez M, Nesman T, Mowery D, Acevedo-Polakovich ID, Callejas LM. Cultural competence: a literature review and conceptual model for mental health services. Psychiatr Serv. 2009;60(8):1046–50.
118. Rochlen AB, Hoyer WD. Marketing mental health to men: theoretical and practical considerations. J Clin Psychol. 2005;61(6):675–84.
119. Griner D, Smith TB. Culturally adapted mental health intervention: A meta-analytic review. Psychother Theory Res Pract Train. 2006;43(4):531.
120. Hammer JH, Vogel DL. Men's help seeking for depression: the efficacy of a male-sensitive brochure about counseling. Couns Psychol. 2010;38(2):296–313.

121. Fortney JC, Harman JS, Xu S, Dong F. The association between rural residence and the use, type, and quality of depression care. J Rural Health. 2010;26(3):205–13.
122. Thornicroft G, Tansella M. The balanced care model for global mental health. Psychol Med. 2013;43(4):849–63.
123. Settlement UNCfH. Urbanization: Facts and Figures 2001 [cited 2017 04/08/2017]. Available from: http://www.un.org/ga/Istanbul+5/bg10.htm.
124. Peters DH, Garg A, Bloom G, Walker DG, Brieger WR, Hafizur RM. Poverty and access to health care in developing countries. Ann N Y Acad Sci. 2008; 1136(1):161–71.
125. Obrist B, Iteba N, Lengeler C, Makemba A, Mshana C, Nathan R, et al. Access to health care in contexts of livelihood insecurity: a framework for analysis and action. PLoS Med. 2007;4(10):e308.
126. Philo C. Across the water: reviewing geographical studies of asylums and other mental health facilities. Health Place. 1997;3(2):73–89.
127. Shannon GW, Bashshur RL, Lovett JE. Distance and the use of mental health services. The Milbank Quarterly. 1986:302–30.
128. Zulian G, Donisi V, Secco G, Pertile R, Tansella M, Amaddeo F. How are caseload and service utilisation of psychiatric services influenced by distance? A geographical approach to the study of community-based mental health services. Soc Psychiatry Psychiatr Epidemiol. 2011;46(9):881–91.
129. Sohler KB, Clapis JA. Jarvis' law and the planning of mental health services. HSMHA health reports. 1972;87(1):75.
130. Davey S, Giles G. Spatial factors in mental health care in Tasmania. Soc Sci Med Med Geogr. 1979;13(2):87–94.
131. Hunter JM, Shannon GW, Sambrook SL. Rings of madness: service areas of 19th century asylums in North America. Soc Sci Med. 1986;23(10):1033–50.

14

Evaluation of attitudes and knowledge toward mental disorders in a sample of the Chinese population using a web-based approach

Juan Li[1], Meng-meng Zhang[1], Lin Zhao[1], Wen-qiang Li[1,3], Jun-lin Mu[1,4] and Zhao-hui Zhang[1,2,3,4*]

Abstract

Background: People with mental disorders often encounter stigmatizing attitudes related to their conditions. Stigma often represents one of the critical obstacles that stand in the way of delivering mental health care. The main aim of the study was to assess the knowledge and attitudes toward mental disorders in a sample of the Chinese population; furthermore, we also aimed to identify and explore the socio-demographic characteristics associated with specific knowledge and attitudes towards psychiatric disorders.

Methods: A cross-sectional survey was created and delivered through an Internet chat application over the period June–December 2017. The Mental Health Knowledge Questionnaire and the Perceived Devaluation and Discrimination Scale were used to evaluate the participants' mental health knowledge and attitudes toward mental disorders.

Results: A total of 1087 participants were recruited in for our survey. The mean score of the MHKQ and PDD were (15.89 ± 2.69) and (33.77 ± 6.66), respectively. Univariate analyses showed that young people and rural residents tended to show more positive attitudes toward mental disorders with respect to older people and urban residents ($P < 0.05$). People with higher education levels, those who had contact with people with mental disorders, and those who learned about mental disorders by personal encounter resulted to have had higher MHKQ scores ($P < 0.05$).

Conclusions: In our sample of the Chinese population, negative attitudes toward mental disorders were often reported. General education programs may not be an effective way to decrease stigma, while anti-stigma campaigns targeted for specific groups, such as urban residents and the older people, should be carried out in the future in China.

Keywords: Mental health knowledge, Stigma, Discrimination, Mental disorders, China

Background

Although there are now a variety of effective treatments for mental disorders, still a significant number of people do not receive proper treatment for mental disorders [1]. Even those who receive care and assistance from mental health services often tend to exhibit a significant delay between symptoms' onset and seeking treatment and this can exacerbate their conditions and increase the psychological and financial burdens [2]. The fear of being discriminated against has been reported to play a significant role in creating barriers and increasing the delay in seeking treatment [3]. Stigma and discrimination are widely experienced by people with mental disorders in many domains of their daily life, such as in employment, social activities, personal relationships, housing, marriage, and so on [4–8]. In China, words like "violent," "crazy," "strange", and "useless" are often used to describe people with mental disorders [9, 10]. Stigma and discrimination surrounding mental disorders represent not only factors that hamper treatment-seeking [11], but may also delay the healing process for people with mental disorders [12] and prevent people with mental disorders from achieving their social rights and full participation in the life of their community.

* Correspondence: zzhui816@126.com
[1]The Second Affiliated Hospital of Xinxiang Medical University, 388# Jianshe Road, Muye, Xinxiang, China
[2]Xinxiang Medical University, 601# Jinsui Road, Hongqi, Xinxiang, China
Full list of author information is available at the end of the article

Moreover, the family members of people with mental disorders are often blamed by the public [13]. Empirical evidence showed that families of people with mental disorders are likely to ignore the problem when their family members experience discrimination: they may hide them from public life, delay treatment seeking, or even reject professional help. Such attitudes and behaviors may determine a pejorative illness course and increase the psychological and financial burdens on the families [14–16].

In order to reduce the treatment gap and provide more consistent and accessible mental health services, the World Health Organization (WHO) has encouraged countries to integrate mental health services into their primary care systems. However, negative attitudes toward mental disorders among the general population are likely to represent an obstacle to the development of more efficient community mental health services [17].

Additionally, the general public could, through greater social engagement and more acceptance of mental disorders, play an essential role in rehabilitating the mentally ill. This is no easy task, since people with mental disorders have often been labeled as "violent" and "dangerous", and the attitudes of the general public have contributed to exacerbating the conditions of people with mental disorders [18].

Thornicroft et al. [19] defined stigma as an overarching term that refers to three main elements: problems of knowledge (ignorance), problems of attitude (prejudice), and problems of behavior (discrimination). It has been reported that lack of accurate mental health knowledge may be one of the leading factors that may contribute to stereotyping people with mental disorders [20]. However, it has also been found that health professionals, who are supposed to have greater knowledge concerning mental health issues with respect to the general population, often have more negative attitudes toward mental disorders than the general public [21–23]. This finding contradicts a common assumption that greater knowledge of mental disorders results in less of a discriminatory attitude, and thus it throws into question the, supposedly positive, relationship between mental health knowledge and discriminatory attitudes.

The main aims of this study were to evaluate attitudes and knowledge about mental disorders in a sample of the Chinese general population and to explore their relationships with socio-demographic characteristics. Results from this study could yield some applications: first, it could help in designing programs that would aim to reduce public stigma against mental disorders; second, it could provide guidance for the government to undertake further strategic action.

Methods

Participants

A "snowball" sampling method was used to recruit participants. A digital version of a self-made schedule and of two standardized questionnaires was sent to 50 people known to the study authors (including families, friends, and other acquaintances), who previously agreed to participate in the study and to share the digital questionnaires through the Internet chat application "We-Chat", which has over 800 million active members in China. A standardized statement accompanying the questionnaire encouraged all the participants to transmit the electronic questionnaire to their friends or family members. Participants were informed, at the beginning of the survey, that expression "mental disorders" in the questionnaire referred to schizophrenia, depression, and bipolar disorder. All potential participants were also informed that they had a chance to win a raffle prize as a reward.

Participants were finally asked to provide anonymous informed consent in electronic format, before taking part in the survey. The survey was conducted from June to December 2017. The study protocol was approved by the Research Ethics Committee of the Second Affiliated Hospital of Xinxiang Medical University.

Instruments

A self-made questionnaire was used to collect participants' basic demographic data (including age, gender, level of education, and place of residence).

The Mental Health Knowledge Questionnaire (MHKQ) was developed to evaluate public knowledge and awareness of mental health by the Chinese Ministry of Health (MOH) in 2009. It contains 20 self-administered items. Items 1–16 (the first section) require participants to select "true," "false," or "unknown" about statements concerning mental health. For items 1, 3, 5, 7, 8, 11, 12, 15 and 16, a "true" answer corresponded to a 1-point score, while a "false" or "unknown" answer corresponded to score of 0. By contrast, for items 2, 4, 6, 9, 10, 13 and 14, a "false" answer gave a score of 1, while "true" or "unknown" answers corresponded to score of 0. Finally, items 17–20 (the second section) are statements concerning previous knowledge about the "four mental health promotion days". Total scores range from 0 to 20, with higher scores indicating greater knowledge of mental health issues. The Cronbach's coefficient of MHKQ was reported to be 0.61 [24].

The Perceived Devaluation and Discrimination Scale (PDD) [25] was used to assess the degree of stigmatizing attitudes toward people with mental disorders. It contains 12 items and each item is rated on a 5-point scale, ranging from 1 (totally agree) to 5 (totally disagree). Items 1, 2, 3, 4, 8 and 10 required reverse scoring. Total scores ranged from 12 to 60, with higher scores indicating lower levels of stigma. The Chinese version of the PDD has been reported to have strong internal consistency (Cronbach's $\alpha = 0.70$).

Participants were also requested to answer three additional questions concerning their source of information about mental disorders (i.e., portrayals in mass media vs. direct encounter), level of contact with mentally ill people, and their attitude toward psychotropic drugs (with the following four response options: "Effective", "They make people worse", "Ineffective" and "Likely to lead to dependency").

Data analysis

Descriptive statistics were used to explore basic socio-demographic data. The scores obtained from PDD and MHKQ were then compared among sample subgroups, created according to demographic characteristics, using one-way analysis of variance. The demographic information used to create subgroups included gender, age, education, place of residence, sources of information, and level of contact with people with mental disorders. The correlation between knowledge about mental disorders and attitudes toward those disorders was examined by the Pearson's correlation coefficient. For all statistical analyses SPSS v18 was used and the level of significance was set at $P < 0.05$.

Results

Sample characteristics

A total of 1104 participants finished the questionnaires, but 15 participants were excluded because they reported having been diagnosed with mental disorders in the past and two participants were excluded because they were below legal age for providing informed consent (i.e., 16 years). A total of 1087 participants were finally included in our survey and their mean (±SD) age was 33.93 (±9.76) years, within a range of 16–67 years. Our participants were predominantly female ($N = 693$; 63.8%). The socio-demographic characteristics are summarized in Table 1.

Contact with and general knowledge about mental disorders

The majority of our respondents declared previous contact with people suffering from mental disorders (64.9%; $n = 706$), although 59.7% ($n = 649$) of participants reported that they learned about mental disorders from portrayals in mass media, while 40.3% ($n = 438$) had personal encounters with mentally ill people as a primary source of knowledge about mental disorders. With respect to the participants' attitudes toward psychotropic drugs, 66.9% ($n = 727$) of them considered them effective, 3.7% ($n = 40$) of participants believed that they would lead to a worse outcome, 25.8% ($n = 280$) envisaged the risk to lead to dependency, and 3.7% ($n = 40$) considered them "ineffective".

Table 1 Characteristics of the participants ($n = 1087$)

Variable	N	%
Gender		
Male	394	36.2
Female	693	63.8
Age (years)		
16–24	114	10.5
25–34	558	51.3
35–44	235	21.6
45 and above	180	16.6
Education		
Junior high school or less	97	8.9
Senior high school	160	14.7
College degree/undergraduate	608	55.9
Postgraduate or above	222	20.4
Place of residence		
Urban area	901	82.9
Rural area	186	17.1

Responses frequencies for the PDD and MHKQ

The mean total score for the PDD was 33.77 (SD = 6.66), and scores ranged from 12 to 57. The answer for each item is displayed in Table 2.

As for the MHKQ, the total scores ranged from 5 to 20 with a mean score of 15.89 (±2.69). The mean score for the first section (true vs. false questions) was 13.50 (± = 2.17), and 159 (14.6%) participants got a score of 16.

For the second section of MHKQ, there were 258 (23.7%) participants who recognized all four mental health promotion days. The rate of correct responses is displayed in Table 3.

PDD and demographic variables

Table 4 shows the mean PDD scores for different subgroups of participants, stratified according to basic socio-demographic characteristics. There were statistically significant differences in the scores that matched with age and place of residence. Analysis of variance showed that those under 25 years old scored higher than those above that age, but the difference was significant only with respect to those aged 35–44 years ($F = 5.37$, $P = 0.001$). Participants from rural areas scored significantly higher than those from cities ($t = -2.42$, $P = 0.016$). Differences in the stigma level according to participants' gender, educational level, sources of information about mental disorders, and contact levels with people with mental disorders were not statistically significant.

MHKQ and demographic variables

Table 5 shows the mean MHKQ scores for different demographic groups of participants. The impact of

Table 2 The results of PDD (n = 1087)

Items	Strongly agree (n, %)	Agree (n, %)	Unsure (n, %)	Disagree (n, %)	Strongly disagree (n, %)
1. Most people would accept a former mental patient as a close friend.	49 (4.5)	149 (13.7)	545 (50.1)	253 (23.3)	91 (8.4)
2. Most people believe that a person who has been in a mental hospital is just as intelligent as the average person.	123 (11.3)	300 (27.6)	418 (38.5)	187 (17.2)	59 (5.4)
3. Most people believe that a former mental patient is just as trustworthy as the average citizen.	92 (8.5)	259 (23.8)	422 (38.8)	249 (22.9)	65 (6.0)
4. Most people would accept a fully recovered former mental patient as a teacher of young children in a public school.	98 (9.0)	285 (26.2)	286 (26.3)	258 (23.7)	160 (14.7)
5. Most people believe that entering a mental hospital is a sign of personal failure.	23 (2.1)	120 (11.0)	213 (19.6)	357 (32.8)	374 (34.4)
6. Most people would not hire a former mental patient to take care of their children, even if he or she had been well for some time.	360 (33.1)	421 (38.7)	169 (15.5)	96 (8.8)	41 (3.8)
7. Most people think less of a person who has been in a mental hospital.	116 (10.7)	397 (36.5)	256 (23.6)	233 (21.4)	85 (7.8)
8. Most employers will hire a former mental patient if he or she is qualified for the job.	73 (6.7)	198 (18.2)	455 (41.9)	268 (24.7)	93 (8.6)
9. Most employers will pass over the application of a former mental patient in favor of another applicant.	199 (18.3)	496 (45.5)	256 (23.6)	101 (9.3)	35 (3.2)
10. Most people in my community would treat a former mental patient just as they treat anyone.	83 (7.6)	311 (28.6)	440 (40.5)	209 (19.2)	44 (4.0)
11. Most young women would be reluctant to date a man who has been hospitalized for serious mental disorder.	365 (33.6)	443 (40.8)	208 (19.1)	53 (4.9)	18 (1.7)
12. Once they know a person was in a mental hospital, most people will take his or her opinions less seriously.	124 (11.4)	430 (39.6)	342 (31.5)	162 (14.9)	29 (2.7)

participants' ages, educational level, areas of residence, sources of information about mental disorders, and level of contact with mentally ill people was significant over the MHKQ scoring. The analysis of variance showed that those aged 25–44 years had significantly higher MHKQ total scores than those above 45 years old. Participants with higher education levels had higher MHKQ scores (F = 65.72, P < 0.001). Urban residents had higher MHKQ scores than rural residents (t = 7.32, P < 0.001). Those who had previous contact with people with mental disorders (t = – 4.85, P < 0.001) and who had learned about mental disorders with personal encounters (t = – 2.10, P = 0.036) had higher MHKQ scores.

The relationship between PDD and MHKQ

We didn't find any statistically significant relationship between the total scores of the PDD and MHKQ scales (r = – 0.032, P = 0.293).

Discussion

To the best of our knowledge, this is the first study to evaluate the general public knowledge of and attitudes toward mental disorders through a web-based survey in China. Although our samples couldn't represent the entire Chinese population, we can still provide a reliable account of attitudes and knowledge toward mental health in China. Compared with previous studies [26–28], our results showed that mental health knowledge has improved recently, while most people's attitudes toward mental disorders are still negative. Hence, it is vital to further discuss how to improve mental health knowledge and what might be the impact of such programs on people's attitudes toward mental disorders.

In terms of knowledge on mental disorders and stigmatizing attitudes, we didn't find any differences with respect to participants' gender, in line with previous studies [20, 24]. However, there were also studies that investigated such measures in medical students and mental health staff that demonstrated that women tend to have greater knowledge about mental health and that they were more willing to interact with people with mental disorders [29, 30]. In our survey, we did not report such significant differences and thus this issue should be further explored in order to properly discuss the need of developing gender-specific anti-stigma interventions in China.

In contrast to other studies [26], our study also found that residents in rural areas had more positive attitudes toward people with mental disorders than those who lived in urban areas. One possible explanation for this evidence is that rural communities may be more tolerant of unusual behaviors, typical of people with mental disorders. However, evidence from previous studies provided rather mixed results. Girma et al. [20] found that living in rural places was the strongest predictor of families holding stigmatizing attitudes toward their mentally ill relatives. Authors reported that rural

Table 3 The correct response rate of MHKQ ($n = 1087$)

Item	n	Percent (%)
1. Mental health is a component of health. (true)	1047	96.3
2. Mental disorders are caused by incorrect thinking. (false)	596	54.8
3. Many people have mental problems but do not realise it. (true)	1052	96.8
4. All mental disorders are caused by external stressors. (false)	653	60.1
5. Components of mental health include normal intelligence, stable mood, a positive attitude, quality interpersonal relationship and adaptability. (true)	1035	95.2
6. Most mental disorders cannot be cured. (false)	742	68.3
7. Psychological or psychiatric services should be sought if one suspects the presence of psychological problems or a mental disorder. (true)	969	89.1
8. Psychological problems can occur at almost any age. (true)	1049	96.5
9. Mental disorders and psychological problems cannot be prevented. (false)	825	75.9
10. Even for severe mental disorders (eg, schizophrenia), medications should be taken for a given period of time only; there is no need to take them for a long time. (false)	887	81.6
11. Positive attitudes, good interpersonal relationships and healthy life style can help maintain mental health. (true)	1046	96.2
12. Individuals with a family history of mental disorders are at a higher risk for psychological problems and mental disorders. (true)	981	90.2
13. Psychological problems in adolescents do not influence academic grades. (false)	964	88.7
14. Middle-aged or elderly individuals are unlikely to develop psychological problems and mental disorders. (false)	957	88.0
15. Individuals with a bad temperament are more likely to have mental problems. (true)	838	77.1
16. Mental problems or disorders may occur when an individual is under psychological stress facing major life events (eg, death of family members). (true)	1031	94.8
17. Have you heard about International Mental Health Day? (yes)	613	56.4
18. Have you heard about the International Day against Drug Abuse and Illicit Drug Trafficking? (yes)	947	87.1
19. Have you heard about the International Suicide Prevention Day? (yes)	345	31.7
20. Have you heard about World Sleep Day? (yes)	694	63.8

residents showed significantly higher stigmatizing attitudes than urban residents, perhaps because of lower mental health literacy. However, we didn't find a significant relationship between mental health literacy and discriminatory attitudes.

Our analyses did not yield any significant relationship between educational level and discrimination, but we found that participants with higher levels of education were more likely to have greater mental health knowledge. Some studies reported that lower education levels were more strongly associated with negative attitudes toward mental disorders [31, 32], but others found the inverse to be also true [33, 34]. These studies indicated that highly educated people had higher expectations of social responsibility and functioning than those with less education, and that they associated people with mental disorders with lower levels of responsibility and functioning.

Today, more and more educational initiatives and informational campaigns have been implemented to improve the public's mental health knowledge, in order to change negative opinions toward people with mental disorders. Some of the interventions yielded positive results, as expected [35, 36]. But in our study, we didn't find any relationship between mental health knowledge and stigmatizing attitudes. In accordance with other studies, our data tend to support the idea that the public's mental health knowledge might not represent a highly effective remedy against discrimination [37]. As some studies have shown, health care staff with supposedly greater knowledge about mental health issues are likely to hold more negative attitudes toward mental disorders than the general population [21, 22]. Moreover, many people with mental disorders have been unfairly treated by health professionals when they have sought help for medical diseases [23]. Altogether, these findings suggest that other ways to decrease stigma against mental disorders are still to be pursued.

Exposing the general public to people with mental disorders has been a method used by many anti-stigma campaigns as an effective way to improve attitudes towards mental disorders among the target group [36, 38–40]. However, in our survey we didn't find any significant difference in the attitudes of subgroups who had or had no previous contact with people with mental disorders. Participants who reported having had contact with people with mental disorders also showed greater mental health knowledge. Once again, such findings are in line with the idea that there is no correlation between knowledge of mental disorders and positive attitudes towards them.

In our study, while 64.9% of participants reported having had direct contact with people with mental disorders, most of our respondents (59.7%) acquired their understanding of mental disorders from portrayals in mass media. For people who had no direct contact with people suffering from mental disorders, mass media may be a relevant source of information which may strongly influence their perceptions and attitudes about mental disorders. However, mass media often portray people with mental disorders as dangerous, strange, unpredictable, and violent [9], which could further lead the general public to fear people with mental disorders, cause

Table 4 Associations between PDD and demographic variables

Item	n	Mean score	t/F	P
Gender			0.67	0.500
Male	394	33.96 ± 7.24		
Female	693	33.66 ± 6.31		
Age (years)			5.37	0.001
16–24	114	35.11 ± 5.48		
25–34	558	34.03 ± 6.69		
35–44	235	32.37 ± 7.11		
45 and above	180	33.92 ± 6.39		
Education			0.13	0.942
Junior high school or less	97	33.90 ± 6.76		
Senior high school	160	33.82 ± 6.77		
College/undergraduate	608	33.83 ± 6.58		
Postgraduate or above	222	33.52 ± 6.79		
Place of residence			−2.42	0.016
Urban area	901	33.56 ± 6.74		
Rural area	186	34.78 ± 6.20		
Sources of information about mental disorders			1.31	0.192
Mass media	649	33.99 ± 6.44		
Personal encounters	438	33.44 ± 6.97		
Contact level			1.40	0.161
No	381	34.15 ± 6.54		
Yes	706	33.56 ± 6.72		

people with mental disorders to feel isolated and rejected, create greater discrimination and prevent people with mental disorders from fully integrating into society [41]. Interventions aimed at changing portrayals of mental disorders in mass media might represent a valid means to induce a significant positive change in public attitudes toward people with mental disorders.

Finally, we didn't find an increased risk for stigmatizing attitudes except for the age and place of residence factors. A German study found that gender, age, education level, and place of residence only accounted for 1.4% of the variance [42].

There are some limitations to our study. First, the survey was based on a cross-sectional sampling strategy and on self-reported measures, so it might be difficult to make reliable inferences about the correlations or causal relationships between attitudes and knowledge. Second, since our study was a web-based survey, we couldn't provide the participants with in-person explanations of the questions and this might influence their responses. On the other hand, using a web-based strategy allowed participants to participate in the study without feeling socially pressured or guided to respond in one way or another. Finally, since included participants represented a convenience sample, it could not fully represent the Chinese population. The latter consideration coupled with some imbalance in terms of socio-demographic characteristics of our sample (e.g., greater ratio of female respondents) might imply that our study should be replicated in a larger and more representative sample of the Chinese population.

Conclusions

Our findings suggested that overall mental health knowledge may have improved in the Chinese population over the years, but that most Chinese people still hold negative attitudes toward mental disorders. According to our data, this tendency seems to be more relevant in urban areas. It is important to carry out anti-stigma campaigns for the future progress of mental health in China. Although some campaigns aim to improve the public's mental health knowledge, it is still a matter of open debate whether increasing mental health knowledge may actually decrease people's discriminatory attitudes toward people with mental disorders or not. Finally, although we did not find a positive correlation between participants' levels of

Table 5 Associations between MHKQ and demographic variables

Item	n	Mean score	t/F	*P*
Gender			−1.02	0.310
Male	394	15.78 ± 2.80		
Female	693	15.95 ± 2.63		
Age (years)			4.56	0.003
16–24	114	15.82 ± 2.16		
25–34	558	15.93 ± 2.86		
35–44	235	16.27 ± 2.52		
45 and above	180	15.30 ± 2.61		
Education			65.72	< 0.001
Junior high school or less	97	13.36 ± 2.28		
Senior high school	160	14.69 ± 2.36		
College/undergraduate	608	16.17 ± 2.51		
Postgraduate or above	222	17.08 ± 2.58		
Place of residence			7.32	< 0.001
Urban area	901	16.15 ± 2.62		
Rural area	186	14.60 ± 2.65		
Sources of information about mental disorders			−2.10	0.036
Mass media	649	15.74 ± 2.54		
Personal encounters	438	16.10 ± 2.89		
Contact level			−4.85	< 0.001
No	381	15.35 ± 2.56		
Yes	706	16.18 ± 2.72		

contact with people with mental illness and their attitudes toward people with mental disorders, we did find similar evidence in other studies. Thus, we should further explore the hypothesis that more frequent contact with people with mental disorders may change negative attitudes towards mental disorders.

Abbreviations

MHKQ: The Mental Health Knowledge Questionnaire (MHKQ); MOH: Ministry of Health; PDD: Perceived Devaluation and Discrimination Scale; WHO: World Health Organization

Acknowledgements

We are very grateful Umberto Volpe (Polytechnic University of Marche) who commented on the manuscript. We also would like to thank Xiaodan Li (Xinxiang Medical University), Hui-cong Ren and Shi-na Gu (The Second Affiliated Hospital of Xinxiang Medical University) who helped in the data collection.

Funding

This study was funded by Xinxiang Medical University Educational Reform Program Foundation (Number2017-XYJG-26), National Natural Science Foundation of China (Number81471349) and Natural Science Foundation of Henan province (Number162300410224).

Authors' contributions

JL designed and led the study, drafted the manuscript. MMZ and LZ contributed to the study design, helped with data collection and conducted the main analysis. WQL and JLM contributed to the study design and critically appraised the manuscript. ZHZ was involved in the data collection and editing the manuscript. All authors read and approved the final manuscript.

Consent for publication

Not applicable.

Competing interests

The authors declare that they have no competing interests.

Author details

[1]The Second Affiliated Hospital of Xinxiang Medical University, 388# Jianshe Road, Muye, Xinxiang, China. [2]Xinxiang Medical University, 601# Jinsui Road, Hongqi, Xinxiang, China. [3]Henan Key Laboratory of Biological Psychiatry (Xinxiang Medical University), 388# Jianshe Road, Muye, Xinxiang, China. [4]Xinxiang Key Laboratory of Electrophysiology, 388# Jianshe Road, Muye, Xinxiang, China.

References

1. Patel V, Maj M, Flisher AJ, De Silva MJ, Koschorke M, Prince M. Reducing the treatment gap for mental disorders: a WPA survey. World Psychiatry. 2010;9(3):169–76.
2. Girma E, Tesfaye M. Patterns of treatment seeking behavior for mental illnesses in Southwest Ethiopia: a hospital based study. BMC Psychiatry. 2011;11:138.

3. Brown NB, Bruce SE. Stigma, career worry, and mental illness symptomatology: factors influencing treatment-seeking for Operation Enduring Freedom and Operation Iraqi Freedom soldiers and veterans. Psychol Trauma. 2016;8(3):276–83.
4. Webber M, Corker E, Hamilton S, Weeks C, Pinfold V, Rose D, Thornicroft G, Henderson C. Discrimination against people with severe mental illness and their access to social capital: findings from the viewpoint survey. Epidemiol Psychiatr Sci. 2014;23(2):155–65.
5. Lasalvia A, Zoppei S, Van Bortel T, Bonetto C, Cristofalo D, Wahlbeck K, Bacle SV, Van Audenhove C, van Weeghel J, Reneses B, Germanavicius A, Economou M, Lanfredi M, Ando S, Sartorius N, Lopez-Ibor JJ, Thornicroft G, ASPEN/INDIGO Study Group. Global pattern of experienced and anticipated discrimination reported by people with major depressive disorder: a cross-sectional survey. Lancet. 2013;381(9860):55–62.
6. Thornicroft G, Brohan E, Rose D, Sartorius N, Leese M. Global pattern of experienced and anticipated discrimination against people with schizophrenia: a cross-sectional survey. Lancet. 2009;373(9661):408–15.
7. Stuart H. Fighting the stigma caused by mental disorders: past perspectives, present activities, and future directions. World Psychiatry. 2008;7(3):185–8.
8. Corker EA, Beldie A, Brain C, Jakovljevic M, Jarema M, Karamustafalioglu O, Marksteiner J, Mohr P, Prelipceanu D, Vasilache A, Waern M, Sartorius N, Thornicroft G, FEDORA Study Group. Experience of stigma and discrimination reported by people experiencing the first episode of schizophrenia and those with a first episode of depression: the FEDORA project. Int J Soc. Psychiatry. 2015;61(5):438–45.
9. Chan SKW, Ching EYN, Lam KSC, So HC, Hui CLM, Lee EHM, Chang WC, Chen EYH. Newspaper coverage of mental illness in Hong Kong between 2002 and 2012: impact of introduction of a new Chinese name of psychosis. Early Interv Psychiatry. 2017;11(4):342–5.
10. Pescosolido BA, Monahan J, Link BG, Stueve A, Kikuzawa S. The public's view of the competence, dangerousness, and need for legal coercion of persons with mental health problems. Am J Public Health. 1999;89(9):1339–45.
11. Al-Darmaki F, Thomas J, Yaaqeib S. Mental health beliefs amongst Emirati female college students. Community Ment Health J. 2016;52(2):233–8.
12. Oexle N, Müller M, Kawohl W, Xu Z, Viering S, Wyss C, Vetter S, Rüsch N. Self-stigma as a barrier to recovery: a longitudinal study. Eur Arch Psychiatry Clin Neurosci. 2018;268(2):209–12.
13. Tawiah PE, Adongo PB, Aikins M. Mental health-related stigma and discrimination in Ghana: experience of patients and their caregivers. Ghana Med J. 2015;49(1):30–6.
14. Larson JE, Corrigan P. The stigma of families with mental illness. Acad Psychiatry. 2008;32(2):87–91.
15. Shibre T, Negash A, Kullgren G, Kebede D, Alem A, Fekadu A, Fekadu D, Madhin G, Jacobsson L. Perception of stigma among family members of individuals with schizophrenia and major affective disorders in rural Ethiopia. Soc Psychiatry Psychiatr Epidemiol. 2001;36(6):299–303.
16. Ohaeri JU, Fido AA. The opinion of caregivers on aspects of schizophrenia and major affective disorders in a Nigerian setting. Soc Psychiatry Psychiatr Epidemiol. 2001;36(10):493–9.
17. Kohls E, Coppens E, Hug J, et al. Public attitudes toward depression and help-seeking: impact of the OSPI-Europe depression awareness campaign in four European regions. J Affect Disord. 2017;217:252–9.
18. Corrigan PW, Watson AC. Understanding the impact of stigma on people with mental illness. World Psychiatry. 2002;1(1):16–20.
19. Thornicroft G, Rose D, Kassam A, Sartorius N. Stigma: ignorance, prejudice or discrimination. Br J Psychiatry. 2007;190:192–3.
20. Girma E, Tesfaye M, Froeschl G, Möller-Leimkühler AM, Müller N, Dehning S. Public stigma against people with mental illness in the Gilgel Gibe Field Research Center (GGFRC) in Southwest Ethiopia. PLoS One. 2013;8(12):e82116.
21. Adewuya AO, Oguntade AA. Doctors' attitude towards people with mental illness in Western Nigeria. Soc Psychiatry Psychiatr Epidemiol. 2007;42(11):931–6.
22. Schulze B. Stigma and mental health professionals: a review of the evidence on an intricate relationship. Int Rev Psychiatry. 2007;19(2):137–55.
23. Harangozo J, Reneses B, Brohan E, Weeks C, Pinfold V, Rose D, Thornicroft G, Henderson C. Stigma and discrimination against people with schizophrenia related to medical services. Int J Soc Psychiatry. 2014;60(4):359–66.
24. Björkman T, Svensson B, Lundberg B. Experiences of stigma among people with severe mental illness. Reliability, acceptability and construct validity of the Swedish versions of two stigma scales measuring devaluation/discrimination and rejection experiences. Nord J Psychiatry. 2007;61(5):332–8.
25. Liu J, Yao MJ, Lu YY, Li YH, Lv QJ. Attitude to mental disorder among residents in Zhengzhou city: a cross-sectional survey. Chin J Public Health. 2015;31(8):987–9 (in Chinese).
26. Yao MJ, Yan XF, Chang ZJ, Liu J, Yan L, Gao Q, Lv QJ. Awareness rate of mental health knowledge in residents in Zheng Zhou City. Chin Ment Health J. 2013;27(9):682–5 (in Chinese).
27. Hu HY, Yan YZ, Chen LM, Pu WJ, Liao W, Li J. Knowledge about mental health and attitude to mental disorder in urban and rural residents in Guangzhou. Chin Ment Health J. 2012;26(1):30–5 (in Chinese).
28. Yu Y, Liu ZW, Hu M, Liu XG, Liu HM, Yang JP, Zhou L, Xiao SY. Assessment of mental health literacy using a multifaceted measure among a Chinese rural population. BMJ Open. 2015;5(10):e009054.
29. Rong Y, Glozier N, Luscombe GM, Davenport TA, Huang Y, Hickie IB. Improving knowledge and attitudes towards depression: a controlled trial among Chinese medical students. BMC Psychiatry. 2011;11:36.
30. Li J, Li J, Thornicroft G, Huang YG. Levels of stigma among community mental health staff in Guangzhou, China. BMC Psychiatry. 2014;14:231.
31. Cook TM, Wang J. Descriptive epidemiology of stigma against depression in a general population sample in Alberta. BMC Psychiatry. 2010;10:29.
32. Reta Y, Tesfaye M, Girma E, Dehning S, Adorjan K. Public stigma against people with mental illness in Jimma Town, Southwest Ethiopia. PLoS One. 2016;11(11):e0163103.
33. Bedaso A, Yeneabat T, Yohannis Z, Bedasso K, Feyera F. Community attitude and associated factors towards people with mental illness among residents of Worabe Town, Silte Zone, southern nation's nationalities and people's region, Ethiopia. PLoS One. 2016;11(3):e0149429.
34. Song LY, Chang LY, Shih CY, Lin CY, Yang MJ. Community attitudes towards the mentally ill: the results of a national survey of the Taiwanese population. Int J Soc Psychiatry. 2005;51(2):162–76.
35. Li J, Li J, Huang Y, Thornicroft G. Mental health training program for community mental health staff in Guangzhou, China: effects on knowledge of mental illness and stigma. Int J Ment Health Syst. 2014;8(1):49.
36. Hansson L, Stjernswärd S, Svensson B. Changes in attitudes, intended behaviour, and mental health literacy in the Swedish. population 2009–2014: an evaluation of a national antistigma programme. Acta Psychiatr Scand. 2016;134(Suppl 446):71–9.
37. Weisman HL, Kia-Keating M, Lippincott A, Taylor Z, Zheng J. Mental health stigma prevention: pilot testing a novel, language arts curriculum-based approach for youth. J Sch Health. 2016;86(10):709–16.
38. Clement S, van Nieuwenhuizen A, Kassam A, Flach C, Lazarus A, de Castro M, McCrone P, Norman I, Thornicroft G. Filmed v. live social contact interventions to reduce stigma: randomised controlled trial. Br J. Psychiatry. 2012;201(1):57–64.
39. Evans-Lacko S, London J, Japhet S, Rüsch N, Flach C, Corker E, Henderson C, Thornicroft G. Mass social contact interventions and their effect on mental health related stigma and intended discrimination. BMC Public Health. 2012;12:489.
40. Klarić M, Lovrić S. Methods to fight mental illness stigma. Psychiatr Danub. 2017;29(Suppl 5):910–7.
41. Schomerus G, Stolzenburg S, Bauch A, Speerforck S, Janowitz D, Angermeyer MC. Shifting blame? Impact of reports of violence and mental illness in the context of terrorism on population attitudes towards persons with mental illness in Germany. Psychiatry Res. 2017;252:164–8.
42. Angermeyer MC, Beck M, Matschinger H. Determinants of the public's preference for social distance from people with schizophrenia. Can J Psychiatry. 2003;48(10):663–8.

15

The prevalence of psychiatric disorders among students aged 6-16 years old in central Hunan, China

Yan-Mei Shen[1,2], Bella Siu Man Chan[3], Jian-Bo Liu[1,2], Yuan-Yue Zhou[4], Xi-Long Cui[1,2], Yu-Qiong He[1,2], Yu-min Fang[1,2], Yu-Tao Xiang[5] and Xue-Rong Luo[1,2*]

Abstract

Background: Though several epidemiological surveys of psychiatric disorders have been carried out in China, only a few of them are concerned about the prevalence of psychiatric disorders in central Hunan and reveal the distribution of common psychiatric disorders and their comorbidities.

Methods: Achenbach's Child Behavior Checklist (CBCL), the Mini International Neuropsychiatric Interview for Children and Adolescents (MINI-KID), and Diagnostic and Statistical Manual of Mental Disorders, 4th Edition (DSM-IV) were administered to a stratified sample of 17,071 participants aged 6 to 16 years old from two cities in the central part of Hunan province. Twelve-month prevalence rates were calculated.

Results: Twelve-month prevalence of the population was 9.74%. The most common psychiatric disorders were attention deficit hyperactivity disorder (ADHD) (4.96%), oppositional defiant disorder (ODD) (2.98%) and generalized anxiety disorder (GAD) (1.77%). Of those with a 12-month prevalence diagnosis, 34.6% had one or more comorbid psychiatric disorders. Most notably, ADHD had comorbidity rates of 25.15% with ODD, 18.18% with CD, 6.38% with GAD, and 3.66% with MDD.

Conclusions: Psychiatric disorders are common in Chinese children and adolescents. Being the most prevalent mental disorder, ADHD requires continued focus and support in awareness and education.

Keywords: Psychiatric disorder, Prevalence, Comorbidity, Gender, Epidemiology, ADHD

Background

Studies focusing on mental disorders of children and adolescents have increased in recent decades [1]. The effect resulting from a psychological disorder not only impacts their quality of life but also predicts a higher chance of developing psychiatric disorders as they enter adulthood [2]. Children and youth with psychiatric disorders are six times more likely to experience health, legal, financial, and social problems as adults [3]. Numerous studies have indicated that children currently in treatment are less than the number of children with mental disorders, and underdiagnosis and undertreatment are major public health problems around the world [4–6]. Despite the critical need for information on the mental health of children and youth, research is scarce. The prevalence of mental health disorders among children and youth varies greatly in different parts of the world, ranging from 3.5 to 40.3% [7, 8]. This wide variation indicates great heterogeneity, which might result in a disparity of study goals, selection of study population, and criteria used to confirm the diagnoses of disorders [9]. China has a population of 1.3 billion, of which 238 million are children under 15 years of age [10]). Research on the prevalence of mental health disorders in children and youth across China is sorely lacking. Of the few epidemiological studies, they were all conducted in Hunan, Liaoning, and

* Correspondence: luoxuerong@csu.edu.cn
[1]Department of Psychiatry, The Second Xiangya Hospital, Central South University, Changsha 410011, Hunan, China
[2]Mental Health Institute of Central South University, China National Clinical Research Center on Mental Disorders (Xiangya), China National Technology Institute on Mental Disorders, Hunan Technology Institute of Psychiatry, Hunan Key Laboratory of Psychiatry and Mental Health, Changsha 410011, Hunan, China
Full list of author information is available at the end of the article

Sichuan provinces, which had a prevalence of 16.22% [11] (2005), 15.24% (2015) [12], and 9.15%(2007) [13], respectively. In the recent 10 years of China, the gross domestic product (GDP) had increased drastically from 18,731.89 billion to 68,905.21 billion RMB. The GDP of Hunan province is 2890.221 billion RMB, which is four times more than that in 2005 (659.61 billion RMB). The huge change suggested that an update in the prevalence rate of mental disability in health care is necessary. The purpose of this study is to investigate the prevalence, distribution, and comorbidities of common psychiatric disorders after 10 years of economic growth. Up-to-date prevalence estimates are vital for service delivery, resource provision, and research developments [14]. Likewise, identifying accurate prevalence variability can help to address queries about etiology and advise the design of future studies.

Methods

Samples and procedure

Hunan province is located in South China, with an area of 21.18 million square kilometers, accounting for 2.2% of China's land area. It consists of 13 cities and 1 autonomous prefecture, with an overall population of 67.8 million in 2015. Two cities located in the central part of Hunan province, Changsha (population of 7 million) and Yiyang (population of 4.8 million), were selected for the study. The sample size of this study was based on the sample size of the national investigation of psychiatric disorder in China held by Beijing Anding Hospital, which was originally supposed to be 14,000. However, our study included 17,000 participants to ensure that we can obtain an adequate number in case of participation refusal. Thirteen schools, including two urban middle schools, four urban primary schools, three rural middle schools, and four rural primary schools, were selected at random. Approximately 18,778 students were enrolled, of which 17,071 participants (90.9%) gave consent to participate. Of the eligible participants, 782 refused or did not complete their questionnaire, and of those who completed, 522 contained missing data (over 10% incomplete on the questionnaire), and 403 were outside the age range. This was a two-stage study that used Achenbach's Child Behavior Checklist (CBCL) as a screening tool, the Mini International Neuropsychiatric Interview for Children and Adolescents (MINI-KID), and the DSM-IV criteria to establish the final diagnosis. Questionnaires were sent to the students, and they brought the scale home for their parents to fill. Of the 17,071 qualified participants who completed the questionnaires, 13,606 participants scored negative to diagnosis, and 3465 scored positive, hinting a potential diagnosis of a disorder. Ten percent of the students with negative scores were selected randomly as controls. All of the 3465 participants with positive scores were given a full diagnostic interview using the MINI-KID (Sheehan et al., 2010) (parent and child versions). For those participants whose parents were unable to perform the diagnostic interview, the teachers were interviewed as alternative informants. Each interview lasted 15–40 min. For any participant with at least one diagnosis or a suspected diagnosis – based on either the parent or the child version of the MINI-KID – a diagnosis would be confirmed using the DSM-IV criteria. Through this procedure, 1663 participants were verified as having a diagnosis of at least one mental health disorder (see Fig. 1).

Eligible subjects were invited to participate in this study based on the following criteria: 1) enrolled students aged 6–16 years; 2) whose parents or guardians have given consent to participate; and 3) who had been living in the investigated sites for at least six months with household municipal registration. Exclusion criteria included the following: 1) informed consent not obtained, 2) students in special schools or not attending school, or 3) students could not be located after at least three attempts to visit at different times. The research protocol was approved by the Ethics Committee of the Second Xiangya Hospital, Central South University, China.

Screening tool

The CBCL is a parent–/caregiver-completed questionnaire that assesses behavioral problems, emotional difficulties, and social competencies of a child. This standardized and objective measurement tool has been revised and widely used by child psychiatrists, pediatricians, developmental psychologists, and other mental health professionals for clinical and research purposes [15]. The Chinese version of CBCL (1991) has demonstrated to have high psychometric properties as a screening tool [16]. The CBCL has 113 items, providing scores for three broad-band scales: internalizing (sum of withdrawn, somatic complaints, and anxious/depressed subscales), externalizing (sum of attention problems and aggressive and delinquent behavior subscales), and total behavior problems. The subscales differ depending on age and gender. Each item is scored on a three-point Likert scale (0 = not true, 1 = somewhat or sometimes true, or 2 = very true or often true). Participants were asked to choose the scale point that best described their child's behavior in the preceding six months [17]. The threshold value of the CBCL used in this study was based on the model for Chinese children and adolescents, and participants were considered to be screened positive when their score meet the criteria of each subscale [18] (see Additional file 1).

Diagnostic criteria and tools

The MINI-KID is a guided structured interview that assesses psychiatric disorders based on the DSM-IV and ICD-10 in children and adolescents aged 6 to 17 years in

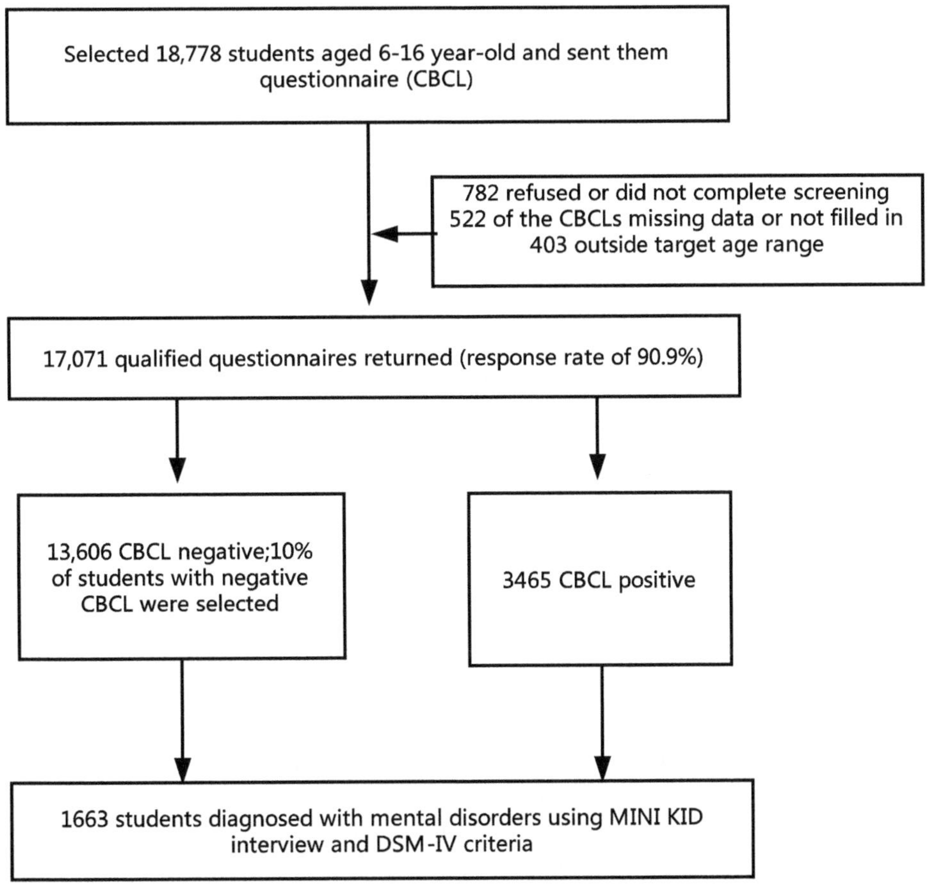

Fig. 1 Procedure of Investigation

a comprehensive and concise way. Both the parent and child participated in the interview, although it can also be administered solely to the children themselves [19]. The MINI-KID, which follows the structure and format of the adult version of the interview (MINI), was designed based on the Structured Clinical Interview for DSM-III-R [20] and the World Health Organization-designed Composite International Diagnostic Interview [21]. The assessment tool is divided into diagnostic sections or modules. It uses two to four questions that screen the respondent for each corresponding disorder. Additional questions of each disorder in a yes or no format will be used further if screened questions are positive. In response to discrepancies, further information will be obtained and concluded through clinical judgement. At the end of the assessment, a summary of the diagnostic criteria will be provided based on each disorder section. The instrument also screens for 24 DSM-IV and ICD-10 psychiatric disorders and suicidality of the target individual. Research had shown that the use of standardized structured and semi-structured diagnostic interviews reduce the risk of inadequate assessment in children and adolescents [22–24]. One down side of these previously used diagnostic instruments is being time consuming and lengthy to complete; each diagnosis requires 2 to 3 h to administer [25]. The MINI-KID is a reasonably accurate and reliable tool that greatly reduces the length and complexity of administration that serves the same psychometric property of the original form [19]. Our study used the validated Chinese version of the MINI-KID. Both the parent and child versions of the Chinese version of the MINI-KID had been proven to be reliable and valid [26, 27]. Potential diagnoses were considered present when they met the criteria on either the parent or child version. The diagnosis established by the MINI-KID was verified by trained psychiatrists following the DSM-IV criteria.

Statistical analysis

Data analyses were performed using SPSS version 18. To estimate the prevalence rate of mental health disorders and comorbidity, frequencies and 95% confidence intervals were calculated. Differences in the prevalence of mental health disorders between different genders and age groups were assessed using the Chi-square (χ^2) test. All statistical tests were two tailed, with 0.05 as the significance level.

Quality control

Quality control for the MINI-KID

Eighteen psychiatrists and 10 graduate students had 6 h of MINI-KID administration training. Two children and parents were interviewed using the MINI-KID, and consistency checks were conducted after the training, with a Kappa of 0.774.

Quality control for the diagnoses

Twelve registered psychiatrists received 8 h of training using the DSM-IV criteria for mental health disorders in children and youth. Two patients were interviewed for the 24 psychiatric disorders using the MINI-KID, and consistency check was conducted after the training, with a Kappa between 0.77 and 0.91.

Results

This study comprised of 4468 urban and 12,603 rural students, with a gender distribution of 8841 males and 8230 females. The 12-month prevalence of mental health disorders was 9.74%. The prevalence (11.79%) in boys was significantly higher than that (7.55%) in girls ($P < 0.05$; Table 1). The prevalence rate was 9.33% in ages under 11 years, 10.11% in 12–14 years, and 9.98% above 15 years ($P > 0.05$; Table 1). The prevalence difference between rural and urban areas (9.70% vs 9.85%) was not significant ($P > 0.05$; Table 1).

Attention deficit hyperactivity disorder (ADHD) ranked the highest with a prevalence of 4.96%, followed by oppositional defiant disorder (ODD) at 2.98%, generalized anxiety disorder (GAD) at 1.77%, and conduct disorder (CD) at 1.39%. Boys showed a significantly higher prevalence than girls in terms of ADHD, ODD, and CD, whereas girls showed a higher prevalence in terms of GAD and major depressive disorder (MDD). Participants aged ≤11 years showed the highest prevalence in ADHD, CD, and ODD (see Table 2).

Table 1 Twelve-month Prevalence, gender, age and urban-rural distribution of mental disorders among children and adolescents

Variable	Sample Rate (%)	95% CI	χ^2	P
Prevalence	17,071(9.74%)	9.30~ 10.18%		
Gender				
Boys	8841(11.79%)	11.12~ 12.46%	87.165	<0.001
Girls	8230(7.55%)	6.98~ 8.12%		
Age				
≤ 11 year	7689(9.33%)	8.68~ 9.98%	2.796	0.247
12–14 year	7198(10.11%)	9.41~ 10.81%		
≥ 15 year	2184(9.98%)	8.72~ 11.24%		
Community				
Rural	12,603(9.70%)	9.18~ 10.22%	0.078	0.781
Urban	4468(9.85%)	8.98~ 10.72%		

Nearly one third of the participants showed at least one psychiatric comorbidity; girls and those aged 12–16 years showed a higher proportion of comorbidity than the other groups (see Table 3). ADHD is most frequently comorbid with ODD (25.15%), CD (18.18%), and GAD (6.38%). In addition, GAD is most likely comorbid with ADHD (17.88%), ODD (17.88%), and MDD (16.56%), whereas MDD with GAD (48.08%) and tic disorder (47.12%) (see Table 4).

Discussion

Prevalence

The 12-month prevalence of any type of psychiatric disorders (9.74%) was within the range of 3.5–40.3% as reported previously [7, 8]. The prevalence in this study was higher than that in Ethiopia (3.5%) [7], Italy (8.2%) [28], Norway (7.0%) [29], and Malaysia (6.1%) [30], but similar to that in Mexico (9.1%) [31], Northeast China (9.49%) [32], and India (12.5%) [33] and lower than that in Russia (15.3%) [34], the Netherlands (22.0%) [35], Ireland (27.4%) [36], America (21.6%) [37], and Chile (38.3%) [38]. The discrepancy between studies may have been caused by several factors. First, various screening and diagnostic tools and different versions of the same instrument used contribute to the fluctuation in the prevalence rate [39]. For instance, a survey conducted in the United Arab Emirates found a prevalence of 15.6% using the Self-Reporting Questionnaire but reported a prevalence of 8.2% using the Composite International Diagnostic Interview [40]. Second, sampling methods may result in inconsistent rates. A meta-analysis reported that prevalence rate following no requirement of impairment was 27.1%, whereas it was 14.0% when disorder-specific impairment was defined by the diagnostic interview [9]. This survey was a standard two-stage study involving the criteria of social impairment, which may lead to low prevalence rate. Third, as much stigma is associated with mental illness in traditional Chinese culture, many Chinese patients tend to deny mental disorders [41]. Many Chinese patients will either avoid seeking medical help for mental health issues or may only bring forward complaints of somatic symptoms. All these factors can result in under- or misdiagnosis [42].

The prevalence of psychiatric disorder was lower than the pooled prevalence of 13.4%. The prevalence of GAD, MDD, and CD was also lower than the pooled prevalence of each kind of disorder reported in a meta-analysis, which indicated a prevalence of 6.5% (anxiety disorder), 2.6% (depressive disorder), and 5.7% (disruptive disorder). By contrast, ADHD was higher than the pooled prevalence of ADHD. One explanation for this perhaps would be that the prevalence rate reported in the meta-analysis study included all types of depressive and anxiety symptoms,

Table 2 Prevalence of common disorders and their distribution among gender, different age group and district

Disorders	Total N(%)	95%CI	Boys N(%)	Girls N(%)	≤11 year N(%)	12–14 year N(%)	≥15 year N(%)	Rural N(%)	Urban N(%)
ADHD	847(4.96)	4.64%--5.29%	628(7.1)	219(2.66)	438(5.7)	331(4.6)	78(3.57)	623(4.94)	224(5.01)
ODD	508(2.98)	2.72%--3.23%	309(3.5)	199(2.42)	240(3.12)	212(2.95)	56(2.56)	378(3.00)	130(2.91)
GAD	302(1.77)	1.57%--1.97%	114(1.29)	188(2.28)	65(0.85)	169(2.35)	68(3.11)	216(1.71)	86(1.92)
CD	237(1.39)	1.21%--1.56%	187(2.12)	50(0.61)	110(1.43)	93(1.29)	34(1.56)	193(1.53)	44(0.98)
SPP	126(0.74)	0.61%--0.87%	59(0.67)	67(0.81)	35(0.46)	60(0.83)	31(1.42)	100(0.79)	26(0.58)
TD	105(0.62)	0.50%--0.73%	43(0.49)	62(0.75)	23(0.3)	65(0.9)	17(0.78)	75(0.60)	30(0.67)
MDD	104(0.61)	0.49%--0.73%	30(0.34)	74(0.9)	17(0.22)	71(0.99)	16(0.73)	75(0.60)	29(0.65)
OCD	98(0.57)	0.46%--0.69%	45(0.51)	53(0.64)	25(0.33)	53(0.74)	20(0.92)	69(0.55)	29(0.65)
Dysthymia	29(0.17)	0.11%--0.23%	9(0.1)	20(0.24)	7(0.09)	19(0.26)	3(0.14)	22(0.17)	7(0.16)
Mania	25 (0.15)	0.10%--0.22%	22 (0.25)	3 (0.04)	13 (0.17)	9(0.13)	3(0.14)	14(0.11)	11(0.25)
SOP	12(0.07)	0.03%--0.11%	6(0.07)	6(0.07)	4(0.05)	7(0.1)	1(0.05)	10(0.08)	2(0.04)
PDD	12(0.07)	0.03%--0.11%	8 (0.09)	4 (0.05)	5 (0.07)	5(0.07)	2(0.09)	9(0.07)	3(0.07)
PTSD	4(0.02)	0.00%--0.05%	1(0.01)	3(0.04)	2(0.03)	0(0)	2(0.09)	4(0.03)	0(0)
SAD	3(0.02)	0.00%--0.04%	0(0)	3(0.04)	3(0.04)	0(0)	0(0)	2(0.02)	1(0.02)

ADHD Attention deficit hyperactive disorder, *ODD* oppositional defiant disorder, *CD* conduct disorder, *GAD* generalized anxiety disorder, *PTSD* post-traumatic stress disorder, *OCD* obsessive compulsive disorder, *SOP* social phobia, *SPP* specific phobia, *SAD* separation anxiety disorder, *MDD* major depressive disorder, *TD* tic disorder, *PDD* pervasive developmental disorders

whereas our study reported on the prevalence of GAD and MDD. Another reason would be the pressure from public discrimination and stigmatization because Chinese individuals feel ashamed to disclose affective symptoms [43]. Furthermore, our study reported higher prevalence rate than the pooled prevalence rate. One reason for this discrepancy might be that parents often consider mild to moderate intensity of oppositional and problem behaviors as symptoms of ADHD, whereas moderate to severe behaviors are considered to be ODD and CD [44].

The prevalence of psychiatric disorders is 9.7% among children and adolescents in our study was lower than the prevalence reported in 2005. There are several reasons contributing to this phenomenon. Firstly, the diagnostic tool is different; in 2005, the diagnostic tool used was Kiddie Schedule for Affective Disorders and Schizophrenia Present and Lifetime Version (K-SADS-PL), and in this study, we used MINI-KID as the diagnostic tool. Secondly, the prevalence of 16.2% reported in 2005 included more psychiatric disorders than this study. In addition to the psychiatric disorders included in MINI-KID, their study also included acute stress disorder, communication disorder (including expressive language disorder, phonological disorder, stutter, and mixed receptive-expressive language disorder), sleep disorders (including dyssomnia, nightmare disorder, sleep terror disorder, and sleep walking disorder), elimination disorders (including encopresis and enuresis), and elective mutism. This broader spectrum of disorders may have resulted in a higher prevalence. Thirdly, though psychiatric disorders remained prevalent, given the rapid economic growth in China, mental health services were improved [45], and several studies have reported that mental health problems have been negatively associated with economic growth in China [46, 47].

Gender difference

The current study shows significant gender differences, i.e., prevalence of ADHD, ODD, and CD in boys was higher than that in girls, which is consistent with other

Table 3 Distribution of comorbidities among different gender, age group and district

	Diagnosed with only 1 kind of Disorder	Comorbid with 1 kind of disorder	Comorbid with 2 kinds of disorder	Comorbid with 3 or more kinds of disorder	χ^2	*p*
Total	1087(65.4%)	391(23.5%)	123(7.4%)	62(3.7%)		
Boys	699(67.1%)	263(25.2%)	57(5.5%)	23(2.2%)	36.11	< 0.001
Girls	388(62.5%)	128(20.6%)	66(10.6%)	39(6.3%)		
6–11 years old	503(68.5%)	182(24.8%)	39(5.3%)	10(1.4%)	30.37	< 0.001
12–16 years old	584(62.9%)	209(22.5%)	84(9.0%)	52(5.6%)		
Urban	293(66.6%)	100(22.7%)	31(7.0%)	16(3.6%)	0.408	0.939
Rural	794(64.9%)	291(23.8%)	92(7.5%)	46(3.8%)		

Table 4 Comorbidity of several common mental disorders with other kinds of common DSM-IV mental disorders

	ADHD(%)	ODD(%)	GAD(%)	CD(%)	SPP(%)	TD(%)	MDD(%)	OCD(%)	Dysthymia(%)	Mania(%)
ADHD	/	213(25.15)	54(6.38)	154(18.18)	26(3.07)	14(1.65)	31(3.66)	27(3.19)	3(0.35)	2(0.24)
ODD	213(41.93)	/	54(10.63)	/	16(3.15)	9(1.77)	12(2.36)	23(4.53)	3(0.59)	2(0.39)
GAD	54(17.88)	54(17.88)	/	23(7.62)	22(7.28)	38(12.58)	50(16.56)	1(0.33)	12(3.97)	/
CD	154(64.98)	/	23(9.7)	/	15(6.33)	5(2.11)	19(8.02)	14(5.91)	2(0.84)	1(0.42)
SPP	26(20.63)	16(12.7)	22(17.46)	15(11.9)	/	7(5.56)	12(9.52)	6(4.76)	9(7.14)	/
TD	14(13.33)	9(8.57)	38(36.19)	5(4.76)	7(6.67)	/	49(46.67)	10(9.52)	20(19.05)	/
MDD	31(29.81)	12(11.54)	50(48.08)	19(18.27)	12(11.54)	49(47.12)	/	15(14.42)	/	/
OCD	27(27.55)	23(23.47)	1(1.02)	14(14.29)	6(6.12)	10(10.2)	15(15.31)	/	7(7.14)	/

studies [11, 48]. Various theories were associated with gender differences. First, the current diagnostic criteria could not fully cover all relevant symptoms in female patients. For example, one study [49] found that a group of untreated girls who did not meet the DSM criteria presented pronounced ODD symptoms and were almost as functionally impaired as girls who met the diagnostic criteria. Interestingly, no boys were found to meet the functional impairment criteria using the same method. This finding suggested the potential underdiagnoses in girls. Second, as symptoms in boys tend to be external problem behaviors, such as hyperactivity, compulsivity, and aggressive behaviors, they are easy to identify. Girls, however, were more likely to exhibit subtle internal problem behaviors, which were more likely to be overlooked [50]. Furthermore, previous studies found biological factors associated with the gender differences in the prevalence of disruptive behavior disorders and externalizing problems [51]. Specifically, Y-linked variants play a role in impulsivity and aggression in boys with ADHD [52]. Approximately half of the variance related to the development of externalizing behaviors are accounted for by biological factors [53].

We also found that girls tend to suffer from GAD and MDD, which is consistent with previous findings [54]. When confronted with stressors, females are likely to be negatively affected [55]. This gender-specific risk might be caused by the inability to regulate negative emotional responses of stress and fear [56]. Generally, females and males confront similar stressors differently, with females being more vulnerable to developing depression and related anxiety disorders than males [57]). Moreover, the hypothalamic–pituitary–adrenal (HPA) axis affects the levels of various hormones, including cortisol. Individuals with mood disorders often show elevated cortisol responses to stress, indicating dysregulation in the HPA. Ovarian hormones found in females also modulate HPA regulation [58]. Symptoms of emotional disorders may be more predominant during rapid changes in levels of ovarian hormones, such as in puberty, as hormonal fluctuation triggers dysregulation of the stress response.

Comorbidity

Our study found that ADHD is the most common comorbid disorder, which is consistent with previous findings [59]. Our study showed that ADHD patients have comorbidity rates of 48.2% with at least one psychiatric disorder, 36.4% with one psychiatric disorder, 8.5% with two kinds of psychiatric disorders, and 3.3% with three or more kinds of psychiatric disorders, which was similar to the rate of 52% reported in Denmark in a large sample [60] and lower than the rate of 66% reported in Italy [61]. Jensen and Steinhausen suggested that a smaller sample size and the absence of an assessment of impaired functioning may have contributed to a higher comorbidity rate [60]. Contrastingly, both our study and the study conducted in Denmark [60] had large samples and included an assessment of impaired functioning, and thus resulted in lower comorbidity rates. Also, the comorbidity of ADHD is considered to be developmental and dynamic [60]; because our study was a cross-sectional study, the participants might have not yet developed a comorbid psychiatric disorder when they were investigated, which might also have resulted in a lower comorbidity rate being presented. The mechanism behind the high comorbidity rate of ADHD and psychiatric disorders remains unclear. Heidbreder (2015) has suggested that, because of the considerable overlapping symptoms between ADHD and its comorbid psychiatric disorders, ADHD should be considered as a spectrum disorder using a dimensional rather than categorical diagnosis [62]. Other studies have also suggested that ADHD and psychiatric disorders might share similar brain regions [63].

Disruptive behavior disorders including ODD and CD remain the most common comorbid disorders; our study reported a comorbidity rate of 25.15% with ODD, which lies in the range of 20~ 60% as reported by other studies [61, 64], and a comorbidity rate of 18.8% with CD, which is slightly lower than the rate of 20% reported by Biederman [64], but higher than the rate of 16.5% reported by Jensen and Steinhausen [60]. Several reasons might contribute to this high comorbidity rate between ADHD and disruptive disorders. First, the symptoms of ADHD and ODD/CD are often correlated and change concurrently over time, and perhaps may be different manifestations or intensities of a similar disorder [65]. Reiff and Stein [44] have proposed that mild to moderate intensity of oppositional behaviors is likely to be a component of ADHD, whereas moderate to severe intensity is more likely to represent ODD/CD. Changes in the symptoms of ADHD, ODD, and CD over time are all correlated [66, 67]. Second, comorbidity could be linked to genetic dispositions; ADHD and disruptive disorders may be a result of shared genetic liabilities and similar interactions between genes and the environment [68].

Our study reported a comorbidity rate of 12.64% in anxiety disorders (including GAD, SPP and OCD), which was higher than the rate reported in Denmark [60], and lies within the range of 15~35% reported by Pliszka et al. [69]. Also, our study found that the comorbidity rate of MDD (3.66%) in ADHD patients is lower than the rate of 5% reported in Italy [61], and higher than that reported in Denmark [60] The comorbidity rate of affective disorder varied substantially, which might be related to epidemiological method and the population enrolled in the study [70].

Strengths and limitations

The strengths of this study included the use of the two-stage method, standardized diagnostic tool, and large sample size. However, this study has several limitations. First, only students enrolled in mainstream schools were included, and children in special schools or who did not go to school were not included. Thus, the findings cannot represent all children and adolescents. Second, we failed to record the number of children with a diagnosis from the MINI-KID but did not meet the criteria of DSM-IV. We considered the diagnosis only made from both the MINI-KID and the DSM-IV criteria. Third, the prevalence of pervasive developmental health disorder was relatively low due to the use of the MINI-KID. The MINI-KID consists of four brief questions on the child's social skills, repetitive interests, and behaviors. Finally, autism spectrum disorder (ASD) is a significant mental health disorder that we did not examine in this study. Future studies should examine the prevalence and distribution of ASD.

Conclusion

Our study revealed that nearly one tenth of Chinese children and adolescents suffer from at least one type of mental health disorder, with a higher prevalence in boys than in girls. Early diagnosis and intervention can help young children when they are most vulnerable to minimize or overcome mental health disorders as they grow older. Over the course of childhood, for those who have a diagnosis, caregivers should be aware of comorbid disorder(s) – either present or potential – and take preventive measures and perform early screening. Doing so can detect underlying or emerging disorders early and help to alleviate a difficult transition into adolescence and adulthood.

Abbreviations

ADHD: Attention deficit hyperactivity disorder; CBCL: Achenbach's Child Behavior Checklist; CD: Conduct disorder; DSM-IV: Diagnostic and Statistical Manual of Mental Disorders, 4th Edition; GAD: Generalized anxiety disorder; MDD: Major depressive disorder; MINI-KID: The Mini International Neuropsychiatric Interview for Children and Adolescents; OCD: Obsessive compulsive disorder; ODD: Oppositional defiant disorder; PDD: Pervasive developmental disorders; PTSD: Post-traumatic stress disorder; SAD: Separation anxiety disorder; SOP: Social phobia; SPP: Specific phobia; TD: Tic disorder

Funding

This study was supported by the National Science and Technology Ministry (ID 2012BAI01B02).

Authors' contributions

All authors have contributed to the research. All authors have contributed significantly in the research, and are all in agreement with the content of the manuscript. XL designed the study, conducted the study and provided guidance on the data analysis. YS conducted the study, did the data analysis and drafted the manuscript of the study. BSMC and YX provided guidance on the study idea and revised the manuscript, YZ, XC, YH and YF contributed to conducting the study and data preparation. JL provided guidance on the data analysis. All authors have read and approved the final manuscript to be submitted.

Consent for publication

All participants and their parents or legal guardians signed the consent form for publication of this study.

Competing interests

The authors declare that they have no competing interests.

Author details

[1]Department of Psychiatry, The Second Xiangya Hospital, Central South University, Changsha 410011, Hunan, China. [2]Mental Health Institute of Central South University, China National Clinical Research Center on Mental Disorders (Xiangya), China National Technology Institute on Mental Disorders, Hunan Technology Institute of Psychiatry, Hunan Key Laboratory of Psychiatry and Mental Health, Changsha 410011, Hunan, China. [3]The Department of Educational and Counselling Psychology, and Special Education, The University of British Columbia, Vancouver, Canada. [4]Mental Health Zhejiang University School of Medicine Hangzhou Seventh People's Hospital, Hangzhou 310013, China. [5]Unit of Psychiatry, Faculty of Health Sciences, University of Macau, Macao SAR, China.

References

1. Achenbach TM, Rescorla LA, Ivanova MY. International epidemiology of child and adolescent psychopathology I: diagnoses, dimensions, and conceptual issues. J Am Acad Child Adolesc Psychiatry. 2012;51(12):1261–72.
2. Hofstra MB, van der Ende J, Verhulst FC. Child and adolescent problems predict DSM-IV disorders in adulthood: a 14-year follow-up of a Dutch epidemiological sample. J Am Acad Child Adolesc Psychiatry. 2002;41(2):182–9.
3. Copeland WE, Wolke D, Shanahan L, Costello EJ. Adult Functional Outcomes of Common Childhood Psychiatric Problems: A Prospective, Longitudinal Study. JAMA Psychiatry. 2015;72(9):892.

4. Belfer ML. Child and adolescent mental disorders: the magnitude of the problem across the globe. J Child Psychol Psychiatry. 2008;49(3):226–36.
5. Merikangas KR, He J-P, Rapoport J, Vitiello B, Olfson M. Medication use in US youth with mental disorders. JAMA Pediatr. 2013;167(2):141–8.
6. Morris J, Belfer M, Daniels A, Flisher A, Villé L, Lora A, Saxena S. Treated prevalence of and mental health services received by children and adolescents in 42 low-and-middle-income countries. J Child Psychol Psychiatry. 2011;52(12):1239–46.
7. Ashenafi Y, Kebede D, Desta M, Alem A. Prevalence of mental and behavioural disorders in Ethiopian children. East Afr Med J. 2001;78(6):308–11.
8. Colonna M, Mitton N, Schott AM, Remontet L, Olive F, Gomez F, Iwaz J, Polazzi S, Bossard N, Trombert B. Prevalence, persistence, and sociodemographic correlates of DSM-IV disorders in the National Comorbidity Survey Replication Adolescent Supplement. Arch Gen Psychiatry. 2012;69(4):372–80.
9. Polanczyk GV, Salum GA, Sugaya LS, Caye A, Rohde LA. Annual research review: a meta-analysis of the worldwide prevalence of mental disorders in children and adolescents. J Child Psychol Psychiatry. 2015;56(3):345–65.
10. Zheng Y, Zheng X. Current state and recent developments of child psychiatry in China. Child Adolesc Psychiatr Ment Health. 2015;9(1):10.
11. Guan B, Luo X, Deng Y, WEI Z, Ye H, Yuan X, Ning Z, Yang W, Ding J. Prevalence of mental disorders among primary and middle school students in Hunan province. J Chin Contemp Pediatr. 2010;12(2):123–7.
12. Qu Y, Jiang H, Zhang N, Wang D, Guo L. Prevalence of mental disorders in 6-16-year-old students in Sichuan province, China. Int J Environ Res Public Health. 2015;12(5):5090–107.
13. Wen P. Epidemiological investigation of mental disorders in children and adolescents in Liaoning province. J Chin Med Univ. 2008;
14. Costello EJ, Burns BJ, Angold A, Leaf PJ. How can epidemiology improve mental health services for children and adolescents? J Am Acad Child Adolesc Psychiatry. 1993;32(6):1106–17.
15. Achenbach TM, Ruffle TM. The child behavior checklist and related forms for assessing behavioral/emotional problems and competencies. Pediatr Rev. 2000;21(8):265–71.
16. Leung PW, Kwong SL, Tang CP, Ho TP, Hung SF, Lee CC, Hong SL, Chiu CM, Liu WS. Test-retest reliability and criterion validity of the Chinese version of CBCL, TRF, and YSR. J Child Psychol Psychiatry. 2006;47(9):970–3.
17. Achenbach TM: The manual for the child behavior checklist. 1991.
18. SU L, Li X, Luo X, Yang Z, Wan G. The standardization of Achenbach child behavior checklist in hunan. J Clin Psychosom Dis. 1995;2:66–72.
19. Sheehan DV, Sheehan KH, Shytle RD, Janavs J, Bannon Y, Rogers JE, Milo KM, Stock SL, Wilkinson B. Reliability and validity of the Mini international neuropsychiatric interview for children and adolescents (MINI-KID). J Clin Psychiatry. 2010;71(3):313–26.
20. Sheehan DV, Lecrubier Y, Sheehan KH, Amorim P, Janavs J, Weiller E, Hergueta T, Baker R, Dunbar GC. The Mini-International Neuropsychiatric Interview (M.I.N.I.): the development and validation of a structured diagnostic psychiatric interview for DSM-IV and ICD-10. J Clin Psychiatry. 1998;59(Suppl 20):22.
21. Lecrubier Y, Sheehan DV, Weiller E, Amorim P, Bonora I, Sheehan KH, Janavs J, Dunbar GC. The MINI international neuropsychiatric interview (MINI). A short diagnostic structured interview: reliability and validity according to the CIDI. Eur Psychiatry. 1997;12(5):224–31.
22. Mcclellan JM, Werry JS. Evidence-based treatments in child and adolescent psychiatry: an inventory. J Am Acad Child Adolesc Psychiatry. 2003;42(12): 1388–400.
23. Mcclellan JM, Werry JS. Introduction--research psychiatric diagnostic interviews for children and adolescents. J Am Acad Child Adolesc Psychiatry. 2000;39(1):19–27.
24. Hughes CW, Rintelmann J, Mayes T, Emslie GJ, Pearson G, Rush AJ. Structured interview and uniform assessment improves diagnostic reliability. J Child Adolesc Psychopharmacol. 2000;10(10):119–31.
25. Reich W. Diagnostic interview for children and adolescents (DICA). J Am Acad Child Adolesc Psychiatry. 2000;39(1):59–66.
26. Liu YX, Liu J. Beijing: Reliability and validity of Chinese version of the Mini International Neuropsychiatric Interview for Children and Adolescents (Parent Version). Chin Ment Health J. 2010;25(1):921–25.
27. Liu YX, Liu J. Beijing: Reliability and validity of Chinese version of the Mini international neuropsychiatric interview for children and adolescents (child version). Chin Ment Health J. 2011;25(1):8–13.
28. Frigerio A, Rucci P, Goodman R, Ammaniti M, Carlet O, Cavolina P, De Girolamo G, Lenti C, Lucarelli L, Mani E, et al. Prevalence and correlates of mental disorders among adolescents in Italy: the PrISMA study. Eur Child Adolesc Psychiatry. 2009;18(4):217–26.
29. Einar H, Stormark KM, Lundervold AJ, Mikael H, Robert G, Maj-Britt P, Ullebø AK, Plessen KJ, Ingvar B, Lie SA. Psychiatric disorders in Norwegian 8- to 10-year-olds : an epidemiological survey of prevalence, risk factors, and service use. J Am Acad Child Adolesc Psychiatry. 2007;46(4):438–47.
30. Kasmini K, Kyaw O, Krishnaswamy S, Ramli H, Hassan S. A prevalence survey of mental disorders among children in a rural Malaysian village. Acta Psychiatr Scand. 1993;87(4):253–7.
31. Benjet C, Borges G, Medina-Mora ME, Zambrano J, Aguilar-Gaxiola S. Youth mental health in a populous city of the developing world: results from the Mexican adolescent mental health survey. J Child Psychol Psychiatry. 2009;50(4):386–95.
32. Xiaoli Y, Chao J, Wen P, Wenming X, Fang L, Ning L, Huijuan M, Jun N, Ming L, Xiaoxia A, et al. Prevalence of psychiatric disorders among children and adolescents in Northeast China. PLoS One. 2014;9(10):e111223.
33. Srinath S, Girimaji SC, Gururaj G, Seshadri S, Subbakrishna DK, Kumar PBN. Epidemiological study of child & adolescent psychiatric disorders in urban & rural areas of Bangalore, India. Indian J Med Res. 2005;122(12):67–79.
34. Goodman R, Slobodskaya H, Knyazev G. Russian child mental health--a cross-sectional study of prevalence and risk factors. Eur Child Adolesc Psychiatry. 2005;14(1):28–33.
35. Ormel J, Raven D, van Oort F, Hartman CA, Reijneveld SA, Veenstra R, Vollebergh WA, Buitelaar J, Verhulst FC, Oldehinkel AJ. Mental health in Dutch adolescents: a TRAILS report on prevalence, severity, age of onset, continuity and co-morbidity of DSM disorders. Psychol Med. 2015;45(2):345–60.
36. Coughlan H, Tiedt L, Clarke M, Kelleher I, Tabish J, Molloy C, Harley M, Cannon M. Prevalence of DSM-IV mental disorders, deliberate self-harm and suicidal ideation in early adolescence: an Irish population-based study. J Adolesc. 2014;37(1):1–9.
37. Carter AS, Wagmiller RJ, Gray SA, Mccarthy KJ, Horwitz SM, Briggs-Gowan MJ. Prevalence of DSM-IV disorder in a representative, healthy birth cohort at school entry: sociodemographic risks and social adaptation. J Am Acad Child Adolesc Psychiatry. 2010;49(7):686.
38. Vicente B, Saldivia S, de la Barra F, Melipillán R, Valdivia M, Kohn R. Prevalence of psychiatric disorders among Chilean children and adolescents. Rev Med Chil. 2012;140(4):447–57.
39. Anselmi L, Fleitlich-Bilyk B, Menezes AM, Araujo CL, Rohde LA. Prevalence of psychiatric disorders in a Brazilian birth cohort of 11-year-olds. Soc Psychiatry Psychiatr Epidemiol. 2010;45(1):135–42.
40. Abou-Saleh MT, Ghubash R, Daradkeh TK. Al Ain Community Psychiatric Survey. I. Prevalence and socio-demographic correlates. Soc Psychiatry Psychiatr Epidemiol. 2001;36(1):20.
41. Prina AM, Ferri CP, Guerra M, Brayne C, Prince M. Co-occurrence of anxiety and depression amongst older adults in low- and middle-income countries: findings from the 10/66 study. Psychol Med. 2011;41(10):2047–56.
42. Parker G, Gladstone G, Tsee Chee K. Depression in the planet's largest ethnic group: the Chinese. Am J Psychiatr. 2001;158(6):857.
43. Yang LH. Application of mental illness stigma theory to Chinese societies: synthesis and new directions. Singap Med J. 2007;48(11):977–85.
44. Reiff MI, Stein MT. Attention-deficit/hyperactivity disorder evaluation and diagnosis: a practical approach in office practice. Pediatr Clin N Am. 2003;50(5):1019–48.
45. Xu J, Wang J, Liu R, Xing J, Su L, Yu F, Lu M. Mental health inpatient treatment expenditure trends in China, 2005-2012: evidence from Shandong. J Mental Health Policy Econ. 2014;17(4):173–82.
46. Yin H, Xu L, Shao Y, Li L, Wan C. Relationship between suicide rate and economic growth and stock market in the People's republic of China: 2004–2013. Neuropsychiatr Dis Treat. 2016;12:3119.
47. Zhang J, Ma J, Jia C, Sun J, Guo X, Xu A, Li W. Economic growth and suicide rate changes: a case in China from 1982 to 2005. Eur Psychiatry. 2010;25(3):159–63.
48. Demmer DH, Hooley M, Sheen J, Mcgillivray JA, Lum JAG. Sex differences in the prevalence of oppositional defiant disorder during middle childhood: a meta-analysis. J Abnorm Child Psychol. 2017;45(2):1–13.
49. Waschbusch DA, King S. Should sex-specific norms be used to assess attention-deficit/hyperactivity disorder or oppositional defiant disorder? J Consult Clin Psychol. 2006;74(1):179–85.
50. Hasson R, Fine JG. Gender differences among children with ADHD on continuous performance tests: a meta-analytic review. J Atten Disord. 2012;16(3):190.

51. Eme RF. Sex differences in child-onset, life-course-persistent conduct disorder. A review of biological influences. Clin Psychol Rev. 2007;27(5): 607–27.
52. Liu L, Cheng J, Li H, Su Y, Sun L, Yang L, Qian Q, Wang Y. Association of Y-linked variants with impulsivity and aggression in boys with attention-deficit/hyperactivity disorder of Chinese Han descent. Psychiatry Res. 2017;252:185.
53. Derks EM, Dolan CV, Hudziak JJ, Neale MC, Boomsma DI. Assessment and etiology of attention deficit hyperactivity disorder and oppositional defiant disorder in boys and girls. Behav Genet. 2007;37(4):559–66.
54. Donner NC, Lowry CA. Sex differences in anxiety and emotional behavior. Pflugers Arch. 2013;465(5):601–26.
55. Altemus M, Sarvaiya N, Epperson CN. Sex differences in anxiety and depression clinical perspectives. Front Neuroendocrinol. 2014;35(3):320–30.
56. Cover KK, Maeng LY, Lebrónmilad K, Milad MR. Mechanisms of estradiol in fear circuitry: implications for sex differences in psychopathology. Transl Psychiatry. 2014;4(8):e422.
57. Wong CM, Yehuda R, Lewishall F, Williams TS, Panetta JA, Herrera JM: Sex differences in posttraumatic stress disorder. 2002.
58. Young E, Korszun A: Women, stress, and depression: sex differences in hypothalamic-pituitary-adrenal axis regulation. 1999.
59. Spencer TJ. ADHD and comorbidity in childhood. J Clin Psychiatry. 2006;67(Suppl 8):27–31.
60. Jensen CM, Steinhausen H-C. Comorbid mental disorders in children and adolescents with attention-deficit/hyperactivity disorder in a large nationwide study. Atten Defic Hyperact Disord. 2015;7(1):27–38.
61. Reale L, Bartoli B, Cartabia M, Zanetti M, Costantino MA, Canevini MP, Termine C, Bonati M, Lombardy AG. Comorbidity prevalence and treatment outcome in children and adolescents with ADHD. Eur Child Adolesc Psychiatry. 2017;26(12):1443–57.
62. Heidbreder R. ADHD symptomatology is best conceptualized as a spectrum: a dimensional versus unitary approach to diagnosis. Atten Defic Hyperact Disord. 2015;7(4):249–69.
63. Klassen LJ, Katzman MA, Chokka P. Adult ADHD and its comorbidities, with a focus on bipolar disorder. J Affect Disord. 2010;124(1):1–8.
64. Biederman J. Attention-deficit/hyperactivity disorder: a selective overview. Biol Psychiatry. 2005;57(11):1215–20.
65. Connor DF, Doerfler LA. ADHD with comorbid oppositional defiant disorder or conduct disorder: discrete or nondistinct disruptive behavior disorders? J Atten Disord. 2008;12(2):126–34.
66. Burke JD, Loeber R, Lahey BB, Rathouz PJ. Developmental transitions among affective and behavioral disorders in adolescent boys. J Child Psychol Psychiatry. 2005;46(11):1200–10.
67. Lahey BB, Loeber R, Burke J, Rathouz PJ, Mcburnett K. Waxing and waning in concert: dynamic comorbidity of conduct disorder with other disruptive and emotional problems over 7 years among clinic-referred boys. J Abnorm Psychol. 2014;111(4):556–67.
68. Nadder TS, Rutter M, Silberg JL, Maes HH, Eaves LJ. Genetic effects on the variation and covariation of attention deficit-hyperactivity disorder (ADHD) and oppositional-defiant disorder/conduct disorder (Odd/CD) symptomatologies across informant and occasion of measurement. Psychol Med. 2002;32(1):39–53.
69. Pliszka SR, Carlson CL, Swanson JM. ADHD with comorbid disorders: clinical assessment and management. New York: Guilford Press; 1999.
70. Taurines R, Schmitt J, Renner T, Conner AC, Warnke A, Romanos M. Developmental comorbidity in attention-deficit/hyperactivity disorder. Atten Defic Hyperact Disord. 2010;2(4):267–89.

Persistent catatonia following epileptic seizures

Ragnar Verbraeken[1*] and Jurjen J. Luykx[2,3,4,5]

Abstract

Background: Catatonia is frequently associated with mood and psychotic disorders as well as with general medical conditions, especially with seizures. In the case of the latter, catatonia mostly resolves when the seizures respond to the anticonvulsive treatment. We report, to our knowledge, the first case of a patient without affective or psychotic disorder, who developed catatonia in the postictum and whose catatonia did not resolve with anticonvulsive treatment, but did so with lorazepam.

Case presentation: We describe a 36-year-old man, with no psychiatric history, except for a possible disorder in the use of cannabis, who developed catatonia after epileptic seizures. The catatonia did not respond to the anticonvulsant therapy, but did so to lorazepam 17 mg/d. Lorazepam could be tapered slowly and stopped without reemergence of catatonic signs.

Conclusion: Catatonia should be part of the differential diagnosis in patients with bradyphrenia and/or remarkable postictal behavior. This report shows that lorazepam should be taken into consideration (before moving to ECT), in cases of unresolved catatonia, even if the seizures are reduced with anticonvulsants.

Keywords: Postictum, Delirium, Catatonia, Lorazepam

Summary

We describe the first case of persistent catatonia following an epileptic seizure (ES) of a patient without a history of psychotic or affective disorders. The catatonic symptoms did not go into remission until a dose of lorazepam 17 mg daily was reached. We tapered and finally discontinued lorazepam without the patient developing new signs of catatonia.

Background

Catatonia is a psychomotor symptom cluster first described by C. Wernicke (motility psychosis) and by K.L. Kahlbaum in 1874 in his publication 'Die Katatonie oder das Spannungsirresein' in which he regarded 'being extremely tense' as the main characteristic of catatonia [1]. Catatonia is observed in a plethora of psychiatric disorders, primarily mood and psychotic disorders, but sometimes in cases of, for example, autism [2–5] or obsessive compulsive disorder (OCD) [6] as well. In DSM-5 it has become possible to classify catatonia as 'catatonia as specifier' or 'catatonic disorder not otherwise specified' or 'unspecified catatonia'. Furthermore, catatonia also occurs in non-psychiatric disorders such as neurological disorders, in metabolic diseases and intoxications, as a consequence of medication [5, 7–9], postoperatively [5], or after withdrawal of alcohol [10], benzodiazepines [8] or cannabis [11]. To our knowledge, catatonia following an ES had not been described before the current report. Here, by describing a case and a systematic literature search we raise awareness of this possible postictal condition to enable earlier diagnosis and management.

Case presentation

A 38- year-old man, with no psychiatric history, known to suffer from epilepsy but who stopped his antiepileptic drugs (AED) is brought into a community hospital's emergency room by an ambulance after being found in the streets in a confused condition and with reduced

* Correspondence: ragnar.verbraeken@opzgeel.be
[1]OPZ Geel, Geel, Belgium
Full list of author information is available at the end of the article

awareness. The history taking in the emergency room is hampered by bradyphrenia and amnesia. The patient merely relates a vague account of a pub fight. At that instant he does not know where he lives nor is he able to provide any contact information about relatives or friends. General physical examination, neurological examination, urine toxicology, brain CAT and cerebrospinal fluid findings (proteins and cells, mainly to exclude meningitis/encephalitis) are unremarkable. Blood analysis shows slight signs of leukocytosis. The EEG shows general slowing without traces of epilepsy. The patient is admitted to the neurology department for diagnostic work-up.

The next day the patient is somewhat less slow and more aware, although still unaware of the events on the day prior to admission. He believes to have fallen as a consequence of an ES. He indicates he has not been taking his AED for some time. Valproic acid was therefore restarted at a dose of 1500mgs daily. He denies having used any drugs or alcohol, as confirmed by urine toxicology. A new blood analysis is carried out, showing a decrease in leukocytosis, an increase of CK to 521 U/L and a slight increase in CRP to 16.2 mg/L. Brain MRI is unremarkable.

Two days after his admission an ES is observed by nursing staff and is interpreted as tonic-clonic, generalized. No clear underlying cause is identified. Valproic acid blood levels are 54 mg/L (at the time of admission this was < 10 mg/L), leading us to increase the dose to 2x1000mg/d. The EEG is unchanged.

The patient then shows peculiar behaviour: he stares and speaks little, leading the neurologist to suspect a psychotic episode and therefore a psychiatrist is consulted. During the psychiatric history the patient informs him that he does not have any complaints other than noticing being somewhat slow. He himself attributes this to the restarted AED. During psychiatric examination we notice bradyphrenia. The patient does blink his eyes and moves slowly, though fluently. There is no posturing or grimacing. He is friendly and cooperative. His conscienceness is clear and his attention span is undisturbed. He is well-oriented. Perception, memory and mood appear intact. The affect is flattened. He denies having suicidal thoughts.

Given this symptomatology the differential diagnosis at that stage included side effects of the valproic acid and, although there were insufficient DSM-5 criteria for catatonia at the time, catatonia. The attending psychiatrist decided to re-evaluate the patient a few days later.

Upon that re-evaluation, the patient rubs his hands in a stereotypical manner and there is evidence of grimacing and posturing (the patient sits bent over for minutes, with hands, head and shoulders in the same position) and of ambitendency. There is no Gegenhalten, no negativism, no Mitmachen. The Bush Francis catatonia rating scale (BFCRS) scores: 0 1 0 1 2 1 0 2 0 0 0 0 0 0 2 0 0 0 3 0 0 0 = 12 (Table 1). Again, the EEG remains without abnormalities and unchanged. Given the stereotypies, the bradyphrenia, hypoactivity, inappropriate behaviour, ambitendency and posturing combined with a BFCRS score of 12, we concluded the patient was suffering from postictal catatonia becoming more severe within 8 days following a seizure. To confirm this hypothesis, we treated him with lorazepam 3dd1mg and 1dd2.5 mg, without improvement, but the lorazepam didn't bring about any sedation. He was then transferred to the psychiatry department for further diagnostic work-up and treatment. During the first days of his stay at the ward symptoms and signs were unchanged. A fourth EEG showed no change either. Lorazepam was increased by 3 mg every 2 days until at a total dose of 17 mg/d the patient clearly improved: he became more talkative, started moving

Table 1 Overview of the catatonic features during the course of illness. Day numbers refer to the number of days after the epileptic seizure

	Day 8 (0 mg Lorazepam)	Day 12 (11.5 mg Lorazepam)	Day 16 (17 mg Lorazepam)	Day33 (0 mg Lorazepam
Excitement	0	0	0	0
Immobility/stupor	1	1	0	0
Mutism	0	0	0	0
Staring	1	1	0	0
Posturing/catalepsy	2	1	0	0
Grimacing	1	1	0	0
Echopraxie/ echolalia	0	0	0	0
Stereotypy	2	1	0	0
Mannerisms	0	0	0	0
Verbigeration	0	0	0	0
Rigidity	0	0	0	0
Negativism	0	0	0	0
Waxy flexibility	0	0	0	0
Withdrawal	0	0	0	0
Impulsivity	2	1	0	0
Autonomic obedience	0	0	0	0
Mitgehen	0	0	0	0
Gegenhalten	0	0	0	0
Ambitendency	3	0	0	0
Grasp reflex	0	0	0	0
Perseveration	0	0	0	0
Combativeness	0	0	0	0
Autonomic abnormality	0	0	0	0
Total	12	6	0	0

more fluently and has not shown signs of grimacing or posturing since. His mood has remained cheerful. Then, lorazepam was gradually tapered by 1 mg/d until it could be stopped completely, with the patient remaining stable and free of symptoms. On his day of discharge at 0 mg of lorazepam an EEG showed a normal base rhythm with only a couple of short episodes of general slowing.

Discussion

Over forty different catatonic symptoms have been described to date [2, 7, 12]. These may be subdivided into the following four categories: motor phenomena (stupor, catalepsy, rigidity, flexibilitas cerea), withdrawal (mutism, staring gaze, negativism, refusal to eat and drink), excitement (hyperactivity, combativeness, autonomous instability, undirected potentially dangerous aggression) and odd repetitive behaviour (grimacing echolalia, echopraxia, stereotypies, manierisms, perseveration, command-automatism, Mitmachen and Gegenhalten, and ambitendency) [7, 9, 13].

Catatonia can be divided into four types [5, 7, 13, 14]. There is the hyperkinetic type of catatonia, characterized by agitation, combativeness [15], verbigeration, stereotypies, echolalia and echopraxia. The stuporous type is characterized by stupor, mutism, posturing and negativism. A third type is lethal or malignant catatonia: an often acutely emerged state involving alterations in consciousness, fever, severe rigidity and autonomous instability. The fourth type is periodic catatonia, characterized by the cyclic return of symptoms of catatonia. These episodes last an average of four to 10 days and can return within weeks or years [9].

The differential diagnosis may be challenging given the current lack of biomarkers and symptom aspecificity. The following conditions need to be considered in the differential diagnosis: malignant antipsychotic syndrome, extrapyramidal side effects of psychopharmacological medication, hyperammonemic encephalopathy [16], acute dystonia, tardive dyskinesia, akathisia, manic episodes, delirium, compulsory movement disorders, conversion disorder, certain compulsions in OCD, serotonin syndrome, locked-in syndrome, vegetative state and stiff person syndrome, kinetic disorders with hypocalcemia, tetanus, strychnine toxicity, rabies and complex partial epilepsy, nonconvulsive status epilepticus [2, 4, 9, 17–19].

In our differential diagnosis we also considered the following: complex partial epileptic seizures [9, 18, 19], postictal akinesia [20], postictal delirium [19], hypoactive delirium [9], nonconvulsive status epilepticus [4, 9], postictal psychosis [21, 22] and non-psychiatric stupor (characterized by immobility, mutism, absence of response to stimuli; this kind of stupor has other causes than catatonia, such as head trauma, anoxia, epilepsy and encephalopathy of unknown origin) [18].

First we would like to address whether it was an ES and not a psychogenic epileptic seizure (PNES) the patient had suffered from. We could not obtain a video EEG, so there is no certainty since video-EEG is the gold standard for such differentiation. We detected however, after the first and second seizures, the last of which was observed by medical staff, a substantial increase in CK which, according to experts, could be a diagnostic instrument for differentiating between ES and PNES [23, 24]. So there is reason to assume it were ES and not PNES.

Another important distinction that must be made in this case is between postictal delirium (occurring in 35% of seizure cases and reported to last sometimes up to 10 days) [25–27] and postictal catatonia as it may substantially influence treatment decision-making [28–30]. Whereas benzodiazepines are used first in cases of catatonia, in delirium such compounds may aggravate symptoms [28–30]. The distinction between the two may be cumbersome given clinical overlap. According to the DSM-5 it is impossible for the two to co-occur since catatonia cannot be diagnosed in the presence of delirium; others question this notion [30]. In addition, Grover [28] found that 12 to 30% of patients with delirium showed symptoms matching the criteria for catatonia.

Another distinction that has to be made is between postictal catatonia and postictal psychosis [21, 22, 31]. Although psychosis as such can be accompanied by catatonic features, this was not the case here as, firstly, except for the psychomotor symptoms, there were no other symptoms of psychosis. Secondly, postictal psychosis is rarely seen with idiopathic generalized epilepsy [21]. And thirdly, postictal psychosis is mostly characterized by delusions of the grandiose or religious type, aggression, pressured speech and excessive emotional response [31].

In our case a diagnosis of catatonia was considered most plausible based on symptomatology (e.g. lack of day-night differences in symptomatology), absence of adverse effects after the lorazepam 'challenge test' and repetitive EEGs showing no signs of epileptic activity. Moreover, our observation that the patient remained well-oriented and attentive argued against delirium and that in combination with the absence of delusions or hallucinations none of the above mentioned characteristics of postictal psychosis were present, against postictal psychosis.

The treatment of catatonia initially consists of benzodiazepines [4, 5, 7, 9, 13, 14, 18, 32–35] (effective in 70–80% of all cases) and only when this is ineffective ECT. When ECT is of little help, transcranial magnetic stimulation [18] and NMDA antagonists such as amantadine and memantine [33, 36] may be considered. When these are still ineffective, anticonvulsants can be tried. In some cases, atypical antipsychotics are combined with benzodiazepines [33, 36]. Our patient was treated with valproic acid for epilepsy.

In our case, it was necessary to increase the dose of Lorazepam to 17 mg/d. before we saw clear amelioration of the symptoms. Improvement could in theory also have been attributed to simply time or to the restarted AED since AEDs are also effective in catatonia. But we like to mention that when the AEDs were restarted, the catatonia did not go into remission, and only did so when we augmented the lorazepam to 17 mg/d. Moreover, the fact that the symptoms remained unchanged the first days of occurrence without lorazepam pleads against resolving as a natural course.

The question then arises if ECT would also be a treatment option for our patient. We believe this is since ECT can be given when a patient has a status epilepticus and for catatonia, as mentioned above. There are, to our knowledge, however, no reports of ECT treatment for postictal catatonia.

We searched articles written in Dutch or English in pubmed with the terms 'post-ictal catatonia', OR 'ictal catatonia' OR 'catatonia seizures', OR 'catatonia postictal state' OR 'catatonia and delirium' as well as cross-references retrieved by our search. We thus found a case series in which four patients developed catatonia during ECT treatment for affective or psychotic disorders [37, 38]. The cause of the catatonia could have been withdrawal of benzodiazepines, besides affective and psychotic disorders, which is supported by the fact that catatonic symptoms disappeared after reinstating benzodiazepines. Two other case reports describe the development of catatonia after ECT, both in patients with a history of bipolar disorder [39, 40], while our patient had no medical history of other psychiatric disorders, except for drug abuse. It is beyond dispute that there is a clear difference between ECT and ES. ECT occurs in a safe environment under controlled circumstances and under narcosis. Furthermore, ECT is often given for conditions that may themselves be accompanied by catatonia. Finally, we found another case report in which catatonia developed postictally, but this patient was known to suffer from schizophrenia [41]. We also found an article by Herman published in 1942 [42], reporting the case of a man stating himself that he suffers from epilepsy. Seizures were, however, not observed and catatonic symptoms were not described clearly.

Conclusion

To our knowledge, we describe the first case of persistent postictal catatonia, following an observed ES. In this case a daily dose of 17 mg of lorazepam was necessary to attain remission. In patients with bradyphrenia and/or remarkable postictal behaviour we advise to consider not only postictal confusion, but catatonia as well, especially when appearing within 24 h after a seizure. Based on our experience we suggest a gradually increasing dose of lorazepam. This dose of medication should be tapered very gradually as rapid tapering may not only spark catatonia relapse, but a new epileptic seizure too.

Bullets:

1. Catatonia should be considered among those with cognitive and/or movement features that commence postictally.
2. The distinction between delirium and catatonia after an ES may be challenging but has treatment implications.
3. More research into the etiology of catatonia in general and postictal catatonia in particular is highly needed.

Abbrevations

AED: Anti-epileptic drugs; BFCRS: The Bush Francis catatonia rating scale; CAT Scan: Computer Assisted Tomography; CK: Creatinine kinase; CRP: C-reactive protein; dd: Daily dose; DSM-5: 5th edition of Diagnostic and Statistical Manual of Mental Disorders; ECT: Electroconvulsive therapy; EEG: Electroencephalogram; ES: Epileptic seizures; GABAA: Gamma-aminobutyric acid A; MRI: Magnetic resonance imaging; NMDA: N-methyl D-aspartate; OCD: Obsessive compulsive disorder; PNES: Psychogenic non-epileptic seizures; U/L: Units per liter

Acknowledgements

We would like to thank the patient for his collaboration.

Funding

Not applicable.

Authors' contributions

JL was the primary clinician involved in the assessment, management and follow-up of the patient. JL provided overall supervision for this case, including manuscript preparation. RV wrote the manuscript with assistance of JL. Both authors contributed to the literature review and manuscript preparation and approved the final manuscript.

Consent for publication

Written informed consent was obtained from the patient for the publication of this case report.

Competing interests

The authors declare that they have no competing interests.

Author details

[1]OPZ Geel, Geel, Belgium. [2]Department Of Psychiatry, Rudolf Magnus Institute of Neuroscience, Utrecht University, Utrecht, The Netherlands. [3]Department of Translational Neuroscience, Rudolf Magnus Institute of Neuroscience, Utrecht University, Utrecht, The Netherlands. [4]SymforaMeander Hospital, Amersfoort, The Netherlands. [5]Department of Psychiatry, ZNA Hospitals, Antwerp, Belgium.

References

1. Kahlbaum K: Die Katatonie oder das Spannungsirresein; 1874.
2. Dhossche D. Catatonia in psychiatric illnesses. In: The medical basis of psychiatry. 3rd ed; 2008. p. 455–70.
3. Dhossche DM, van der Steen LF, Shettar SM. Catatonia in autism spectrum disorders: review and case-report. Tijdschr Psychiatr. 2015;57(2):89–93.
4. Rasmussen SA, Mazurek MF, Rosebush PI. Catatonia: our current understanding of its diagnosis treatment and pathophysiology. World J Psychiatry. 2016;6(4):391–8.
5. Wijemanne S, Jankovic J. Movement disorders in catatonia. J Neurol Neurosurg Psychiatry. 2015;86(8):825–32.
6. IGG GE, Yosmaoğlu A. Catatonia as a symptom of obsessive compulsive disorder: a case report. Adv Life Sci. 2014;4(5):245–6.
7. Bruijn DJBJ. Katatonie. *nederlands tijdschrift voor geneeskunde.* 2010;154:A2284.
8. Gelenberg AJ. The catatonic syndrome. Lancet. 1976;1(7973):1339–41.
9. van Harten PN. Katatonie een syndroom om te herinneren. Nederlands tijdschrift voor psychiatrie. 2005;47(6):371–82.
10. Oldham MA, Desan PH. Alcohol and sedative-hypnotic withdrawal catatonia: two case reports, systematic literature review, and suggestion of a potential relationship with alcohol withdrawal delirium. Psychosomatics. 2016;57(3):246–55.
11. Caudron M, Rolland B, Deheul S, Geoffroy PA, Thomas P, Amad A. Catatonia and cannabis withdrawal: a case report. Subst Abus. 2016;37(1):188–9.
12. Sahaya K, Lardizabal D. Catatonia in encephalitis and nonconvulsive seizures: a case report and review of the literature. Epilepsy Behav. 2010;17(3):420–5.
13. Barnes MP, Saunders M, Walls TJ, Saunders I, Kirk CA. The syndrome of Karl Ludwig Kahlbaum. J Neurol Neurosurg Psychiatry. 1986;49(9):991–6.
14. Walther S, Strik W. Catatonia. CNS spectrums. 2016;21(4):341–8.
15. Luykx JJ, Post EH, van der Erf M, Van Hecke J. Agitation after minor trauma: combativeness as a cardinal catatonic feature. BMJ case reports. 2013;2013: bcr2012008217.
16. Perez-Esparza R, Onate-Cadena N, Ramirez-Bermudez J, Espinola-Nadurille M. Valproate-induced Hyperammonemic encephalopathy presenting as catatonia. Neurologist. 2018;23(2):51–2.
17. Komatsu T, Nomura T, Takami H, Sakamoto S, Mizuno K, Sekii H, Hatta K, Sugita M. Catatonic symptoms appearing before autonomic symptoms help distinguish neuroleptic malignant syndrome from malignant catatonia. Intern Med (Tokyo, Japan). 2016;55(19):2893–7.
18. Bartolommei N, Lattanzi L, Callari A, Cosentino L, Luchini F, Mauri M. Catatonia: a critical review and therapeutic recommendations. J Psychopathol. 2012;18:234–46.
19. Repchak AT, Quinn DK. Epileptic catatonia: a case series and systematic review. Psychosomatics. 2016;57(2):217–25.
20. Dhossche DM, Sienaert P, van der Heijden FM. Mechanisms of catatonia. Tijdschr Psychiatr. 2015;57(2):99–103.
21. Kanner AM, Rivas-Grajales AM. Psychosis of epilepsy: a multifaceted neuropsychiatric disorder. CNS spectrums. 2016;21(3):247–57.
22. Logsdail SJ, Toone BK. Post-ictal psychoses. A clinical and phenomenological description. Br J Psychiatry. 1988;152:246–52.
23. Nass RD, Sassen R, Elger CE, Surges R. The role of postictal laboratory blood analyses in the diagnosis and prognosis of seizures. Seizure. 2017;47:51–65.
24. Petramfar P, Yaghoobi E, Nemati R, Asadi-Pooya AA. Serum creatine phosphokinase is helpful in distinguishing generalized tonic-clonic seizures from psychogenic nonepileptic seizures and vasovagal syncope. Epilepsy Behav. 2009;15(3):330–2.
25. Ito M. Neuropsychiatric evaluations of postictal behavioral changes. Epilepsy Behav. 2010;19(2):134–7.
26. Krauss G, Theodore WH. Treatment strategies in the postictal state. Epilepsy Behav. 2010;19(2):188–90.
27. Shorvon S, Trinka E. Nonconvulsive status epilepticus and the postictal state. Epilepsy Behav. 2010;19(2):172–5.
28. Grover S, Ghosh A, Ghormode D. Do patients of delirium have catatonic features? An exploratory study. Psychiatry Clin Neurosci. 2014;68(8):644–51.
29. Schieveld JNM, Strik J. Catatonia, delirium, and critical illness: a diagnostic statistical manual 5 mystery partially disentangled. Crit Care Med. 2017; 45(11):1953–4.
30. Wilson JE, Carlson R, Duggan MC, Pandharipande P, Girard TD, Wang L, Thompson JL, Chandrasekhar R, Francis A, Nicolson SE, et al. Delirium and catatonia in critically ill patients: the delirium and catatonia prospective cohort investigation. Crit Care Med. 2017;45(11):1837–44.
31. Sakakibara E, Nishida T, Sugishita K, Jinde S, Inoue Y, Kasai K. Acute psychosis during the postictal period in a patient with idiopathic generalized epilepsy: postictal psychosis or aggravation of schizophrenia? A case report and review of the literature. Epilepsy Behav. 2012;24(3):373–6.
32. Honings ST, Arts BM, van Os J. A case-report on catatonia: a prevalent but under-recognised psychiatric illness. Tijdschr Psychiatr. 2016;58(3):232–6.
33. Sienaert P, Dhossche DM, Vancampfort D, De Hert M, Gazdag G. A clinical review of the treatment of catatonia. Front Psychiatry. 2014;5:181.
34. Walstra AN, den Broek MV, Giltay EJ, van Paassen J, van Noorden MS. Successful amantadine treatment of a patient with ECT-resistant catatonia. Tijdschr Psychiatr. 2016;58(8):599–602.
35. Walther S, Schappi L, Federspiel A, Bohlhalter S, Wiest R, Strik W, Stegmayer K. Resting-state Hyperperfusion of the supplementary motor area in catatonia. Schizophr Bull. 2017;43(5):972–81.
36. Beach SR, Gomez-Bernal F, Huffman JC, Fricchione GL. Alternative treatment strategies for catatonia: a systematic review. Gen Hosp Psychiatry. 2017;48:1–19.
37. Luchini F, Medda P, Mariani MG, Mauri M, Toni C, Perugi G. Electroconvulsive therapy in catatonic patients: efficacy and predictors of response. World J Psychiatry. 2015;5(2):182–92.
38. Malur C, Francis A. Emergence of catatonia during ECT. J ECT. 2001; 17(3):201–4.
39. Pandey RS, Sharma P. E.c.t. induced Catationia: a case report. Indian J Psychiatry. 1988;30:105–7.
40. Tan AH, Low SC, Tan CY, Lim KS, Tan CT, Lim SY. "Ictal catatonia": rare but not to be missed! Parkinsonism Relat Disord. 2016;32:137–9.
41. Gunduz A, Benbir G, Bayar R. Postictal catatonia in a schizophrenic patient and electroconvulsive treatment. J ECT. 2008;24(2):166–7.
42. Herman M. Nonschizophrenic catatonic states. NY State JM. 1942;1:624–7.

17

Evaluation of an interaction-skills training for reducing the burden of family caregivers of patients with severe mental illness: a pre-posttest design

Yasmin Gharavi[1], Barbara Stringer[2,4], Adriaan Hoogendoorn[3], Jan Boogaarts[4], Bas Van Raaij[4] and Berno Van Meijel[3,5,6,7*]

Abstract

Background: Family members who care for patients with severe mental illness experience emotional distress and report a higher incidence of mental illness than those in the general population. They report feeling inadequately prepared to provide the necessary practical and emotional support for these patients. The MAT training, an Interaction-Skills Training program (IST) for caregivers, was developed to meet those needs. This study used a single-arm pretest-posttest design to examine the impact of the training on caregivers' sense of competence (self-efficacy) and burden.

Methods: One hundred family caregivers recruited from three mental health institutions participated in the training. Burden was assessed using the Involvement Evaluation Questionnaire, and self-efficacy using the Self-Efficacy Questionnaire. Analysis of variance with repeated measures was used to investigate whether participation in the training changed the level of family caregivers' burden and self-efficacy. Pearson's correlation was used to examine the relationships between self-efficacy and burden.

Results: Our results indicate that, after the training, self-efficacy increased significantly over time ($p < 0.001$) and that burden decreased significantly ($p < 0.001$). However, the results could not demonstrate the expected association between an increase of self-efficacy and decrease of burden. Caregivers expressed high appreciation for the training.

Conclusions: After following the IST program, family caregivers of patients with severe mental illness experienced a greater sense of competence and a significant decrease in burden. The training was greatly appreciated and satisfied caregivers' need to acquire the skills required in complex caregiving situations.

Keywords: Interaction-skills training, IST, Psycho-education, Family caregivers, Self-efficacy, Burden, Severe mental disorders

* Correspondence: Berno.vanMeijel@inholland.nl
[3]Department of Psychiatry, Amsterdam Public Health research institute, VU University Medical Center, Amsterdam, The Netherlands
[5]Inholland University of Applied Sciences, Amsterdam, The Netherlands
Full list of author information is available at the end of the article

Background

A significant proportion of individuals with a severe mental illness (SMI) are unable to manage the demands of daily life. This is mainly caused by their symptoms and the associated impairments of cognitive and social skills. Informal caregivers therefore play an indispensable role in supporting them in their daily activities [1].

As Ostman & Hansson [2] indicated, approximately 90% of individuals with a severe mental illness are supported practically and emotionally by family caregivers on an almost daily basis. But as many caregivers are not properly prepared for a role as informal caregiver, they experience a great deal of psychological strain and a sense of burden [3, 4]. Up to 50% of informal caregivers report significantly more psychological distress and a higher incidence of mental illness than people in the general population [5]. They report in particular feelings of depression, distress, fatigue and trouble sleeping. The burden they experience also intrudes upon their social lives in ways that makes them feel trapped in their caregiving role and isolated from society [6].

Even though previous studies made it clear that patients' challenging behavior causes caregivers to experience substantial distress and health problems, effective support strategy for reducing the subjective burden are limited [7]. Current interventions to support family caregivers are based mainly on psycho-education [8]. But as caregivers lack the skills and confidence they need to deal effectively with patient's emotions and behavior [9], they also need practical training to increase their interaction and communication skills [9, 10].

There is limited scientific evidence regarding the effects of broader psychosocial intervention strategies aimed at the reduction of caregivers' burden. For example, Martire, Lustig, Schulz, Miller and Helgeson [11] described the positive effects of behavioral family therapy on caregiver burden, depression and anxiety. The psychosocial intervention in this therapy targeted the patient's closest family member or relative. Smeerdijk and colleagues found that the combination of family motivational interventions (MI) and the IST was effective in reducing family members' worrying and burden [12]. A systematic evaluation by Signe & Elmståhl [13] showed that 90% of family caregivers expressed great satisfaction with respect to psychosocial interventions intended to meet caregiver's needs. Caregivers seemed to benefit from the network that was created when information and experiences were shared. There is also evidence that caregivers who were exposed to family interventions targeting their caregiver's needs seemed less disturbed by a patient's disruptive behavior, because they had learned to attribute it to the illness and not to the patient's personality [9].

One explanatory variable with respect to the acquisition of these skills and reduction of caregivers' burden is self-efficacy [14], which concerns people's beliefs that they can produce the desired effects through their actions [15]. Self-efficacy is seen as a crucial determinant of emotional reactions and burden. Research indicates that lower self-efficacy is associated with greater subjective burden [16].

Late last century, we used available knowledge about burden, self-efficacy and behavioral family interventions to develop the MAT training, being an Interaction Skills Training program (IST) for informal caregivers that would serve the needs of family caregivers. In the present study, we investigated the impact of this training program on the levels of self-efficacy and burden experienced by caregivers caring for a family member with a severe mental illness. We hypothesized that the training was effective in increasing caregivers' self-efficacy and reducing their burden. Hereinafter, the training will be referred to as "the IST program".

Method

Design

We used a pretest-posttest design to examine the effect of the IST program on self-efficacy and burden, which were measured on three occasions: at T0 (baseline), T1 (after the training) and T2 (three months after termination of the training). The third measurement also included a brief evaluation of the caregivers' perspective on the training.

Participants

The training program was offered at three mental health institutions in various parts of the Netherlands. Within these three hospitals, there was an open registration for family members to participate in the training. The training was announced through the mental health professionals, local media, or a brochure. The inclusion criteria were as follows: being a family member of, and caring for, a patient with a severe mental illness, defined as not being free of symptoms, having had the mental illness in the long term (> 2 years), and having serious limitations in personal and social functioning [17]. Informed consent was obtained from all participants and confidentiality was assured. One hundred primary caregivers participated in the training, but, due to incomplete data, only 75 were included in the analyses. Twenty-five participants were excluded from the analysis because of missing data at one of the three measurements T0, T1 or T2.

The MAT training

The history of MAT started in 1994 when the development of interaction-skills training programs for use in the mental health sector was initiated by Ypsilon, a Dutch advocacy organization committed to family members and close relatives of people with psychosis. These skill-based programs were intended to serve as a tool to improve the interaction and communication between professionals/informal caregivers and patients with psychosis [18].

Successful versions of the MAT training have since evolved into the current MAT program, which we used in our study. Its purpose is to provide family caregivers with various interaction skills that can support them in their caregiving role. The MAT is used as a tool to demonstrate through role-play whether or not one is having a problem with another person's behavior. This is done either by standing on the green section of a mat, which stands for 'cooperation area', or on the red section, which stands for 'problem area'. Either a fellow family member or a MAT trainer takes the position of the patient in the role-plays. In the training, the mat is used to practice several interaction skills that are important in handling difficult confrontations between a family member and a patient, i.e. when one or both of them are standing on the red section of the mat, see Fig. 1.

The complete training comprises seven 3-h sessions over a 10-week period. Our training was taken by a total of eleven groups, with a minimum of eight and a maximum of sixteen participants. It was provided by certified MAT trainers together with trained professionals from a range of disciplines, who also had personal experience of caring for a family member with a severe mental illness. An overview of the training sessions is provided in Table 1. The sessions have a structure that gradually adds new interaction elements to the training with increasing difficulty of the interaction process. The sessions were accompanied by homework assignments with instructions to practice the specific skills that were central in the successive sessions. The participants' experiences when executing the homework assignments were discussed at the start of the following session.

Data collection

Self-efficacy

Self-efficacy was measured with the Self-Efficacy Questionnaire (SEQ). The SEQ is a questionnaire developed by our research group to measure the extent to which caregivers find themselves competent to interact effectively with a family member with a mental illness. The development process of the SEQ involved the following steps. First, a panel of nine experts, both researchers and MAT trainers, compiled an item pool with items referring to essential competencies of caregivers to effectively interact with the patient with severe mental illness. Next, these items were clustered into meaningful units of caregiver competences. The nine experts participated in four commentary rounds to develop the first version of the questionnaire. This first version of the SEQ was then presented to Ypsilon and five MAT trainers for review with respect to content, formulations and construction. In the last stage, nine caregivers completed the latest version to test its comprehensibility and feasibility. The final version of the SEQ consists of 23 items that are rated on a 4 point Likert scale ranging from '1 = probably not' to '4 certainly'. Examples of items are: 'I think I'm able to make the difference in situations when patient is *not capable* or *not willing* to do something'. Or: 'I think I'm able to align my own behavior to the patient's inabilities'. In our sample, the internal consistency of the SEQ was very high, i.e. 0.94. The SEQ is currently subject to further psychometric evaluation, whose results will be published elsewhere.

Burden

The Involvement Evaluation Questionnaire (IEQ) measures the degree of subjective burden of caregivers of people with schizophrenia, depression and mixed psychiatric disorders [19]. It covers all domains of burden relevant to caregivers. It was shown to be valid, reliable, easy to understand, not time consuming, and sensitive to changes [20]. With a high degree of internal consistency, ranging from 0.74 to 0.85 for the subscales and 0.90 for all items of the instrument, the IEQ has proven to have satisfactory reliability [19].

The original **IEQ** consists of seven modules. As the second module represents the core module, it was the only module used for this study. The questions concern the burden experienced in the preceding 4 weeks. The items are measured on a 5-point Likert-scale ranging from '1 = never' to '5 = (almost) always'. The module contains 31 items which are distributed over the following four subscales:

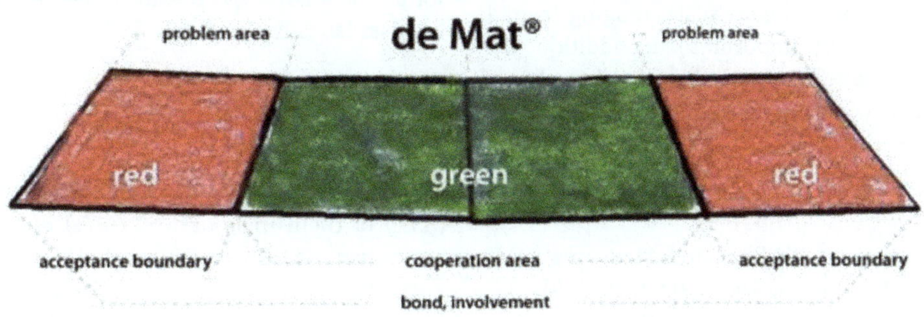

Fig. 1 Illustration of the mat

Table 1 Description of the content of the seventraining sessions

Training meeting	Content of meeting
Meeting 1: Goal-oriented interaction	The meeting started with a personal introduction. To improve caregivers' knowledge of severe mental illness, this was followed by psycho-education and a description of the training program. The participants learned to distinguish between concrete behavior and interpretations. They were also asked to describe specific behaviors of the patient they found hard to deal with. They were then informed about the purpose of the mat in the training. Finally, the participants were asked to formulate their personal learning objectives and were introduced to the homework assignment that would follow each meeting.
Meeting 2: My own life	The homework assignment was discussed. This meeting revolved around challenging the participants to discover how much control they actually had in their own lives. They were asked to write down what they needed in order to feel good, and how much time they needed to perform these activities. If they felt like missing out on these activities, they were asked to draw up a goal plan to serve their needs. Finally, the participants had to come up with three ways of communicating their needs to the patient.
Meeting 3: The communication process	The homework assignment was discussed. The main focus in this meeting, which involved psycho-education, lay on getting a better understanding of transmitting clear messages and listening effectively. The conditions for communicating properly were discussed. Participants practiced their communication skills on the mat.
Meeting 4: My position	After discussion of the homework assignment, the different communication styles and their effect on interaction with the patient were discussed. Participants practiced with the communication styles and with drawing a line when making an issue negotiable. They also learned to make the switch between expressing disagreement properly and listening actively to understand another person's behavior. To achieve an effective strategy for confrontations when the patient showed resistance, they ended the meeting by practicing the switch.
Meeting 5: Dealing with conflicts	After discussing the previous homework assignment, participants discovered the capacities and incapacities of patients with a severe mental illness with regard to solving a conflict or problem effectively. The participants gained a better understanding of the crucial difference between 'cannot cooperate' and 'will not cooperate'. At the end of the meeting, this psycho-educational form of learning was used on the mat to practice situations in which this problem could arise.
Meeting 6: Working together as a strategy	After discussing the previous homework assignment, participants learned how to cope with the patient when he or she 'cannot' cooperate in performing a task, and how to influence the interaction positively. At the end of the meeting, participants were asked to create a management plan to use in teamwork between caregiver, patient and staff as a strategy when contact breaks down.
Meeting 7: Going back home	The last meeting revolved around practicing the skills learnt during the previous six meetings. The learning experiences were translated into real life situations. Finally, the personal learning objectives were discussed and remaining questions were answered.

feelings of tension (9 items), which refer to mental or emotional strain; supervision (6 items), which refer to caregiver's tasks of guarding the patient's needs; worrying (6 items), which covers feelings of concern and unease; and urging (8 items), which relates to the patient's activation and motivation to undertake certain activities [20]. The items 28 and 44 are used in more than one scale.

Appreciation

To evaluate the appreciation of the training, we developed a short survey with 11 statements referring to the central aims and components of the training (see Table 4). These items are rated on a 4 point Likert scale, ranging from 1 ('not important' to 4 ('very important'). In addition, the respondents were requested to score the overall quality of the training regarding content and trainers (10 point scale: 1 = low; 10 = high).

Data-analyses

The Analysis of Variance with Repeated Measures (RM-ANOVA) was used to examine the main hypothesis, i.e. whether the training had a significant effect over time on family caregivers' burden and self-efficacy.

Next, on the assumption that an increase in self-efficacy would result in a decrease in burden, we used linear regression analysis to evaluate the relationship between the increased self-efficacy and decreased burden. Any changes in self-efficacy and burden were calculated using delta scores (endpoint score minus baseline score). Additional exploratory analyses were conducted to investigate the relationship between increased self-efficacy and the different subscales of burden. Finally, we evaluated the relationship between caregivers' appreciation of the training and any changes of burden and self-efficacy.

The SPSS Statistics program version 20.0 [21] was used for all the analyses. A p value of less than 0.05 was considered statistically significant.

Results

Sample characteristics

A total of 75 participants were included in the analyses, 25 (33%) of them male and 50 (67%) of them female. Their age range was 25 to 78 years (*Mean* = 55.4, *SD* = 11.1). Forty-eight percent had a lower level of education; 42% had a medium level (bachelor level); and 10% had attended higher education (master level).

The effect for caregivers' self-efficacy and burden over time

Mauchly's Test of Sphericity indicated that the assumption of sphericity (i.e., homogeneity of variance) had not been violated for self-efficacy ($\chi2(2) = 5.34$, $p = 0.069$), but had been violated for burden ($\chi2(2) = 30.74$, $p < 0.001$). We therefore corrected degrees of freedom using Lower-Bound estimates of sphericity ($\varepsilon = 0.74$) for burden. The results provide good support for the main hypotheses, showing a significant increase in participants' self-efficacy after the training ($F(2,134) = 33.09$, $p < 0.001$) and a significant decrease in their burden ($F(1,70) = 21.37$, $p < 0.001$) (Table 2). Figure 2. illustrates these effects. The effect sizes for these analyses ($d = -0.71$ for self-efficacy, $d = 0.46$ for burden) were classed as large to moderate, in accordance with existing guidelines for interpreting the effect sizes, as offered by Cohen [22].

Correlations between self-efficacy and burden

Pearson's correlation was used to assess the relationship between the change in self-efficacy and the change in level of burden, including the changes in the subscales of burden (see Table 3). There was no significant correlation between the change in self-efficacy and change in burden ($r = 0.03$, $n = 70$, $p = 0.78$). Neither did additional analyses of the relationship between change in self-efficacy and change in the subscales of burden show any significant correlation (see Table 3).

Evaluation of the training

The participants expressed great appreciation for the training: on the 10 point scale, the mean score for training content was 8.4 ($SD = 0.73$); for the trainers it was 8.6 ($SD = 0.85$). There were no significant associations between their appreciation of the training and their decrease in burden ($r(75) = -0.102$, $p = 0.384$), and their increase in self-efficacy ($r(75) = 0.092$, $p = 0.432$). With regard to appreciation of the different components of the training, the highest average score was for 'Determining whose problem it is: mine or his/hers' ($mean = 3.37$, $SD = 0.56$). Table 4 shows the complete list of components, ranked from the highest appreciation to the lowest.

Discussion

In this study, we found that the caregiver's level of self-efficacy after the IST had increased, and that their level of burden had decreased. We may conclude that the training program led to meaningful changes in caregiver's lives. Our results confirm the findings of an earlier study [12] where families who completed the IST reduced burden effectively.

This study did not support Solomon and Draine's hypothesis that higher self-efficacy is associated with decreased subjective burden [16]. Neither was self-efficacy associated with either of the subscales representing burden. One possible explanation for this is that the great reduction in burden may have been due partly to the supporting network created between caregivers who had to cope with the difficulties, see also Signe & Elmståhl [13]. Another possible explanation is that the follow-up period in our study was too short to assess an association between the increase in self-efficacy and decrease in burden. This effect may develop in later stages when the self-efficacy skills learned have been applied for longer. Caregivers in previous successful versions of the MAT training reported not having enough time to practice the skills they learnt during the training; 75% of them asked for follow-up training [18]. The results of a longer follow-up period should either verify or falsify the hypothesis.

Table 2 Repeated Measures Anova: The effect on self-efficacy and burden over time (T0, T1, T2; N self-efficacy = 68, N burden = 71)

	Mean (SD)	*Type III SS*	*df*	*Mean Squared*	*F*	*p*
Self-efficacy						
T0	53.92 (13.91)					
T1	62.24 (12.45)					
T2	63.44 (13.06)					
RM-ANOVA – sphericity assumed:						
within subjects		3652.90	2	1826.45	33.09	< 0.001
error		7395.85	134	55.19		
Burden						
T0	69.29 (12.62)					
T1	63.81 (10.94)					
T2	63.72 (11.55)					
RM-ANOVA – Lower bound corrected:						
within subjects		1448.12	1	1448.12	21.37	< 0.001
error		4743.52	70	67.76		

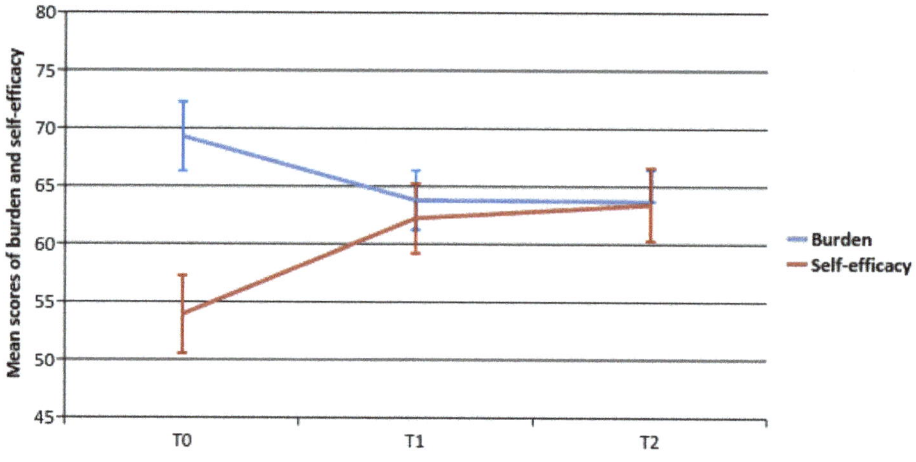

Fig. 2 Illustration of the changes in burden and self-efficacy over time. Error bars indicate 95% confidence confidence intervals of the mean

As the evaluation of caregiver's participation in the training shows, the caregivers regarded the interaction skills training program as very successful, expressing great satisfaction with both its content and the trainers. These results are consistent with the findings of Signe & Elmståhl [13]. With regard to the various training components in our study, caregivers reported great appreciation for 'determining whose problem it is: mine or his/hers', 'dealing with the handicaps' of the person involved and 'insight into the handicap'. They also reported feeling more confident about the appropriate things to say, and more competent in ensuring that elaborative conversations did not turn into endless circular discussions. These findings point out the importance of interventions that train caregivers how to effectively manage the caregiver situation. This is consistent with previous research that examined 'a sense of mastery' as a caregiving concern [3] and how successful daily interactions between family member and patient were a result of the IST [18].

This study has two main strengths. First, the results of our study regarding self-efficacy and burden, in combination with the caregivers' great appreciation of the program, provides evidence of the effectiveness of interactive interventions targeting caregiver self-efficacy and burden. As Rose et al. [9] claimed that providing information and support alone is not enough to improve caregivers' understanding of the mental illness; nor does it increase their sense of competence and confidence in their caregiving ability. Given the current trend in mental health care towards more ambulatory treatment [23] with more caring responsibilities for family members, mental health care should rely less on psycho-educational interventions alone, and more on interaction training programs that include psycho-educational components.

The second strength of our study is that the medium to large effect sizes implicate reliable reduction in burden and improvement of self-efficacy in practical terms for caregivers' daily life.

Our study also has some limitations. The first was our use of a non-experimental design. Therefore, we could not identify desirable between-group effects by contrasting our results with those of a control group. However, in view of

Table 3 Pearson's correlation: The relationship between change in self-efficacy and change in burden and its subscales (N = 70)

	r	95%-Confidence Interval	*p*
Burden	0.03	(−0.20, 0.27)	0.78
Subscales Burden			
Tension	−0.19	(−0.41, 0.06)	0.13
Supervision	0.10	(−0.14, 0.33)	0.40
Worrying	0.07	(−0.17, 0.30)	0.56
Urging	0.15	(−0.09, 0.37)	0.22

Table 4 Appreciation of the components of the training, ranked from highest rated to lowest rated (mean and standard deviations)

1. Determining whose problem it is: his/hers or mine.	3.37	.56
2. Dealing with the handicaps of the person involved.	3.35	.53
3. Insight into the handicaps of the person involved.	3.29	.53
4. Expressing your boundaries.	3.27	.53
5. Recognizing your own boundaries.	3.25	.60
6. Listening attentively: listening to what he/she is trying to tell you.	3.24	.65
7. Listening attentively: actively listening	3.21	.64
8. Practical experience gained by working on the mat.	3.17	.65
9. Formulating your own personal learning objectives.	3.13	.50
10. Guiding your own life.	3.08	.71
11. Confronting the other with his/her behaviour.	3.00	.59

the long-term distress experienced by the family members, spontaneous increase of self-efficacy and decrease of burden over a period of weeks is not very likely [9]. The second limitation is that our findings are based on non-probability sampling. As the caregivers were required to enroll themselves in the training, there may have been selection bias. Similarly, the fact that caregivers were informed about and recruited for the training in various ways may have affected their motivation for signing up for and participating in the training. The third limitation was the relatively small sample size caused by incomplete data; roughly a quarter of our participants were excluded from analyses. Fourth, as there is no follow-up data, we cannot examine the effect over a longer period. Finally, although SEQ showed high face validity, good feasibility and high internal consistancy, further examination of the psychometric properties of the Self-Efficacy Questionnaire (SEQ) is necessary. This psychometric research is currently in progress.

Conclusions

The main purpose of the IST program is to train caregivers in using effective communication and interactive skills when dealing with patients who frequently behave disruptively. After taking the IST program, family caregivers of patients with severe mental illness experienced a greater sense of competence (self-efficacy) and a significant decrease in burden. The training, combining psychoeducation and interactive skills, was greatly appreciated, and satisfied the caregivers' need to acquire the skills they required in complex caregiving situations.

Abbreviations

IST: Interaction-Skills Training; MI: Motivational Interventions

Acknowledgements

We would like to thank all family members for their participation in this study.

Funding

No funding was obtained for this study.

Authors' contributions

YG was the project leader and executive researcher. YG, BS and BvM designed the study and chose together with AH the appropriate statistical methodology to analyze the data. YG conducted the study, performed the literature search, performed the statistical analyses and wrote the manuscript. BS and BvM supervised the study and commented on the draft versions of the manuscript. AH supervised the statistical analyses. AH resolved any practical problems with SPSS and consulted us with his statistical knowledge to interpret the results of the data analysis correctly. JB and BvR were the trainers and performed data collection, together with YG. JB and BvR also provided the information needed to describe the training sessions precisely. All authors had acces to any data and read and approved the final manuscript. Also, all authors agreed to be accountable for the aspect of the work they were responsible for.

Consent for publication

Not applicable.

Competing interests

The authors declare that they have no competing interests.

Author details

[1]GGZ inGeest, Amsterdam, The Netherlands. [2]Research group Recovery and Rehabilitation, GGZ inGeest, Amsterdam, The Netherlands. [3]Department of Psychiatry, Amsterdam Public Health research institute, VU University Medical Center, Amsterdam, The Netherlands. [4]The Mat Training & Education, Amsterdam, The Netherlands. [5]Inholland University of Applied Sciences, Amsterdam, The Netherlands. [6]Parnassia Psychiatric Institute, The Hague, The Netherlands. [7]Academy for Masters in Advanced Nursing Practice, Utrecht, The Netherlands.

References

1. Bentur N, Moualem A. The effect on family members of treating home hospitalized patients. Harefuah. 2001;140(5):386–91.
2. Ostman M, Hansson L. Family burden and care participation: a test-retest reliability study of an interview instrument concerning families with a severely mentally ill family member. Nordic Journal of Psychiatry. 2000;54:327–32.
3. Chang KH, Horrocks S. Lived experiences of family caregivers of mentally ill relatives. J Adv Nurs. 2006;53(4):435–43.
4. Rose L, Mallinson RK, Walton-Moss B. A grounded theory of families responding to mental illness. West J Nurs Res. 2002;24(5):516–36.
5. Shah AJ, Wadoo O, Latoo J. Psychological distress in carers of people with mental disorders. British Journal of Medical Practitioners. 2010;3(3):18.
6. Zarit SH, Reever KE, Bach-Peterson J. Relatives of the impaired elderly: correlates of feelings of burden. Gerontologist. 1980;20(6):649–55.
7. Carter PA. Family caregivers' sleep loss and depression over time. Cancer Nurs. 2003;26(4):253–9.
8. Schulze B, Rössler W. Caregiver burden in mental illness: review of measurement, findings and interventions in 2004–2005. Current Opinion in Psychiatry. 2005;18(6):684–91.
9. Rose LE, Mallinson RK, Gerson LD. Mastery, burden, and areas of concern among family caregivers of mentally ill persons. Arch Psychiatr Nurs. 2006;20(1):41–51.
10. Given B, Sherwood PR, Given CW. What knowledge and skills do caregivers need? AJN The American Journal of Nursing. 2008;108(9):28–34.
11. Martire LM, Lustig AP, Schulz R, Miller GE, Helgeson VS. Is it beneficial to involve a family member? A meta-analysis of psychosocial interventions for chronic illness. Health Psychol. 2004;23(6):599.
12. Smeerdijk M, Keet R, van Raaij B, Koeter M, Linszen D, de Haan L, Schippers G. Motivational interviewing and interaction skills training for parents of young adults with recent-onset schizophrenia and co-occurring cannabis use: 15-month follow-up. Psychol Med. 2015;45(13):2839–48.
13. Signe A, Elmståhl S. Psychosocial intervention for family caregivers of people with dementia reduces caregiver's burden: development and effect after 6 and 12 months. Scand J Caring Sci. 2008;22(1):98–109.
14. Zeiss AM, Gallagher-Thompson D, Lovett S, Rose J, McKibbin C. Self- efficacy as a mediator of caregiver coping: development and testing of an assessment model. Journal of Clinical Geropsychology. 1999;5(3):221–30.
15. Bandura, A. (1994). Self-efficacy. New York City, United States: John Wiley & Sons, Inc.
16. Solomon P, Draine J. Subjective burden among family members of mentally ill adults: relation to stress, coping, and adaptation. Am J Orthopsychiatry. 1995;65(3):419.
17. Delespaul PH, De Consensusgroep EPA. Consensus over de definitie van mensen met een ernstige psychische aandoening (epa) en hun aantal in Nederland. Tijdschrift voor Psychiatrie. 2013;55(6):427–38.

18. Kuipers T, Kuipers-van Bekkum N. Training helpt in dagelijkse omgang. Ypsilon Nieuwsbrief. 2002;100:10–1.
19. Schene AH, van Wijngaarden B. Family members of people with a psychotic disorder; a study among members of Ypsilon. Amsterdam: Department of Psychiatry, University of Amsterdam; 1993.
20. Wijngaarden BV, Schene AH, Koeter MWJ, Vazquez-Barquero JL, Knudsen HC, Lasalvia A, McCrone P. Caregiving in schizophrenia: development, internal consistency and reliability of the involvement evaluation Questionaire-European version. EPSILON study 4. Br J Psychiatry. 2000; 177(S39):21–7.
21. IBM Corp. (2011). Released 2011. IBM SPSS statistics for windows, version 20. 0. Armonk, NY: IBM Corp.
22. Cohen, J. (1988). Statistical power analysis for the behavioral sciences. Hillside, NJ: Lawrence Earlbaum Associates.
23. Bond GR, Drake RE, Mueser KT, Latimer E. Assertive community treatment for people with severe mental illness. Disease Management and Health Outcomes. 2001;9(3):141–59.
24. Centrale Commissie Mensgebonden Onderzoek (CCMO), http://www.ccmo.nl/en/(2015).

18

Psychosocial stress impairs health behavior in patients with mental disorders

Till Fabian Beutel[1,2*], Rüdiger Zwerenz[1] and Matthias Michal[1]

Abstract

Background: It has been shown, that in the general population psychosocial stress affects health behaviors. However similar studies of high risk populations are sparse. Therefore, the aim of this cross-sectional study is to analyze the association between common psychosocial stressors and health behavior in a sample of patients with mental disorders.

Methods: We analyzed data of n = 2326 outpatients from a mental health care department. Severity of psychosocial stress was assessed by the PHQ-stress module of the Patient Health Questionnaire (PHQ). Health behaviors included obesity, uncontrolled eating, smoking and physical inactivity. Multiple binary regression models were conducted for the PHQ-stress score and for each of the ten PHQ-stress items as independent variables.

Results: 'Financial stress' and 'having no one to turn to with problems' were mainly associated with adverse health behaviors after adjustment for multivariate effects. The most affected health behaviors were uncontrolled eating in both sexes and obesity in women.

Conclusion: Our findings indicate specific influences of psychosocial stressors on unhealthy behaviors in a clinical sample. Patients with financial strain and lack of social support might need specific support for improving their health behavior.

Background

Stress is widespread and about a quarter of the US citizens rate their stress levels as "extreme" (8, 9 or 10 on a 10-point scale), with money, work and family responsibilities being the top sources of stress [1]. The concept of stress and its assessment have been viewed from a biomedical, psychological, sociological and environmental perspective [2–4]. Thus it can be operationalized differently and psychosocial stress has been considered for instance as major life events, chronic strains, day-to-day hassles and also as trauma [5].

Commonly analyzed outcomes of stress concern physical and mental health [6], such as cardiovascular disease [7, 8], cancer [9] or depression and anxiety [10, 11].

The complex pathways linking stress to disease and dysfunction are not fully understood [6]. Psychological stress has been linked to health behavior [12–14], which has been demonstrated to be a potential link to health outcomes [15]. Many studies have focused on the relationship between work-related stress and unhealthy lifestyles such as smoking or physical inactivity in healthy subjects [16–19].

The aim of our study is to explore the association between stress factors and health behavior in a clinical sample. Previous research has found significant correlations between stress and health behavior which will be reported below for selective forms. Most studies analyzed subjects from the general population.

Psychosocial stress and health behavior

Smoking

A longitudinal study investigated how psychosocial stressors (e. g. relationship stress, work stress, financial stress and family problems) influence smoking behavior in a general US sample over 9-10 years [12]. After adjustment for age, sex and socioeconomic status, Slopen et al. (2013) found an association between high psychosocial stress and persistence of smoking. However, there is a need for more research concerning the impact of certain psychosocial

* Correspondence: till.beutel@unimedizin-mainz.de
[1]Department of Psychosomatic Medicine and Psychotherapy, University Medical Center of the Johannes Gutenberg University Mainz, Untere Zahlbacher Str. 8, 55131 Mainz, Germany
[2]Institute of Occupational, Social and Environmental Medicine, University Medical Center of the Johannes Gutenberg University Mainz, Obere Zahlbacher Str. 67, 55131 Mainz, Germany

stressors on smoking behavior [12]. Regarding sex issues, it has been found that women were more vulnerable to tobacco use when having stress [20]. Female smokers had greater craving, arousal and stress reactions when confronted with stress cues, compared to male smokers [21, 22].

Different mechanisms are possible by which smoking behavior is influenced through stress. Smoking desire can be activated by acute psychosocial stress [13, 21], which has been shown for the Trier Social Stress Test (TSST) [13] and it can be used as a dysfunctional way to cope with stress [12, 23, 24]. Alternatively, self-regulation can be diminished as a result of stress which leads to smoking [25, 26].

Obesity and eating behavior

The amount of stress in life was associated with obesity in a large sample (N > 112.000) of the general Canadian population in a cross-sectional study [27]. A further study indicated that more than three chronic stressors compared to no stressor were linked to significantly higher odds of obesity (OR = 1.5) and percentage body fat (ß = 1.5) in a Hispanic sample [28]. Harding et al. (2014) [29] analyzed subjects from the general Australian population over five years. Psychosocial stressors were significantly associated with weight gain, but not with weight loss [29]. An association between psychosocial stress and weight gain has also been found in a longitudinal study in the general US population [14]. Relevant stressors were financial problems (difficulty paying bills) and job-related demands in both sexes, in women additionally constraints in life and family strains. Chen & Qian (2012) found a stronger association between stress and obesity in women in their Canadian sample [27].

Psychosocial stress is also associated with more uncontrolled eating [1, 30] and food craving which influences body weight [31]. Only few studies have considered which certain stressors influence eating patterns. Work-related or interpersonal (e.g. family problems, argument with partner) hassles have been associated with unhealthy eating behavior [32]. Significant predictors in terms of binge eating were as different stressors as changes in family or relationship, experiences of abuse, work stress or critical comments about weight or shape [33] and bereavement or separation from a family member [34].

More research is necessary to identify groups that are vulnerable to obesity and dysfunctional eating patterns when being under stress [28].

Physical inactivity

Although measures of stress were different from each other and the quality of the studies varied, in a review [35] a mainly negative impact of stress on physical activity has been found. The authors also reported of some studies that had found a positive impact on physical activity, as some individuals are physical active to cope with stress. A systematic review [36] reported of typical barriers for physical activity. Those were stress and low mood in patients with mental illness. Motivating aspects for physical activity on the other side were reducing stress and improving mood.

Aims and hypothesis

In our study, we want to analyze the association between psychosocial stress and health behavior in patients seeking psychotherapeutic treatment. Moreover, we want to figure out which specific psychosocial stressors are relevant for certain dysfunctional health behaviors. Previous research has found sex differences concerning the impact of stress on health behavior in the general population for instance in terms of smoking [20–22] and obesity [27], whereas women seemed to be more vulnerable. For that reason we want to take sex differences into account. Based on previous literature we suppose to see higher correlations between psychosocial stress and health behaviors in women. To the best of our knowledge this is the first study to analyze the association between psychosocial stress, assessed by the stress module of PHQ, and health behavior in a clinical sample.

Method

Procedure and study sample

We analyzed the medical records of outpatients who had been examined and treated in the Department of Psychosomatic Medicine and Psychotherapy at a university medical center between 01/2010 and 12/2013. Data of N = 2326 patients who were diagnosed and who completed the measures went into the analyses. Informed consent was obtained. The work has been carried out in accordance with the Declaration of Helsinki. The publication of this work has been approved by the Ethics Committee of the State Board of Physicians of Rhineland-Palatinate, Mainz, Germany.

Measures

The medical records contain a comprehensive set of measures which are filled out routinely by patients and by the attending physician or clinical psychologist. The self-reported measures include socio-demographic items, health behaviors and the Patient Health Questionnaire (PHQ-D, German Version). All patients were diagnosed by a clinician according to ICD-10 Chapter V diagnoses.

Health Behaviors

Physical inactivity was determined by one item, which had previously predicted mortality in patients with a history of infarction or cardiovascular disease [37]. The degree of physical activity during the last month ("activities such as

15 to 20 minutes of brisk walking, swimming, general conditioning or recreational sports") was rated according to a 5-point Likert scale: "not at all active" or "a little active (1-2 times per month)" (0), "fairly active (3-4 times per month)" (1), "quite active (1-2 times per week)" (2), "very active (3-4 times per week)" (3) and "extremely active (more than 5 times a week)" (4) [37]. Patients who rated physical activity of 15-20 minutes 3-4 times per month or less were classified as physical inactive. Smoking was asked dichotomously (yes / no). The amount of cigarettes per day was recorded in smokers (continuous). Obesity was categorized according to the body mass index (BMI ≥ 30.0). Control about the amount of food ingested was measured by an item of PHQ-D section assessing symptoms of "binge eating".

Patient Health Questionnaire - stress scale

Stress factors were assessed using the section "PHQ-stress" from the PHQ-D (German Version, [38]). It measures psychosocial strain during the last month by ten items including health, work/financial, social and traumatic stress. Ratings comprise "not at all bothered" (0), "bothered a little" (1) and "bothered a lot" (2). The summation shows cumulative values between "0" and "20" which represent the severity of stress. While validated cut-off scores are available for other scales of PHQ-D [39], no cut-off scores exist for PHQ-stress. We calculated Cronbach's alpha for the PHQ-stress scale, which was acceptable ($\alpha = 0.71$).

Statistical Analyses

Frequencies and descriptive statistics were calculated for all variables. Reliability analysis (Cronbach's alpha) was conducted for the PHQ-stress scale. The relationship between psychosocial stressors and health behavior was calculated using Chi^2-test (nominal / ordinal variables) and F-Test for continuous variables. Effect sizes were calculated using Cohen's d for means and Cramer's V for crosstabs. We computed binary logistic and linear regression analyses (method enter) with health behaviors as dependent variables. Variables were eligible to be entered into the regression model when being significantly associated with health behavior in former analyses. Regression analyses were conducted unadjusted and adjusted to check for an incremental effect of stress factors on health behaviors beyond known variables. Where necessary we adjusted multiple regression analyses for depressive disorders. We categorized depression as "0" (no depressive disorder), "1" (mild depressive disorder; ICD-10 F32.0, F33.0, F31.3), "2" (moderate depressive disorder; ICD-10 F32.1, F33.1) and "3" (severe depressive disorder; ICD-10 F32.2, F33.2). Analyses were additionally adjusted for strong overweight of parents, mainly concerning obesity and uncontrolled eating.

We conducted analyses for the PHQ-stress score and for each of the ten PHQ-stress items. All analyses were stratified by sex. Statistical analyses were carried out using IBM SPSS Statistics 23. Significance level was defined as $p < 0.05$.

Results

Demographic variables & health behavior

Table 1 shows descriptive information. The sample consisted of 56.6% ($n = 1316$) women, the mean age was 39.5 years (SD = 14.1, range = 18-93 years).

38.4% ($n = 851$) of the patients were smokers, among those were significantly ($p < 0.001$) more male (44.0%) compared to female smokers (34.0%). Male smokers consumed a higher number of cigarettes per day ($p < 0.05$). The body mass index (BMI) was higher in men ($p < 0.001$), but women were slightly more likely to be obese (BMI ≥ 30; n. s.). The prevalence of physical inactivity was around 62% (see Table 1).

PHQ-stress

The mean PHQ-stress score was M = 8.08 (SD = 4.26), women had significantly ($p < 0.001$) higher scores than men (see Table 2). The most frequent stressor was *worries about health* affecting about 57% of the patients a lot (women: 61.8%; men: 51.0%; $p < 0.001$). About one third of the patients were bothered a lot by *stress at work or at school* (34.3%), *worries about weight or look* (32.1%) and *financial problems or worries* (30.2%). *Worries about weight or look* were the second most prevalent stressors in women, *financial problems or worries* in men. Male patients were slightly more often bothered a lot by *financial problems* (n. s.), although women were significantly more bothered by all other psychosocial stressors, in terms of *difficulties with partner* only by trend (n. s.). The third most severe stressor was *stress at work or at school*, concerning both men and women.

Associations between PHQ-stress and health behaviors

BMI and obesity

The mean stress score was weakly associated ($r = 0.09$; $p < 0.001$) with BMI (continuous) (see Table 3). Obese (BMI ≥ 30) patients had a higher stress score ($p < 0.001$). Stratified for sex, higher overall stress scores were associated with obesity only in women (see Table 4). This was also significant after adjustment for confounders (adj. OR = 1.07; $p < 0.01$). On item level *worries about weight or look* (adj. OR = 2.02; $p < 0.001$), *financial problems or worries* (adj. OR = 1.64; $p < 0.01$) and *having no one to turn to with problems* (adj. OR = 1.55; $p < 0.05$) were significant predictors for obesity in women. In men *worries about weight or look* (adj. OR = 3.18; $p < 0.001$)

Table 1 Demographic and clinical characteristics, health behavior

	Total	Women	Men	*p*-value
Age Mean (SD; range)	39.5 (14.1; 18-93)	40.4 (14.2; 18-93)	38.3 (13.9; 18-83)	**<0.001**
Sex (%; *n*)		56.6 (1316)	43.4 (1010)	
Marital status (%; *n*)				**<0.001**
single	50,3 (1133)	46.3 (589)	55.6 (544)	
married	33,1 (745)	33.9 (431)	32,1 (314)	
separate living	3,8 (86)	4.4 (56)	3.1 (30)	
divorced	10,4 (234)	11.9 (152)	8.4 (82)	
widowed	2,2 (49)	3.1 (40)	0.9(9)	
School degree (%; *n*)				n.s.
in school	1.2 (27)	0.9 (11)	1.6 (16)	
no or special school degree	1.9 (43)	1.8 (23)	2.0 (20)	
basic school ("Hauptschule")	24.3 (548)	22.8 (292)	26.2 (256)	
secondary school ("Realschule")	29.0 (654)	32.4 (415)	24.4 (239)	
grammar school ("Abitur")	41.7 (941)	40.3 (515)	43.6 (426)	
Vocational degree (%; *n*)				**<0.001**
no vocational degree	15.3 (329)	12.3 (149)	19.2 (180)	
still in vocational training	10.2 (218)	10.1 (122)	10.2 (96)	
apprenticeship	39.3 (844)	43.6 (526)	33.9 (318)	
master craftsman	3.4 (72)	1.7 (20)	5.5 (52)	
university degree	21.0 (451)	20.5 (248)	21.6 (203)	
others	10.8 (232)	11.8 (142)	9.6 (90)	
Vocational position (%; *n*)				**<0.001**
employed full time	33.4 (743)	26.4 (333)	42.4 (410)	
employed part time	16.3 (363)	23.4 (295)	7.0 (68)	
not employed (e.g. housewife)	5.8 (130)	9.5 (120)	1.0 (10)	
vocational training	8.6 (191)	7.9 (100)	9.4 (91)	
unemployed	14.1 (315)	10.8 (136)	18.5 (179)	
retired	9.7 (217)	10.6 (133)	8.7 (84)	
others	12.0 (268)	11.3 (143)	12.9 (125)	
Diagnoses ICD-10 (%; *n*)				
depression (F32, F33, F34) (%)				**<0.001**
no depressive disorder / other	50.0 (1162)	46.4 (610)	54.7 (552)	
mild depressive disorder	8.0 (185)	8.5 (112)	7.2 (73)	
moderate depressive disorder	34.6 (804)	37.1 (488)	31.3 (316)	
severe depressive disorder	7.5 (175)	8.1 (106)	6.8 (69)	
anxiety disorder (F40. F41) (%)	27.3 (634)	29.0 (382)	25.0 (252)	**<0.05**
somatoform disorder (F45) (%)	18.2 (423)	20.7 (272)	15.0 (151)	**<0.001**
number of F-diagnoses/patient	2.0 (2326)	2.0 (1316)	2.0 (1010)	
Health behavior				
smoking (% yes; *n*)	38.4 (851)	34.0% (424)	44.0% (427)	**<0.001**
number of cig./day (M; SD)	11.4 (15.7)	10.5 (16.5)	12.4 (14.9)	**<0.05**

Table 1 Demographic and clinical characteristics, health behavior *(Continued)*

	Total	Women	Men	*p*-value
BMI (M; SD)	25.5 (5.8)	24.9 (6.3)	26.2 (5.1)	**<0.001**
obesity (BMI ≥ 30.0) (%; *n*)	18.5 (377)	19.3 (218)	17.4 (159)	
uncontrolled eating (% yes; *n*)	24.9 (552)	27.3 (341)	21.7 (211)	**<0.001**
physical inactivity (< 2)	61.9 (1345)	62.3 (762)	61.3 (583)	

Significant differences between female (n = 1316) and male (n = 1010) patients were tested by Chi^2-Test for crosstabs and by F-Test for means, significant differences are highlighted in bold and presented as p-value

Table 2 Frequency of psychosocial stress stratified by sex

PHQ-stress scale (M; SD)	M	SD						*p*-value
Total	8.08	4.26						**<0.001**
Women	8.70	4.29						
Men	7.34	4.11						
PHQ-stress items (M; *n*)								
	not bothered		bothered a little		bothered a lot			
Worries about health	15.1	(335)	27.8	(619)	57.1	(1269)		**<0.001**
Women	12.2	(152)	26.0	(325)	61.8	(772)	[1]	
Men	18.8	(183)	30.2	(294)	51.0	(497)	[1]	
Stress at work or at school	43.7	(933)	22.0	(470)	34.3	(732)		**<0.01**
Women	41.9	(501)	20.5	(245)	37.6	(449)	[3]	
Men	46.0	(432)	23.9	(225)	30.1	(283)	[3]	
Worries about weight or look	31.9	(710)	36.0	(802)	32.1	(716)		**<0.001**
Women	27.3	(343)	33.0	(415)	39.6	(498)	[2]	
Men	37.8	(367)	39.8	(387)	22.4	(218)	[6]	
Financial problems or worries	39.6	(877)	30.1	(667)	30.2	(669)		n.s.
Women	41.7	(519)	29.0	(361)	29.4	(366)	[5]	
Men	37.0	(358)	31.6	(306)	31.3	(303)	[2]	
Little or no sexual desire	46.4	(1004)	26.7	(577)	26.9	(582)		**<0.01**
Women	45.1	(543)	24.8	(299)	30.1	(363)	[4]	
Men	48.1	(461)	29.0	(278)	22.9	(219)	[5]	
Difficulties with partner	49.7	(1066)	25.5	(546)	24.8	(532)		n.s.
Women	48.7	(584)	25.1	(301)	26.1	(313)	[7]	
Men	51.0	(482)	25.9	(245)	23.2	(219)	[4]	
Thinking / dreaming about something terrible that happened	56.2	(1236)	18.9	(416)	24.8	(546)		**<0.001**
Women	49.1	(606)	21.6	(266)	29.3	(361)	[6]	
Men	65.3	(630)	15.5	(150)	19.2	(185)	[8]	
Having no one to turn to with problems	47.2	(1041)	29.8	(657)	23.0	(507)		**<0.05**
Women	45.0	(558)	30.4	(377)	24.7	(306)	[8]	
Men	50.1	(483)	29.0	(280)	20.9	(201)	[7]	
Something bad that happened recently	64.4	(1391)	14.7	(317)	20.9	(452)		**<0.001**
Women	60.8	(736)	15.2	(184)	24.0	(291)	[9]	
Men	69.0	(655)	14.0	(133)	17.0	(161)	[9]	
Stress of care taking	61.5	(1336)	20.5	(446)	18.0	(392)		**<0.001**
Women	57.3	(700)	21.6	(264)	21.0	(257)	[10]	
Men	66.7	(636)	19.1	(182)	14.2	(135)	[10]	

Psychosocial stressors are rated "not at all bothered" to "bothered a lot" and presented according to frequency of "bothered a lot", rankings of men and women are presented in square brackets. Sex differences were calculated by Chi^2-Test. Significant differences are highlighted in bold

Table 3 Association between PHQ-stress and health behavior

	BMI					Obesity (BMI ≥ 30)			Uncontrolled eating			Smoking			Cig / day					Physical inactivity		
						no	yes		no	yes		no	yes							no	yes	
PHQ-stress scale (0-20)	r=0.09***					M=7.92	M=8.94	***	M=7.43	M=10.16	***	M=7.85	M=8.47	**	r=0.08**					M=7.40	M=8.52	***
						SD=4.22	SD=4.33		SD=4.13	SD=3.98		SD=4.13	SD=4.37							SD=4.06	SD=4.28	
	BMI (M, SD)					Obesity (% BMI ≥ 30)			Uncontrolled eating (% yes)			Smoking (% yes)			Cig / day (M, SD)					Physical inactivity (% inactive)		
PHQ-stress items (dichotomous)	not/a little bothered		bothered a lot			not/a little bothered	bothered a lot		not/a little bothered	bothered a lot		not/a little bothered	bothered a lot		not/a little bothered		bothered a lot			not/a little bothered	bothered a lot	
					d_{Cohen}			Cramérs V			Cramérs V			Cramérs V					d_{Cohen}			Cramérs V
Worries about health	25.3	(5.4)	25.6	(6.1)		**16.2**	**19.9**	**0.05***	**22.3**	**26.8**	**0.05***	**43.4**	**34.9**	**0.09*****	11.2	(12.6)	10.7	(15.5)		**58.5**	**64.5**	**0.06****
Stress at work or at school	25.3	(5.8)	25.6	(5.9)		**16.6**	**20.6**	**0.05***	**20.8**	**31.9**	**0.12*****	40.1	35.8		**11.5**	**(15.3)**	**9.7**	**(12.9)**	**0.12***	61.7	62.4	
Worries about weight or look	**25.1**	**(4.9)**	**26.4**	**(7.3)**	**0.23*****	**14.3**	**28.0**	**0.16*****	**15.2**	**45.6**	**0.33*****	38.7	38.4		10.8	(13.3)	11.5	(16.5)		60.7	64.5	
Financial problems or worries	**25.1**	**(5.8)**	**26.3**	**(6.0)**	**0.21*****	**16.0**	**24.3**	**0.10*****	**20.7**	**34.4**	**0.15*****	**32.8**	**51.3**	**0.18*****	**9.8**	**(14.7)**	**13.3**	**(13.7)**	**0.24*****	**59.0**	**68.0**	**0.09*****
Little or no sexual desire	25.4	(5.7)	25.6	(6.1)		18.6	17.9		**22.8**	**29.6**	**0.07****	39.2	37.3		10.9	(14.7)	11.5	(14.1)		60.8	65.5	
Difficulties with partner	25.5	(5.8)	25.3	(5.8)		18.7	16.5		**22.4**	**30.4**	**0.08*****	**36.8**	**44.4**	**0.07****	10.9	(15.4)	11.4	(11.7)		61.0	65.3	
Thinking / dreaming about sth terrible	**25.2**	**(5.5)**	**26.4**	**(6.7)**	**0.21*****	**17.0**	**22.7**	**0.06****	**21.0**	**36.6**	**0.16*****	37.4	40.7		10.5	(13.1)	11.8	(16.0)		60.9	64.7	
Having no one to turn to with problems	25.3	(5.7)	25.9	(6.3)		**17.3**	**22.1**	**0.05***	**21.9**	**34.8**	**0.13*****	37.7	40.6		10.7	(14.5)	11.7	(14.3)		**58.7**	**72.0**	**0.12*****
Something bad that happened recently	25.4	(6.0)	25.7	(5.2)		17.9	19.6		24.7	25.7		37.9	40.6		10.7	(13.8)	11.9	(16.7)		**60.4**	**66.9**	**0.06***
Stress of care taking	**25.3**	**(5.7)**	**26.3**	**(6.6)**	**0.17****	**17.3**	**23.2**	**0.06****	**22.7**	**34.3**	**0.10*****	37.9	42.8		10.7	(14.7)	12.4	(13.5)		**60.8**	**68.0**	**0.06****

***$p < 0.001$; **$p < 0.01$; *$p < 0.05$; correlation analyses *r* Pearson's r; *M* mean, *SD* standard deviation. PHQ-stress items: comparison between "not or a little bothered" vs. "bothered a lot". Physical inactivity: patients who rated 3-4 times per month of physical activity or less were classified as physical inactive. Significance level was tested by Chi^2 for crosstabs and F-Test for means
Effect sizes for significant results were calculated using Cohen's d for means and Cramer's V for crosstabs. Significant results are highlighted in bold

Table 4 Multiple regression analyses (binary, linear) between PHQ-stress and health behavior stratified by sex

	Obesity			Uncontrolled eating			Smoking			Cig/day		Physical inactivity		
PHQ-stress - Women	OR	95% CI	Nagelk. R^2	OR	95% CI	Nagelk. R^2	OR	95% CI	Nagelk. R^2	stand. ß	adj. R^2	OR	95% CI	Nagelk. R^2
PHQ-stress scale (0-20) (unadj.)	**1.07****	**1.03-1.11**	**2.0**	**1.18*****	**1.14-1.23**	**13.1**	**1.05****	**1.02-1.08**	**1.3**	n.s.		**1.06*****	**1.03-1.09**	**1.9**
PHQ-stress scale (0-20) (adjusted)	**1.07****	**1.03-1.11**	**11.7**	**1.17*****	**1.12-1.22**	**18.5**	1.03	1.00-1.07	n.s.	n.s.		**1.05***	**1.01-1.08**	**5.5**
PHQ-stress items (dichotomous)														
Worries about health (unadj.)	n.s.			n.s.			**0.77***	**0.59-0.83**	**0.5**	n.s.		n.s.		
adjusted	n.s.			n.s.			0.77	0.57-1.03	n.s.	n.s.		n.s.		
Stress at work or at school (unadj.)	n.s.			**1.75*****	**1.35-2.27**	**2.2**	n.s.			n.s.		n.s.		
adjusted	n.s.			**1.69*****	**1.26-2.27**	**10.4**	n.s.			n.s.		n.s.		
Worries about weight or look (unadj.)	**2.03*****	**1.51-2.74**	**3.0**	**4.86*****	**3.72-6.36**	**15.9**	n.s.			n.s.		n.s.		
adjusted	**2.02*****	**1.46-2.79**	**12.6**	**4.49*****	**3.38-5.97**	**21.7**	n.s.			n.s.		n.s.		
Financial problems or worries (unadj.)	**1.78*****	**1.30-2.43**	**1.9**	**2.15*****	**1.65-2.79**	**3.7**	**1.85*****	**1.43-2.38**	**2.5**	**0.10****	**0.9**	**1.48*****	**1.22-1.80**	**1.0**
adjusted	**1.64****	**1.18-2.31**	**11.3**	**1.79*****	**1.34-2.38**	**11.0**	**1.45***	**1.08-1.93**	**14.1**	**0.09***	**1.9**	**1.34***	**1.01-1.77**	**4.1**
Little or no sexual desire (unadj.)	n.s.			**1.39***	**1.06-1.82**	**0.7**	n.s.			n.s.		n.s.		
adjusted	n.s.			1.30	0.97-1.74	n.s.	n.s.			n.s.		n.s.		
Difficulties with partner (unadj.)	n.s.			**1.59****	**1.20-2.10**	**1.2**	**1.44****	**1.10-1.89**	**0.8**	n.s.		**1.40***	**1.06-1.85**	**0.7**
adjusted	n.s.			1.36	0.99-1.87	n.s.	**1.47***	**1.08-1.99**	**14.3**	n.s.		1.30	0.97-1.76	n.s.
Thinking/dreaming about sth terrible that happened (unadj.)	**1.46***	**1.06-2.00**	**0.8**	**1.98*****	**1.52-2.59**	**2.9**	**1.56*****	**1.20-2.01**	**1.3**	**0.12****	**1.2**	n.s.		
adjusted	1.37	0.98-1.92	n.s.	**1.78*****	**1.34-2.37**	**10.9**	**1.52****	**1.14-2.03**	**15.0**	**0.10****	**2.7**	n.s.		
Having no one to turn to with problems (unadj.)	**1.71****	**1.24-2.37**	**1.5**	**1.96*****	**1.49-2.59**	**2.6**	n.s.			n.s.		**1.67*****	**1.26-2.23**	**1.5**
adjusted	**1.55***	**1.10-2.19**	**10.9**	**1.58****	**1.17-2.15**	**10.1**	n.s.			n.s.		**1.50****	**1.10-2.05**	**4.9**
Something bad that happened recently (unadj.)	n.s.			n.s.			**1.39***	**1.06-1.83**	**0.6**	n.s.		**1.33***	**1.06-1.66**	**0.9**
adjusted	n.s.						1.26	0.91-1.74	n.s.	n.s.		**1.40***	**1.04-1.89**	**4.5**
Stress of care taking (unadj.)	**1.46***	**1.03-2.07**	**0.6**	**1.58****	**1.17-2.13**	**1.0**	n.s.			n.s.		n.s.		
adjusted	1.41	0.97-2.06	n.s.	**1.57****	**1.13-2.18**	**9.9**	n.s.			n.s.		n.s.		
PHQ-stress - Men	OR	95% CI	Nagelk. R^2	OR	95% CI	Nagelk. R^2	OR	95% CI	Nagelk. R^2	stand. ß	adj. R^2	OR	95% CI	Nagelk. R^2
PHQ-stress scale (0-20) (unadj.)	1.03	0.99-1.08	n.s.	**1.13*****	**1.09-1.18**	**6.7**	**1.04***	**1.00-1.07**	**0.7**	**0.12****	**1.2**	**1.07*****	**1.04-1.11**	**2.6**
PHQ-stress scale (0-20) (adj.)	1.02	0.98-1.07	n.s.	**1.14*****	**1.09-1.19**	**9.3**	**1.06****	**1.02-1.10**	**19.8**	**0.10***	**5.7**	**1.06****	**1.02-1.10**	**5.2**

Table 4 Multiple regression analyses (binary, linear) between PHQ-stress and health behavior stratified by sex *(Continued)*

	Obesity			Uncontrolled eating			Smoking			Cig/day		Physical inactivity		
PHQ-stress items (dichotomous)														
Worries about health (unadj.)	n.s.			n.s.			0.69**	0.53-0.89	1.2			1.45**	1.11-1.89	1.1
adjusted	n.s.			n.s.			0.73*	0.55-0.98	19.3			1.33*	1.01-1.75	4.4
Stress at work or at school (unadj.)	n.s.			1.72**	1.24-2.39	1.7	n.s.			n.s.		n.s.		
adjusted	n.s.			1.57**	1.11-2.21	3.9	n.s.			n.s.		n.s.		
Worries about weight or look (unadj.)	2.89***	1.99-4.18	5.4	4.27***	3.05-5.97	10.9	n.s.					n.s.		
adjusted	3.18***	2.15-4.71	13.8	4.05***	2.88-5.68	12.8	n.s.					n.s.		
Financial problems or worries (unadj.)	1.57*	1.10-2.24	1.1	1.87***	1.36-2.57	2.3	2.59***	1.96-3.43	6.2	0.13***	1.5	1.49**	1.11-1.99	1.1
adjusted	1.39	0.95-2.04	n.s.	1.75***	1.26-2.41	4.5	2.25***	1.63-3.09	22.4	0.12**	6.5	1.30	0.96-1.76	n.s.
Little or no sexual desire (unadj.)	n.s.			1.41	0.99-2.01	0.6	n.s.			n.s.		n.s.		
adjusted	n.s.			1.37	0.94-1.99	n.s.	n.s.			n.s.		n.s.		
Difficulties with partner (unadj.)	n.s.			n.s.			n.s.			n.s.		n.s.		
adjusted	n.s.			n.s.			n.s.			n.s.		n.s.		
Thinking/dreaming about sth terrible that happened (unadj.)	n.s.			2.33***	1.63-3.33	3.3	n.s.			n.s.		n.s.		
adjusted	n.s.			2.19***	1.51-3.17	5.5	n.s.			n.s.		n.s.		
Having no one to turn to with problems (unadj.)	n.s.			1.76**	1.23-2.51	1.5	n.s.			n.s.		2.02***	1.42-2.88	2.4
adjusted	n.s.			1.6*	1.11-2.31	3.6	n.s.			n.s.		1.87***	1.30-2.69	5.2
Something bad that happened recently (unadj.)	n.s.			n.s.			n.s.			n.s.		n.s.		
adjusted	n.s.			n.s.			n.s.			n.s.		n.s.		
Stress of care taking (unadj.)	n.s.			2.03***	1.36-3.03	1.9	1.59*	1.10-2.31	0.9	0.09*	0.6	1.72**	1.14-2.60	1.0
adjusted	n.s.			2.00***	1.33-3.03	4.3	1.87**	1.22-2.87	20.2**	0.11*	6.1	1.64*	1.08-2.51	4.2

Each PHQ-stress item was dichotomized in "not or a little bothered (0)" and "bothered a lot (1)". PHQ-stress scale ranges from 0-20. Logistic Regression analyses are presented unadjusted and adjusted for age, education, vocational training, depression

Analyses concerning obesity (BMI>30) and binge eating were adjusted for obesity of parents. Non-significant results from previous analyses were not considered in regression analyses and marked as n.s. *unadj* unadjusted. ***$p < 0.001$; **$p < 0.01$; *$p < 0.05$. *OR* Odds Ratio. Effect sizes (Cohen's d) are calculated for OR. Nagelk. R^2 = explained variance (in %). Significant results are highlighted in bold predicted obesity in an adjusted logistic regression model (see Table 4).

Uncontrolled eating

Higher overall stress scores were associated with a higher chance of uncontrolled eating in women (adj. OR = 1.17; $p < 0.001$) and in men (adj. OR = 1.14; $p < 0.001$) in an adjusted logistic regression model (see Table 4). Women and men showed higher odds of uncontrolled eating when being bothered a lot by *worries about weight or look* (women: adj. OR = 4.49; p < 0.001; men: adj. OR = 4.05; $p < 0.001$), *financial problems* (women: adj. OR = 1.79; $p < 0.001$; men: adj. OR = 1.75; $p < 0.001$), *having no one to turn to with problems* (women: adj. OR = 1.58; $p < 0.01$; men: adj. OR = 1.60; $p < 0.01$), *stress of care taking* (women: adj. OR = 1.57; $p < 0.01$; men: adj. OR = 2.00; $p < 0.001$), *stress at work or at school* (women: adj. OR = 1.69; $p < 0.001$; men: adj. OR = 1.57; $p < 0.01$) and *thinking/dreaming about something terrible that happened* (women: adj. OR = 1.78; $p < 0.001$; men: adj. OR = 2.19; $p < 0.001$).

Smoking and cigarettes per day

Patients with higher stress scores were more likely to be smokers ($p < 0.01$; see Table 3). The overall stress score was - adjusted for multivariate effects - only significant in male patients (see Table 4). Being bothered a lot by *worries about health* had lower odds towards smoking in male (adj. OR = 0.73; $p < 0.05$) and in female patients (adj. OR = 0.77; n. s.). Patients with severe *financial problems* were more likely to smoke, the odds ratio was higher in men (adj. OR = 2.25; $p < 0.001$) compared to women (adj. OR = 1.45; $p < 0.05$). Moreover, male and female smokers fumed significantly more cigarettes when being bothered a lot by *financial problems* (women: stand. ß = 0.09; $p < 0.05$; men: stand. ß = 0.12; $p < 0.01$). *Difficulties with partner* (adj. OR = 1.47; $p < 0.05$) and *thinking/dreaming about something terrible that happened* (adj. OR = 1.52; $p < 0.01$) were further predictors in women. Men were significantly more likely to be smoking when being bothered a lot by *stress of care taking* (adj. OR = 1.87; $p < 0.01$), which was also associated with a higher consumption of cigarettes (stand. ß = 0.11; $p < 0.05$).

Physical inactivity

Higher overall stress scores went along with a higher prevalence of physical inactivity, which was significant as a mean score ($p < 0.001$, see Table 3) and in an adjusted regression model for men ($p < 0.01$) and women ($p < 0.05$; see Table 4). On item-level, both male and female patients had a higher prevalence of physical inactivity when being bothered a lot by *having no one to turn to with problems* (men: adj. OR = 1.87; $p < 0.001$; women: adj. OR = 1.50; $p < 0.01$). Men also showed a higher prevalence of physical inactivity when being bothered a lot by *stress of care taking* (adj. OR = 1.64; $p < 0.05$) and *worries about health* (adj. OR = 1.33; $p < 0.05$). Female patients who were bothered a lot by *something bad that happened recently* (adj. OR = 1.40; $p < 0.05$) and by *financial problems or worries* (adj. OR = 1.34; $p < 0.05$) were more likely to be physical inactive.

Discussion

The overall stress score in our sample (M = 8.08) was much higher compared to primary care patients (PHQ-stress: M = 2.3 for older and M = 4.7 for younger patients; [40]. Women were significantly more bothered by psychosocial stress than men. This sex difference has also been found in previous studies [1, 28, 40]. The most frequent stressor by which both male and female patients were bothered a lot by was worries about health in almost 60% of our sample. The second most severe stressor was worries about weight or look in women and financial problems in men. However, stress at work or at school was common in both. Those were also frequent stressors found in former studies [1, 40], although differences in the order existed.

The global PHQ-stress score was significantly associated with health behaviors. After adjustment for further variables the stress score was associated with obesity, uncontrolled eating and physical inactivity in women and concerning men with smoking, uncontrolled eating and physical inactivity.

The focus on specific stressors made clear, that the associations between the stress score and health behaviors were based on certain stressors. Some specific stressors were not at all associated with health behavior. This is similar to a study by Slopen et al. (2013). The authors focused on smoking and concluded that the cumulative stress score did not predict smoking behavior better in the general population, as some stressors were not associated with it at all (such as neighborhood stress or work-family conflict) [12].

Hereafter, relevant stressors and health behaviors from our findings will be emphasized.

Financial problems or worries as well as social support ("having no one to turn to with problems") have been identified as important stress factors being associated with health behaviors in a clinical sample.

In terms of financial problems, the adjusted regression model showed higher chances of uncontrolled eating and obesity as well as smoking and physical inactivity in women having great financial worries. Male patients had higher chances of smoking and uncontrolled eating. Financial problems showed incremental explanation of variance in health behaviors beyond known factors such as sociodemographic variables (age, education) as well as depression, which the regression model has been adjusted for. A negative effect of financial problems on smoking behavior [12] and on weight gain respectively obesity [14] has been reported in previous studies concerning the general population. Indeed, findings were not fully consistent as high financial stress has also led to higher odds of quitting smoking [12].

Another important stressor being associated with adverse health behavior was lack of social support. Being bothered a lot by having no one to turn to with problems was associated with obesity, uncontrolled eating and physical inactivity in women. In men having no one to turn to with problems was associated with uncontrolled eating and physical inactivity. A laboratory study with female students also indicated the relevance of social stress on health behavior [41]. The students showed a higher caloric intake when being confronted with an induced social stressor compared to an academic stressor. Another study found a positive association of social support with better dietary quality in persons from the general population [42]. This goes inversely in line with our findings according to eating behavior.

Interestingly, being bothered a lot by worries about health was associated with lower chances of being a smoker. Adjusted for covariates, this was only significant in men. It corresponds with a finding that many smokers do not consider themselves to be a high risk group in terms of cancer or cardiovascular disease [43]. Also, health-related worries were not associated with obesity or physical inactivity although those lifestyle behaviors have higher health risks as well. We also found stress factors that were not associated with health behaviors at all. Those were little or no sexual desire concerning both sexes. Furthermore, regarding men difficulties with partner and something bad that happened recently had no impact on health behavior. In sum, we found health behaviors to be influenced selectively by certain psychosocial stressors. Concerning health behaviors, mostly associated with psychosocial stress were uncontrolled eating in both sexes and obesity in women. Especially uncontrolled eating was mostly associated with the considered psychosocial stress factors and showed the highest effect sizes. This goes in line with previous research. The majority of previous studies reported that stress predicted uncontrolled eating [30], binge eating [33, 34] and worse dietary habits such as the intake of high caloric food [32, 44, 45]. Some studies also reported findings to predominantly eat less in stress (so called "stress-undereaters") or found no effect on eating behavior [41, 46, 47]. Also, in previous studies [14, 27] obesity has been linked to stress rather in women than in men. Contrary to studies from the general population [20–22] we did not see that women were more vulnerable to smoking when having stress.

We only found marginal sex differences. Financial stress was associated with health behaviors in both, men and women. However, having no one to turn to was clearer associated with health behaviors in women, while stress of care taking was clearer in men. This is interesting, as women were much more often bothered by stress of care taking. Nonetheless, this psychosocial stressor seemed to affect health behavior of men more negatively. In sum and contrary to our hypothesis, sex differences were not that distinctive concerning the associations between psychosocial stress and health behaviors. One potential reason might be due to differences in the measurement as different studies measured psychosocial stress differently. It is also possible, that this illustrates differences between persons from the general population and the considered sample of patients. Further research should clarify this. Sex differences were only clear on descriptive level, where women were consistently more burdened by psychosocial stress, which goes in line with previous research [11, 28, 40, 48].

Influences on health behavior are multifactorial and we could indicate that psychosocial stress has small, but significant associations with health behaviors in a clinical sample.

Limitations & strengths

One of the limitations of our study is the cross-sectional design which is not able to allow statements towards causality and which does not provide information on how long patients have been bothered by certain stressors. Although associations between psychosocial stress and health behaviors have been highly significant, we have mainly found low effect sizes. This has been shown for instance by the explained variance and goes in line with previously reported studies. Still we found an incremental effect of stress on health behavior beyond known factors such as demographic and socio-economic variables.

Although we considered psychosocial stress to affect health behavior, influences can be reverse as well. Moreover, limitations concerning the measurement of health behaviors should be pointed out. Due to the limitations of clinical records we were only able to conduct basic measures of health behaviors. Moreover, all measurements are self-rated, which might be a source of error. A further aspect refers to physical inactivity, which has been measured only by one item. For this reason it can only be considered as a rough screening. More detailed instruments (e.g. International Physical Activity Questionnaire, IPAQ; [49]) would have been more sophisticated. On the other side, longer scales do not seem to have an added value compared to one item scales [50, 51]. Stress-related eating for instance can include different aspects as the amount and type of food [30, 52]. We cannot answer if patients eat more or less when being bothered by psychosocial stress. We can only conclude that patients seem to eat uncontrolled when being bothered by certain stressors. The measurement of psychosocial stress is complex as different concepts exist and many assessments are available

[4, 5, 53]. We measured psychosocial stress via the PHQ-stress module which includes ten major stressors. In contrast to more detailed scales [5, 54], the PHQ-stress module can only be considered as a screening instrument. It is useful to quickly identify important psychosocial stress factors in patients. The items are heterogeneous, nonetheless the scale's reliability is still acceptable ($\alpha = 0.71$).

Still, we wanted to screen for specific stressors contrary to e.g. the Perceived Stress Scale (PSS-10; [55]) which does not name particular stressors. We showed the usability of PHQ-stress being part of the most important comprehensive clinical measure (PHQ) with the external criterion of health behavior. While the Patient Health Questionnaire is a well validated instrument [56–59], the module PHQ-stress has been neglected. To our knowledge the PHQ-stress module has not been validated, however it has been used in different studies [40, 60–63]. Efforts to validate PHQ-stress would be helpful.

Health behavior is influenced by different factors, amongst others by somatic and mental illness. We did not control for comorbid somatic diseases as it is almost impossible to conclude on functional aspects just from the ICD-10 diagnosis, which can be seen as a limitation. However, health behavior is strongly affected by mental illness as depression [64–66]. In order to reduce this bias, we adjusted our analyses where necessary for depressive disorders, which were diagnosed by a clinician for all patients. We consider this as a strength of our study as we were able to adjust for the severity of depression. Where elsewhere necessary, besides demographic variables we adjusted for strong overweight of parents. By this, we roughly took genetic and environmental factors into account. A further strength is our large clinical sample and the consideration of different health behaviors. Many studies analyzed samples from the general population and we were able to close a gap for a clinical sample which is generally at high risk for maladaptive health behaviors.

Conclusions

Longitudinal studies are necessary to further research the impact of psychosocial stress on health behaviors in mental health patients. Presumably, greater associations between those variables would be found in a longitudinal design. The duration and the severity of different stress factors as well as coping strategies should be taken into account. In addition, it would be important to consider sex differences which we found on descriptive level significantly, but not in terms of associations. These findings might be different in longitudinal studies.

As a clinical implication, specific trainings can be tested for certain clusters of psychosocial stress. For example, to reduce psychosocial stress resulting from relationships (e.g. having no one to turn to) an additional treatment to improve social skills for those patients can be beneficial. Especially, patients with financial strain and lack of social support might need specific assistance to improve their health behavior.

It would be helpful to assist patients in developing functional coping strategies which enable them to reduce unhealthy behaviors for emotional regulation. In the recent years, different ways to include treatment of unhealthy behaviors into psychotherapy were presented [67–69]. Moreover, a more holistic model of the patient's disorder is necessary, as psychosocial stress, psychopathology and health behavior presumably influence each other mutually. This might be the case in patients seeking psychotherapeutic treatment in particular as these are more often affected by psychosocial stress than for instance primary care patients. The improvement of health behaviors should be part of the treatment in general as these patients are more likely to show unhealthy behaviors [70–72], which contribute to a worse somatic health status [73–76]. Furthermore, the improvement of health behaviors can have positive effects on mental disorders. For instance, a recent review has shown antidepressant effects of physical activity [77].

Abbreviations

BMI: Body mass index; OR: Odds ratio; PHQ: Patient Health Questionnaire; SD: Standard deviation; ß: standardized beta; TSST: Trier Social Stress Test

Acknowledgements

Not applicable.

Funding

This research did not receive any specific grant from funding agencies in the public, commercial, or not-for-profit sectors.

Authors' contributions

TB is the main author of this article. He planned this work, calculated the statistics and wrote all chapters. RZ supported in providing the data. MM contributed ideas. Both RZ and MM provided this work with proof reading. All authors have approved of the submission of the manuscript to the journal.

Consent for publication

Not applicable.

Competing interests

The authors declare that they have no competing interests.

References

1. American Psychological Association. Stress in America: The impact of discrimination. Stress in America™ Survey; 2016.
2. Cohen S, Kessler RC, Gordon LU. Measuring stress: A guide for health and social scientists: Oxford University Press; 1995.
3. McEwen BS, McEwen CA. Response to Jerome Kagan's Essay on Stress (2016). Perspect Psychol Sci. 2016;11:451–5. https://doi.org/10.1177/1745691616646635.

4. Cohen S, Gianaros PJ, Manuck SB. A Stage Model of Stress and Disease. Perspect Psychol Sci. 2016;11:456–63. https://doi.org/10.1177/1745691616646305.
5. Thoits PA. Stress and health: major findings and policy implications. J Health Soc Behav. 2010;51(Suppl):S41–53. https://doi.org/10.1177/0022146510383499.
6. Cohen S, Janicki-Deverts D, Miller GE. Psychological stress and disease. JAMA. 2007;298:1685–7. https://doi.org/10.1001/jama.298.14.1685.
7. Aboa-Eboule C, Brisson C, Maunsell E, Masse B, Bourbonnais R, Vezina M, et al. Job strain and risk of acute recurrent coronary heart disease events. JAMA. 2007;298:1652–60. https://doi.org/10.1001/jama.298.14.1652.
8. de Bacquer D, Pelfrene E, Clays E, Mak R, Moreau M, de Smet P, et al. Perceived job stress and incidence of coronary events: 3-year follow-up of the Belgian Job Stress Project cohort. Am J Epidemiol. 2005;161:434–41. https://doi.org/10.1093/aje/kwi040.
9. Chida Y, Hamer M, Wardle J, Steptoe A. Do stress-related psychosocial factors contribute to cancer incidence and survival? Nat Clin Pract Oncol. 2008;5:466–75. https://doi.org/10.1038/ncponc1134.
10. Hammen C. Stress and depression. Annu Rev Clin Psychol. 2005;1:293–319. https://doi.org/10.1146/annurev.clinpsy.1.102803.143938.
11. Wiegner L, Hange D, Bjorkelund C, Ahlborg G Jr. Prevalence of perceived stress and associations to symptoms of exhaustion, depression and anxiety in a working age population seeking primary care--an observational study. BMC Fam Pract. 2015;16:38. https://doi.org/10.1186/s12875-015-0252-7.
12. Slopen N, Kontos EZ, Ryff CD, Ayanian JZ, Albert MA, Williams DR. Psychosocial stress and cigarette smoking persistence, cessation, and relapse over 9-10 years: a prospective study of middle-aged adults in the United States. Cancer Causes Control. 2013;24:1849–63. https://doi.org/10.1007/s10552-013-0262-5.
13. Childs E, de Wit H. Effects of acute psychosocial stress on cigarette craving and smoking. Nicotine Tob Res. 2010;12:449–53. https://doi.org/10.1093/ntr/ntp214.
14. Block JP, He Y, Zaslavsky AM, Ding L, Ayanian JZ. Psychosocial stress and change in weight among US adults. Am J Epidemiol. 2009;170:181–92. https://doi.org/10.1093/aje/kwp104.
15. Robert Koch-Institut. Gesundheit in Deutschland. Gesundheitsberichterstattung des Bundes: RKI-Bib1 (Robert Koch-Institut); 2015.
16. Fransson EI, Heikkila K, Nyberg ST, Zins M, Westerlund H, Westerholm P, et al. Job strain as a risk factor for leisure-time physical inactivity: an individual-participant meta-analysis of up to 170,000 men and women: the IPD-Work Consortium. Am J Epidemiol. 2012;176:1078–89. https://doi.org/10.1093/aje/kws336.
17. Kivimäki M, Nyberg ST, Fransson EI, Heikkilä K, Alfredsson L, Casini A, et al. Associations of job strain and lifestyle risk factors with risk of coronary artery disease: A meta-analysis of individual participant data. CMAJ. 2013;185:763–9. https://doi.org/10.1503/cmaj.121735.
18. Kouvonen A, Vahtera J, Oksanen T, Pentti J, Vaananen AKP, Heponiemi T, et al. Chronic workplace stress and insufficient physical activity: a cohort study. Occup Environ Med. 2013;70:3–8. https://doi.org/10.1136/oemed-2012-100808.
19. Griep RH, Nobre AA, MGdM A, MdJM d F, LdO C, Giatti L, et al. Job strain and unhealthy lifestyle: results from the baseline cohort study, Brazilian Longitudinal Study of Adult Health (ELSA-Brasil). BMC Public Health. 2015;15:309. https://doi.org/10.1186/s12889-015-1626-4.
20. Torres OV, O'Dell LE. Stress is a principal factor that promotes tobacco use in females. Prog Neuropsychopharmacol Biol Psychiatry. 2016;65:260–8. https://doi.org/10.1016/j.pnpbp.2015.04.005.
21. Wray JM, Gray KM, McClure EA, Carpenter MJ, Tiffany ST, Saladin ME. Gender differences in responses to cues presented in the natural environment of cigarette smokers. Nicotine Tob Res. 2015;17:438–42. https://doi.org/10.1093/ntr/ntu248.
22. Saladin ME, Gray KM, Carpenter MJ, LaRowe SD, DeSantis SM, Upadhyaya HP. Gender differences in craving and cue reactivity to smoking and negative affect/stress cues. Am J Addict. 2012;21:210–20. https://doi.org/10.1111/j.1521-0391.2012.00232.x.
23. McGee R, Williams S, Nada-Raja S, Olsson CA. Tobacco smoking in adolescence predicts maladaptive coping styles in adulthood. Nicotine Tob Res. 2013;15:1971–7. https://doi.org/10.1093/ntr/ntt081.
24. Khantzian EJ. The self-medication hypothesis of substance use disorders: A reconsideration and recent applications. Harv Rev Psychiatry. 1997;4:231–44. https://doi.org/10.3109/10673229709030550.
25. Baumeister RF, Vonasch AJ. Uses of self-regulation to facilitate and restrain addictive behavior. Addict Behav. 2015;44:3–8. https://doi.org/10.1016/j.addbeh.2014.09.011.
26. Daly M, Delaney L, Baumeister RF. Self-control, future orientation, smoking, and the impact of Dutch tobacco control measures. Addict Behav Rep. 2015;1:89–96. https://doi.org/10.1016/j.abrep.2015.07.002.
27. Chen Y, Qian L. Association between lifetime stress and obesity in Canadians. Prev Med. 2012;55:464–7. https://doi.org/10.1016/j.ypmed.2012.08.013.
28. Isasi CR, Parrinello CM, Jung MM, Carnethon MR, Birnbaum-Weitzman O, Espinoza RA, et al. Psychosocial stress is associated with obesity and diet quality in Hispanic/Latino adults. Ann Epidemiol. 2015;25:84–9. https://doi.org/10.1016/j.annepidem.2014.11.002.
29. Harding JL, Backholer K, Williams ED, Peeters A, Cameron AJ, Hare MJ, et al. Psychosocial stress is positively associated with body mass index gain over 5 years: evidence from the longitudinal AusDiab study. Obesity (Silver Spring). 2014;22:277–86. https://doi.org/10.1002/oby.20423.
30. Järvelä-Reijonen E, Karhunen L, Sairanen E, Rantala S, Laitinen J, Puttonen S, et al. High perceived stress is associated with unfavorable eating behavior in overweight and obese Finns of working age. Appetite. 2016;103:249–58. https://doi.org/10.1016/j.appet.2016.04.023.
31. Chao A, Grilo CM, White MA, Sinha R. Food cravings mediate the relationship between chronic stress and body mass index. J Health Psychol. 2015;20:721–9. https://doi.org/10.1177/1359105315573448.
32. O'Connor DB, Jones F, Conner M, McMillan B, Ferguson E. Effects of daily hassles and eating style on eating behavior. Health Psychol. 2008;27:S20–31. https://doi.org/10.1037/0278-6133.27.1.S20.
33. Pike KM, Wilfley D, Hilbert A, Fairburn CG, Dohm F-A, Striegel-Moore RH. Antecedent life events of binge-eating disorder. Psychiatry Res. 2006;142:19–29. https://doi.org/10.1016/j.psychres.2005.10.006.
34. Degortes D, Santonastaso P, Zanetti T, Tenconi E, Veronese A, Favaro A. Stressful life events and binge eating disorder. Eur Eat Disord Rev. 2014;22:378–82. https://doi.org/10.1002/erv.2308.
35. Stults-Kolehmainen MA, Sinha R. The effects of stress on physical activity and exercise. Sports Med. 2014;44:81–121. https://doi.org/10.1007/s40279-013-0090-5.
36. Firth J, Rosenbaum S, Stubbs B, Gorczynski P, Yung AR, Vancampfort D. Motivating factors and barriers towards exercise in severe mental illness: a systematic review and meta-analysis. Psychol Med. 2016;46:2869–81. https://doi.org/10.1017/S0033291716001732.
37. Whooley MA, de Jonge P, Vittinghoff E, Otte C, Moos R, Carney RM, et al. Depressive symptoms, health behaviors, and risk of cardiovascular events in patients with coronary heart disease. JAMA. 2008;300:2379–88. https://doi.org/10.1001/jama.2008.711.
38. Löwe B, Spitzer RL, Zipfel S, Herzog W. Gesundheitsfragebogen für Patienten (PHQ D). Komplettversion und Kurzform. 2. Auflage. Karlsruhe: Pfizer; 2002.
39. Gräfe K, Zipfel S, Herzog W, Löwe B. Screening psychischer Störungen mit dem "Gesundheitsfragebogen für Patienten (PHQ-D)". Diagnostica. 2004;50:171–81. https://doi.org/10.1026/0012-1924.50.4.171.
40. Klapow J. Psychological Disorders and Distress in Older Primary Care Patients: A Comparison of Older and Younger Samples. Psychosomatic Med. 2002;64:635–43. https://doi.org/10.1097/01.PSY.0000021942.35402.C3.
41. Emond M, ten Eycke K, Kosmerly S, Robinson AL, Stillar A, van Blyderveen S. The effect of academic stress and attachment stress on stress-eaters and stress-undereaters. Appetite. 2016;100:210–5. https://doi.org/10.1016/j.appet.2016.01.035.
42. Ferranti EP, Dunbar SB, Higgins M, Dai J, Ziegler TR, Frediani JK, et al. Psychosocial factors associated with diet quality in a working adult population. Res Nurs Health. 2013;36:242–56. https://doi.org/10.1002/nur.21532.
43. Ayanian JZ. Perceived Risks of Heart Disease and Cancer Among Cigarette Smokers. JAMA. 1999;281:1019. https://doi.org/10.1001/jama.281.11.1019.
44. Ng DM, Jeffery RW. Relationships between perceived stress and health behaviors in a sample of working adults. Health Psychol. 2003;22:638–42. https://doi.org/10.1037/0278-6133.22.6.638.
45. Barrington WE, Beresford SAA, McGregor BA, White E. Perceived stress and eating behaviors by sex, obesity status, and stress vulnerability: Findings from the vitamins and lifestyle (VITAL) study. J Acad Nutr Diet. 2014;114:1791–9. https://doi.org/10.1016/j.jand.2014.03.015.
46. Macht M. How emotions affect eating: A five-way model. Appetite. 2008;50:1–11. https://doi.org/10.1016/j.appet.2007.07.002.
47. Stone AA, Brownell KD. The stress-eating paradox: Multiple daily

measurements in adult males and females. Psychol Health. 1994;9:425–36. https://doi.org/10.1080/08870449408407469.
48. Cohen S, Janicki-Deverts D. Who's Stressed?: Distributions of Psychological Stress in the United States in Probability Samples from 1983, 2006, and 20091. J Appl Soc Psychol. 2012;42:1320–34. https://doi.org/10.1111/j.1559-1816.2012.00900.x.
49. Craig CL, Marshall AL, Sjöström M, Bauman AE, Booth ML, Ainsworth BE, et al. International physical activity questionnaire: 12-country reliability and validity. Med Sci Sports Exerc. 2003;35:1381–95. https://doi.org/10.1249/01.MSS.0000078924.61453.FB.
50. Jackson AW, Morrow JR, Bowles HR, FitzGerald SJ, Blair SN. Construct validity evidence for single-response items to estimate physical activity levels in large sample studies. Res Q Exerc Sport. 2007;78:24–31. https://doi.org/10.1080/02701367.2007.10599400.
51. Bowles HR, FitzGerald SJ, Morrow JR, Jackson AW, Blair SN. Construct validity of self-reported historical physical activity. Am J Epidemiol. 2004;160:279–86. https://doi.org/10.1093/aje/kwh209.
52. Morris MJ, Beilharz JE, Maniam J, Reichelt AC, Westbrook RF. Why is obesity such a problem in the 21st century? The intersection of palatable food, cues and reward pathways, stress, and cognition. Neurosci Biobehav Rev. 2015;58:36–45. https://doi.org/10.1016/j.neubiorev.2014.12.002.
53. Taylor SE. Health psychology. New York: McGraw-Hill Education; 2015.
54. Turner RJ, Wheaton B, Lloyd DA. The Epidemiology of Social Stress. Am Sociol Rev. 1995;60:104. https://doi.org/10.2307/2096348.
55. Cohen S, Kamarck T, Mermelstein R. A global measure of perceived stress. J Health Soc Behav. 1983;24:385–96.
56. Löwe B, Kroenke K, Herzog W, Gräfe K. Measuring depression outcome with a brief self-report instrument: Sensitivity to change of the Patient Health Questionnaire (PHQ-9). J Affect Disord. 2004;81:61–6. https://doi.org/10.1016/S0165-0327(03)00198-8.
57. Kroenke K, Spitzer RL, Williams JBW. The PHQ-9. J Gen Intern Med. 2001;16:606–13. https://doi.org/10.1046/j.1525-1497.2001.016009606.x.
58. Löwe B, Spitzer RL, Williams JBW, Mussell M, Schellberg D, Kroenke K. Depression, anxiety and somatization in primary care: Syndrome overlap and functional impairment. Gen Hosp Psychiatry. 2008;30:191–9. https://doi.org/10.1016/j.genhosppsych.2008.01.001.
59. Löwe B, Decker O, Müller S, Brähler E, Schellberg D, Herzog W, Herzberg PY. Validation and standardization of the Generalized Anxiety Disorder Screener (GAD-7) in the general population. Med Care. 2008;46:266–74. https://doi.org/10.1097/MLR.0b013e318160d093.
60. Michal M, Wiltink J, Grande G, Beutel ME, Brähler E. Type D personality is independently associated with major psychosocial stressors and increased health care utilization in the general population. J Affect Disord. 2011;134:396–403. https://doi.org/10.1016/j.jad.2011.05.033.
61. Zilz C, Blaas SH, Pfeifer M, Jörres RA, Budweiser S. Mental health, serum biomarkers and survival in severe COPD: A pilot study. Multidiscip Respir Med. 2015;11:3. https://doi.org/10.1186/s40248-016-0041-8.
62. Sommerer C, Feuerstein D, Dikow R, Rauch G, Hartmann M, Schaier M, et al. Psychosocial and physical outcome following kidney donation-a retrospective analysis. Transpl Int. 2015;28:416–28. https://doi.org/10.1111/tri.12509.
63. Hausteiner C, Huber D, Bornschein S, Grosber M, Bubel E, Groben S, et al. Characteristics of oligosymptomatic versus polysymptomatic presentations of somatoform disorders in patients with suspected allergies. J Psychosom Res. 2010;69:259–66. https://doi.org/10.1016/j.jpsychores.2010.03.006.
64. Michal M, Wiltink J, Reiner I, Kirschner Y, Wild PS, Schulz A, et al. Association of mental distress with smoking status in the community: Results from the Gutenberg Health Study. J Affect Disord. 2013;146:355–60. https://doi.org/10.1016/j.jad.2012.09.019.
65. Khaled SM, Bulloch AG, Williams JVA, Hill JC, Lavorato DH, Patten SB. Persistent heavy smoking as risk factor for major depression (MD) incidence--evidence from a longitudinal Canadian cohort of the National Population Health Survey. J Psychiatr Res. 2012;46:436–43. https://doi.org/10.1016/j.jpsychires.2011.11.011.
66. Teychenne M, Ball K, Salmon J. Sedentary behavior and depression among adults: A review. Int J Behav Med. 2010;17:246–54. https://doi.org/10.1007/s12529-010-9075-z.
67. Michal M, Subic-Wrana C, Beutel ME. Psychodynamische Psychotherapie, Lebensstil und Prävention. Z Psychosom Med Psychother. 2014;60:350–67. https://doi.org/10.13109/zptm.2014.60.4.350.
68. Sallis R, Franklin B, Joy L, Ross R, Sabgir D, Stone J. Strategies for promoting physical activity in clinical practice. Prog Cardiovasc Dis. 2015;57:375–86. https://doi.org/10.1016/j.pcad.2014.10.003.
69. Stonerock GL, Blumenthal JA. Role of Counseling to Promote Adherence in Healthy Lifestyle Medicine: Strategies to Improve Exercise Adherence and Enhance Physical Activity. Prog Cardiovasc Dis. 2017;59:455–62. https://doi.org/10.1016/j.pcad.2016.09.003.
70. Ye S, Muntner P, Shimbo D, Judd SE, Richman J, Davidson KW, Safford MM. Behavioral mechanisms, elevated depressive symptoms, and the risk for myocardial infarction or death in individuals with coronary heart disease: The REGARDS (Reason for Geographic and Racial Differences in Stroke) study. J Am Coll Cardiol. 2013;61:622–30. https://doi.org/10.1016/j.jacc.2012.09.058.
71. Lederbogen F, Schwarz P, Häfner S, Schweiger U, Bohus M, Deuschle M. Kardiale und metabolische Risikofaktoren bei schweren psychischen Erkrankungen. Aufgaben eines Präventionsmanagers. Nervenarzt. 2015;86:866–71. https://doi.org/10.1007/s00115-014-4232-2.
72. Bonnet F, Irving K, Terra J-L, Nony P, Berthezène F, Moulin P. Anxiety and depression are associated with unhealthy lifestyle in patients at risk of cardiovascular disease. Atherosclerosis. 2005;178:339–44. https://doi.org/10.1016/j.atherosclerosis.2004.08.035.
73. Moussavi S, Chatterji S, Verdes E, Tandon A, Patel V, Ustun B. Depression, chronic diseases, and decrements in health: Results from the World Health Surveys. Lancet. 2007;370:851–8. https://doi.org/10.1016/S0140-6736(07)61415-9.
74. Novak M, Mucsi I, Rhee CM, Streja E, Lu JL, Kalantar-Zadeh K, et al. Increased Risk of Incident Chronic Kidney Disease, Cardiovascular Disease, and Mortality in Patients With Diabetes With Comorbid Depression. Diabetes Care. 2016;39:1940–7. https://doi.org/10.2337/dc16-0048.
75. Hert MD, Correll CU, Bobes J, Cetkovich-Bakmas M, Cohen DAN, Asai I, et al. Physical illness in patients with severe mental disorders. I. Prevalence, impact of medications and disparities in health care. World Psychiatry. 2011;10:52–77.
76. Penninx BWJH. Depression and cardiovascular disease: Epidemiological evidence on their linking mechanisms. Neurosci Biobehav Rev. 2017;74:277–86. https://doi.org/10.1016/j.neubiorev.2016.07.003.
77. Hallgren M, Herring MP, Owen N, Dunstan D, Ekblom O, Helgadottir B, et al. Exercise, Physical Activity, and Sedentary Behavior in the Treatment of Depression: Broadening the Scientific Perspectives and Clinical Opportunities. Front Psychiatry. 2016;7:36. https://doi.org/10.3389/fpsyt.2016.00036.

19

Prevalence and stability of mental disorders among young adults: findings from a longitudinal study

Kristin Gustavson[1,5*], Ann Kristin Knudsen[2,3], Ragnar Nesvåg[1,4], Gun Peggy Knudsen[6], Stein Emil Vollset[2] and Ted Reichborn-Kjennerud[1,7]

Abstract

Background: Mental disorders often have onset early in life, contribute substantially to the global disease burden, and may interfere with young people's ability to complete age-relevant tasks in important developmental periods. However, knowledge about prevalence and course of mental disorders in young adulthood is sparse. The aim of the current study was to estimate prevalence and stability of mental disorders from the twenties to the thirties/forties.

Methods: DSM-IV mental disorders were assessed with the Composite International Diagnostic Interview in two waves (1999–2004 and 2010–2011) in 1623 young adult Norwegian twins (63.2% women, aged 19–29 years in wave 1).

Results: In wave 1, the 12-month prevalence of any mental disorder among people in the twenties was 19.8% (men) and 32.4% (women), anxiety disorders: 9.6% (men) and 26.7% (women), anxiety disorders excluding specific phobias: 2.5% (men) and 6.9% (women), major depressive disorder (MDD): 4.4% (men) and 7.2% (women), and alcohol use disorder (AUD): 8.7% (men) and 4.4% (women). The prevalence of any mental disorder decreased from the twenties to the thirties/forties. This was due to a decrease in AUD and specific phobias. Anxiety disorders in the twenties predicted anxiety disorders and MDD ten years later, even when controlling for the association between these disorders in the twenties. MDD in the twenties predicted MDD ten years later. At both ages, two-week and 12-month prevalence estimates differed markedly for MDD - indicating an episodic course.

Conclusions: Common mental disorders are highly prevalent among young adults in the twenties, and somewhat less prevalent in the thirties/forties. Those who suffer from one mental disorder in the twenties are at considerably increased risk for suffering from a disorder ten years later as well. This may have significant implications for young people's ability to attain education, establish a family, and participate in occupational life.

Keywords: Mental disorders, Young adulthood, Health surveys, Prevalence, Stability

Background

Mental disorders are among the most prevalent health problems affecting the adult population [1]. The Global Burden of Disease Study 2015 (GBD 2015) estimated that seven of the top 25 causes of years lived with disability (YLD) globally were mental disorders, with major depressive disorder (MDD) ranked second and anxiety disorders ranked ninth [2]. The high rankings were a result of both high prevalence and the disability associated with these disorders. Estimates of 12-month prevalence of mental disorders vary between 9.6 and 27.8% in the general adult population [3–8]. Mood disorders, anxiety disorders (including specific phobias), and alcohol use disorders (AUD) are the most prevalent disorders and are included in all the above-mentioned studies.

* Correspondence: krbr@fhi.no
[1]Department of mental disorders, Norwegian Institute of Public Health, Oslo, Norway
[5]Department of Psychology, University of Oslo, Oslo, Norway
Full list of author information is available at the end of the article

Young adulthood

The shift in recent decades toward longer educations and higher age when committing to stable relationships and having children, has led researchers to aknowledge the age between 18 and 29 as an important developmental period [9]. It is characterized by changes in love and work life, and frequent residental change [9, 10]. Completing education and building a stable life structure are important developmental tasks in this period, while raising children is an important task for later periods [9, 10].

Mental health problems are associated with poor educational attainment as well as work and interpersonal problems [11–18]. Research results indicate that half of US adolescents' failure to complete secondary school is attributable to mental disorders [19]. Mental disorders are also associated with maladaptive parenting behaviors, such as low affection toward the child and inconsistent enforcement of rules [20]. Because mental disorders may interfere with developmental tasks in different periods, we need to increase our knowledge about the prevalence and stability of such disorders at different ages to be able to correctly assess the magnitude of this problem.

Prevalence of mental disorders in young adulthood

Findings from the New Zealand Mental Health Survey (NZMHS), the Dutch Tracking Adolescents' Individual Lives Survey (TRAILS), the US National Comorbidity Survey (NCS) and its replication (NCS-R), and the Children in the Community Study (CICS) from the US, show 12-month prevalence estiatmes of MDD between 8.3 and 12.4% among people between 18 and 33 years [16, 21–23]. The 12-month prevalence was between 19.4 and 22.3% for anxiety disorders (including specific phobias), between 2.5 and 10.3% for acohol dependence, and between 7.1 and 18.4% for alcohol abuse [21–23].

Stability of mental disorders in young adulthood

Previous studies indicate that the prevalence of depression is stable over the earliest part of adulthood, whereas AUD decreases, and findings regarding anxiety disorders are mixed [21, 24]. In the Dunedin study from New Zealand, the 12-month prevalence of MDD was 16.8% at age 21 years and 16.3% at 32 years [21]. The 12-month prevalence of any anxiety disorder (including specific phobias) was 20.3% at 21 years and 22.2% at 32 years. In the Simmons Longitudinal Study from the US, prevalence estiamtes of MDD showed a weak and not statistically significant increase from age 21 to 30 (from 5.4 to 8.0%), while there was a decline in the 12-month prevalence for phobia (including specific phobias) (from 16.8 to 2.3%) [24]. The prevalence of alcohol dependence declined (from 18.4 to 8.1%) from age 21 to 32 in the Dunedin study, and the prevalence of AUD declined from 26.7 to 6.0% in the Simmons Longituidnal Study [21, 24].

Some people have long-lasting and/or recurrent episodes of mental disorders [25, 26]. In the general adult population, about 40% of those who have depression or anxiety at one time point, have been found to have at least one of these disorders 7 years later [27]. Having a disorder or mental health problems in adolescence increases the risk of such disorders/problems in early adulthood [18, 28–30]. Findings from the NCS follow-up (NCS-2) showed that having MDD or generalized anxiety disorder (GAD) in the twenties and thirties predicted having any of these disorders eleven years later [31]. Depression seems to be more episodic than anxiety disorders among adolescents, as shown by higher 12-month to 30-day prevalence ratios of mood than anxiety disorders [22].

Comorbidity

Comorbidity between mental disorders is extensive with up to 50% of those who have one mental disorder also having at least one additional comorbid mental disorder [4, 7, 32]. This is also reported among young people [33]. Comorbidity seems to a large degree to be due to common liablity factors for several disorders [34, 35] and is related to severity and chronicity [27, 33, 36, 37]. Hence, estimates of comorbidity in different developmental periods may increase our understanding of the potential effects of common mental disorders on young adults.

Need for further knowledge

Current knowledge on prevalence and stability of mental disorders among young adults relies heavily on results from the US and New Zealand. Longitudinal studies from several different countries are needed to inform policy makers in different parts of the world and to estimate global disease burden in this age period.

Previous prevalence estiamtes of any mental disorder or any anxiety disorder typically include specific phobias, which by definiton involves imapirment in circumscribed situations and can sometimes be treated in a single therapy session [38]. Prevalence estiamtes both including and excluding such phobias are therefore needed to plan mental health services for young adults.

Findings are divergent with regards to whether or not anxiety disorders become less prevalent during young adulthood. Previous studies have included different anxiety disorders when examining this. There is a lack of studies tracking the episodic versus chronic nature of MDD and anxiety disorders across young adulthood. If depression tends to get more or less episodic over time, the burden of recurrent depression will decrease or increase as people get older. More knowledge about the stability of anxiety disorders and MDD from the twenties to the thirties/forties may increase our understanding of the potential impact of such disorders on young adult development. This is important for planning mental health services for young adults.

A limitation in several previous studies of AUD is different diagnostic criteria across waves and use of alcohol abuse as a screen for alcohol dependence [39]. This may affect estimates of prevalence and stability of this disorder [24, 39].

To the best of our knowledge, no previous studies have examined prevalence and stablity in common mental disorders by both: Following the same individuals from the twenties to the thirties/forties, estimating prevalence of anxiety disorders at the different ages including as well as excluding specific phobias, comparing the episodic versus chronic nature of disorders at both ages, and examining comorbidity between disorders at both ages.

Aims of the study

The overall aim of the current study was to address limitations in previous literature on prevalence and stability of common mental disorders from the twenties to the thirties/forties. More specifically, the aims were to: 1) Estimate the 12-month prevalence of anxiety disorders (with and without specific phobias), mood disorders, and AUD among people aged 19 to 29, 2) Compare these estimates to prevalence estimates ten years later, 3) Compare 12-month to two-week prevalence estimates to examine the episodic nature of disorders across these two developmental periods, 4) Examine the degree to which those who have an anxiety disorder or MDD in the twenties, are at increased risk of having these disorders ten years later, 5) Examine comorbidity of common mental disorders among people in the twenties and ten years later.

Methods

Sample

Data came from the Norwegian Institute of Public Health Twin Panel (NIPHTP), which includes health questionnaires at two time points (Q1 and Q2), and diagnostic interviews at two later time points (wave 1 and wave 2). The current study used data from the two interviews. The NIPHTP is described thoroughly elsewhere [40–44], and recruitment is illustrated in Fig. 1.

The first wave of the interview study (wave 1) took place between 1999 and 2004, and 2801 individuals (44% of the invited) were interviewed. All twins who had participated in wave 1 were invited for a re-interview between 2010 and 2011 (wave 2). The follow-up participation rate from

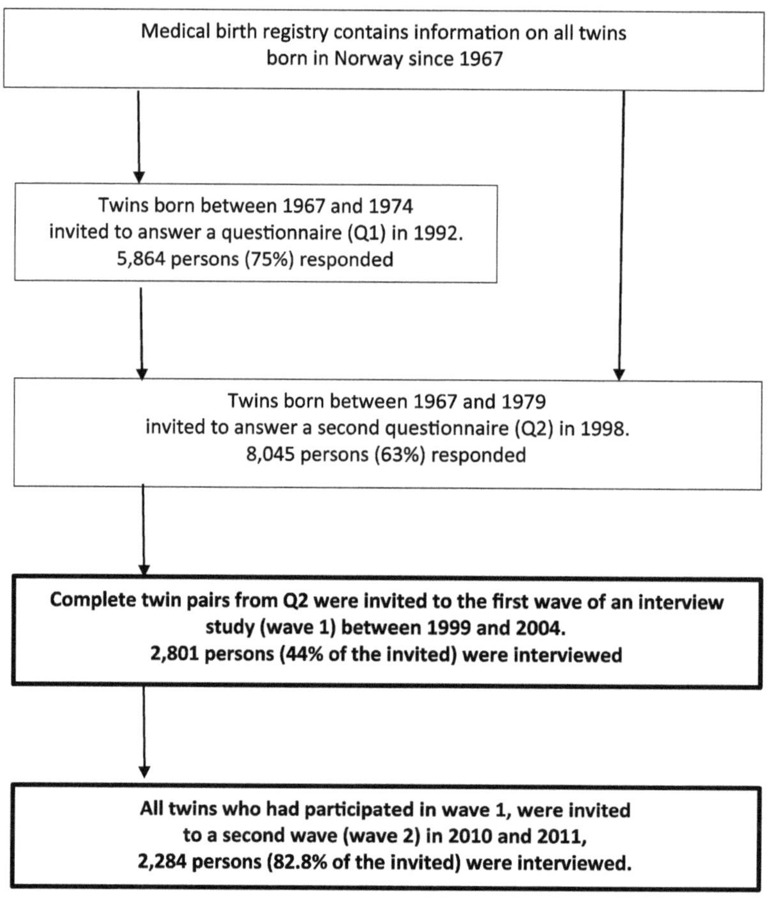

Fig. 1 Flow-chart of recruitment to the study. The current study used data from the two interview studies, indicated with bold font

wave 1 to wave 2 was 82.8% ($n = 2284$) [41]. Mean age was 28.3 years (range 19–36 years) in wave 1 and 37.9 years (range 30–44 years) in wave 2. Mean time between interviews was 9.6 years (range 7–13 years). Participation in wave 1 was predicted by increasing age and monozygosity, but not by any indicator of mental health [42]. Participation in wave 2 was predicted by high education, female sex, and monozygosity. Neither the total number of mental disorders nor any specific disorder in wave 1 predicted participation in wave 2 [41].

The current study aimed to examine mental disorders in a specific developmental period (19–29 years of age) and follow these individuals over time. Hence, only participants below age 30 in wave 1 were included in the main analyses. This resulted in a sample of 597 men and 1026 women in wave 1, and 457 men and 850 women in wave 2. Mean age in wave 1 was 25.4 years (range 19 to 29), and mean age in wave 2 was 35.3 years (range 30 to 42). Mean time between the two interviews was 9.6 years. Prevalence estimates for the wider age range of the entire sample were also calculated and are presented in Additional file 1: Tables S1 and S2, for readers who are interested in prevalence of mental disorders in a wider age group.

Measures

A Norwegian version of the computerized Munich Composite International Diagnostic Interview (M-CIDI), originally developed by the World Health Organization, was employed in both interview waves [45]. Diagnoses were coded according to the Diagnostic and Statistical Manual of Mental Disorders, Fourth Edition (DSM-IV). The interview was mainly administered face-to-face in wave 1. For practical reasons, 231 interviews (8.3%) were conducted by telephone. To maximize response rate, all the interviews were conducted by telephone in wave 2. Interviewers were mostly psychology graduate students or experienced psychiatric nurses who had received standardized training by certified instructors. Each twin in a pair was interviewed by a different interviewer.

Respondents answered one question about when they last experienced symptoms of each of the disorders. The response categories were "Within the last two weeks", "Two weeks to less than a month", "One to five months", "6 to 12 months", "Last 12 months, but cannot remember exactly when", and "More than one year". Endorsement of the first option was used to estimate 2-week prevalence, endorsement of any of the first two options to estimate 4-week prevalence, endorsement of any of the first three options to estimate 5(6) month-prevalence, and endorsement of any of the first five options to estimate 12-month-prevalence. Hence, individuals contributing to two-week prevalence estimates were a sub-group of those contributing to all other prevalence estimates of each disorder.

Table 1 shows an overview of combined categories of diagnoses. *AUD* consisted of alcohol abuse and alcohol dependence. *Any mood disorder* consisted of MDD and dysthymia. *Any anxiety disorder W1* consisted of panic disorder, agoraphobia without a history of panic disorder, specific phobias, social phobia, GAD, obsessive-compulsive disorder (OCD), and post-traumatic stress

Table 1 Overview of disorders included in the combined categories

Combined category	Includes	Constructed for wave
Any mood disorder	MDD, Dysthymia	1 and 2
Any anxiety disorder W1	Panic disorder, Agoraphobia without a history of panic disorder, Specific phobias, Social phobia, GAD, OCD, PTSD.	1
Any Anxiety disorder W1–2	Panic disorder, Agoraphobia without a history of panic disorder, Specific phobias, Social phobia, GAD.	1 and 2
Any anxiety disorder W1–2 excluding specific phobias	Panic disorder, Agoraphobia without a history of panic disorder, Social phobia, GAD.	1 and 2
AUD	Alcohol abuse, Alcohol dependence.	1 and 2
Any mental disorder W1	Any mood disorder, Any anxiety disorder W1, AUD.	1
Any mental disorder W1–2	Any mood disorder, Any anxiety disorder W1–2, AUD.	1 and 2
Any mental disorder W1–2 excluding specific phobias	Any mood disorder, Any anxiety disorder W1–2 excluding specific phobias, AUD.	1 and 2
Categories only presented in Supplementary table		
Drug use disorder	Drug abuse, drug dependence.	1
Any substance use disorder	Drug use disorder, AUD.	1
Any disorder W1- supplement	Any mood disorder, Any anxiety disorder W1, Any substance use disorder	1

Legends: *MDD* Major depressive disorder, *GAD* Generalized anxiety disorder, *OCD* Obsessive-compulsive disorder, *PTSD* Post-traumatic stress disorder, *AUD* Alcohol use disorder
W1 Wave 1, *W2* wave 2

disorder (PTSD). In wave 2, OCD and PTSD were not assessed. These two disorders are no longer classified as anxiety disorders in DSM-5 [46]. *Any anxiety disorder W1–2* did not include these two disorders, and was constructed for both waves to allow comparison of anxiety disorders across age. *Any anxiety disorder W1–2 excluding specific phobias* consisted of all anxiety disorders measured in both waves except specific phobias. *Any mental disorder W1* consisted of *Any mood disorder, Any anxiety disorder W1*, and *AUD*. *Any mental disorder W1–2* consisted of *Any mood disorder, Any anxiety disorder W1–2*, and *AUD*. *Any mental disorder W1–2 excluding specific phobias* consisted of *Any mood disorder, Any anxiety disorder W1–2 excluding specific phobias*, and *AUD*.

Total as well as sex-stratified prevalence estimates are presented for MDD, *Any mood disorder, Any anxiety disorder (W1, W1–2,* as well as *W1–2 excluding specific phobias), AUD,* and *Any mental disorder (W1, W1–2,* and *W1–2 excluding specific phobias)*. Prevalence estimates for low frequent specific disorders (e.g. panic disorders and dysthymia) are only presented for both genders together. Drug use disorders (drug addiction and drug abuse) were only assess in wave 1, and are presented in Additional file 1: Table S1.

We report 12-month and 2-week prevalence estimates. The other two measured prevalences (5(6)-month and four-week) are presented in Additional file 1: Tables S1 and S2. Interested readers may use those estimates to compare findings with other studies that have used estimates between 12-month and two-week (as for example [22, 47]).

Statistical analyses

Analyses were performed in Stata version 15. Testing all the prevalence estimates for statistically significant gender differences would imply a large number of tests, thus increasing the risk of random findings. Such testing was therefore only performed for the following estimates: 12-month *Any mental disorder W1–2*, 12-month *Any mood disorder*, 12-month *Any anxiety disorder W1–2*, and 12-month *AUD*.

The 12-month and 2-week prevalence estimates were compared for MDD and *Any anxiety disorder W1–2*. Episodic disorders are expected to show higher 12-month than 2-week prevalences whereas the prevalences are expected to be more similar for more chronic disorders.

Absolute stability was examined by comparing prevalence estimates at the two waves. Only those who participated in wave 2, were included in significance testing of change in prevalence estimates, thus reducing the risk of bias du to potential selective attrition. Relative stability refers to the degree to which it is the same or different people who have a diagnosis across ages [48]. This was examined with logistic regression for MDD, *Any anxiety disorder W1–2*, and *AUD*, adjusted for age in wave 1. We also examined the degree to which MDD in wave 1 predicted having *Any anxiety disorder W1–2* in wave 2, and vice versa, controlled for age. Because of low number of cases and thus low statistical power, *AUD* was not included. Men and women were collapsed in these analyses to increase statistical power.

Comorbidity within each wave was examined with tetrachoric correlations between MDD, *Any anxiety disorders W1–2*, and *AUD*. Comorbidity was also examined by showing the proportion of people with one disorder, who also had another disorder, and by illustrating how many of a hypothetical sample of 100 individuals who would have either one disorder, or a combination of two or three disorders. Men and women were collapsed.

The concordance between twins may affect results. First, standard errors may be too small due to clustering effects [49–51]. This was adjusted for by drawing clusters (twin-pairs) rather than individuals in the bootstrapping/jackknife process and by using the robust estimator for standard errors in logistic regression [49–51]. Second, sensitivity analyses were performed including only one twin from each pair, to see if this affected results.

Results

Prevalence estimates

We report results for 597 men and 1026 women (63.2%) who participated in wave 1 (Table 2) and 457 men and 850 women (65.0%) who also participated in wave 2 (Table 3).

In wave 1, when the participants were in the twenties, *Any anxiety disorder W1* was the most prevalent combined category of disorders for both men and women (see Table 2). The 12-month prevalence for *Any anxiety disorder W1* was 9.6% (95% confidence interval (CI) = 7.0–12.4) for men and 26.7% (95% CI = 23.7–29.7) for women. For *Any anxiety disorder W1–2*, the 12-month prevalence was 9.3 (95% CI = 7.0–12.3) for men and 26.0% (95% CI = 23.1–29.0) for women. *AUD* ranked second among men (8.7% 12-month prevalence, 95% CI = 6.5–11.3), and *Any mood disorder* ranked second among women (8.7% 12-month prevalence, 95% CI = 6.7–10.6). Specific phobias were highly prevalent among men and women (12-month prevalence = 7.6% with 95% CI = 5.5–10.2 for men and 22.3% with 95% CI = 19.5–25.0 for women). *AUD* and *Any mood disorder* were the most common groups of disorders for men, and *Any mood disorder* was the most common group of disorders for women when specific phobias were excluded. Results from significance testing of gender

Table 2 Prevalence of mental disorders in wave 1 (age 19–29 years, $n = 597$ men and 1026 women)

	Men and women		Men		Women		Ratio (women/men) of 12-month prevalence estimates (95% CI)
	12 month prevalence (95% CI)	Two-week prevalence (95% CI)	12 month prevalence (95% CI)	Two-week prevalence (95% CI)	12 month prevalence (95% CI)	Two-week prevalence (95% CI)	
MDD	6.2 5.0–7.4	1.3 0.7–1.8	4.4 2.8–6.3	0.8 0.2–1.6	7.2 5.5–8.8	1.6 0.9–2.4	
Dysthymia	1.7 1.1–2.4	1.4 0.8–2.0					
Any mood disorder [a]	7.3 5.9–8.6	2.3 1.5–3.0	4.9 3.2–6.8	1.2 0.4–2.2	8.7 6.7–10.6	2.9 1.9–4.0	1.79*** 1.19–2.68
Any anxiety disorder W1 [b]	20.4 18.3–22.7	15.2 13.5–17.3	9.6 7.0–12.4	5.9 4.2–8.2	26.7 23.7–29.7	20.7 18.1–23.5	
Any anxiety disorder W1–2 [c]	19.8 17.7–22.0	14.8 13.0–16.7	9.3 7.0–12.3	5.7 4.0–7.9	26.0 23.1–29.0	20.1 17.4–22.7	2.80*** 2.13–3.68
Any anxiety disorder W1–2 excluding specific phobias [d]	5.3 4.2–6.6	3.2 2.3–4.1	2.5 1.3–4.2	1.3 0.5–2.6	6.9 5.3–8.7	4.2 3.0–5.7	
Specific phobias	16.9 14.9–19.0	12.4 10.8–14.1	7.6 5.5–10.2	4.9 3.3–6.9	22.3 19.5–25.0	16.8 14.5–19.2	
Panic disorder	1.5 1.0–2.2	0.4 0.1–0.7					
Agoraphobia without panic	1.4 0.9–2.0	1.1 0.6–1.7					
Social phobia	2.3 1.7–3.3	1.8 1.2–2.7					
GAD	1.2 0.7–1.9	0.4 0.1–0.7					
CCD	0.3 0.1–0.6	0.2 0.1–0.4					
PTSD	1.2 0.7–1.8	0.7 0.4–1.2					
Alcohol abuse	2.8 2.0–3.7	0.9 0.5–1.5					
Alcohol Dependence	4.7 3.6–5.8	2.1 1.4–2.8					
AUD	6.0 4.8–7.3	2.7 1.9–3.6	8.7 6.5–11.3	3.7 2.3–5.4	4.4 3.2–5.7	2.0 1.2–3.0	0.50*** 0.34–0.74

Table 2 Prevalence of mental disorders in wave 1 (age 19–29 years, $n = 597$ men and 1026 women) *(Continued)*

	Men and women		Men		Women		Ratio (women/men) of 12-month prevalence estimates (95% CI)
	12 month prevalence (95% CI)	Two-week prevalence (95% CI)	12 month prevalence (95% CI)	Two-week prevalence (95% CI)	12 month prevalence (95% CI)	Two-week prevalence (95% CI)	
Any mental disorder W1 [e]	27.8 25.4–30.3	18.6 16.7–20.6	19.8 16.4–23.4	9.7 7.3–12.4	32.4 29.4–35.7	23.8 21.1–26.6	
Any mental disorder W1–2 [f]	27.6 25.3–30.2	18.2 16.2–20.1	19.8 16.4–23.4	9.5 7.1–12.2	32.2 29.2–35.4	23.3 20.7–26.0	1.63*** 1.35–1.96
Any mental disorder W1–2 excluding specific phobias [g]	15.3 13.5–17.5	7.3 6.0–8.8	14.3 11.2–17.3	5.6 3.7–7.7	15.9 13.6–18.5	8.3 6.5–10.3	

Legends: *** $p < 0.001$, *MDD* Major depressive disorder, *GAD* Generalized anxiety disorder, *OCD* Obsessive-compulsive disorder, *PTSD* Post-traumatic stress disorder, *AUD* Alcohol use disorders, i.e. alcohol dependence or alcohol abuse

CI Confidence interval. 95% CIs are based on standard errors obtained from bootstrapping (1000 replications), bias corrected for skewness in the bootstrap distribution, and adjusted for cluster-effects among twins

[a]MDD and/or dysthymia

[b]Panic disorder, agoraphobia without panic, specific phobias, social phobia, GAD, OCD, and/or PTSD

[c]Panic disorder, agoraphobia without panic, specific phobias, social phobia and/or GAD

[d]Panic disorder, agoraphobia without panic, social phobia and/or GAD

[e]Any mood disorder, Any anxiety disorder W1, AUD

[f]Any mood disorder, Any anxiety disorder W1–2, AUD

[g]Any mood disorder, Any anxiety disorder W1–2 excluding specific phobias, AUD

Table 3 Prevalence of mental disorders in wave 2 (age 30–42 years, $n = 457$ men and 850 women)

	Men and women		Men		Women		Ratio (women/men) of 12-month prevalence estimates (95% CI)
	12 month prevalence (95% CI)	Two-week prevalence (95% CI)	12 month prevalence (95% CI)	Two-week prevalence (95% CI)	12 month prevalence (95% CI)	Two-week prevalence (95% CI)	
MDD	5.0 3.8–6.3	1.1 0.6–1.7	3.3 1.9–5.2	0.9 0.2–1.9	5.9 4.3–7.5	1.2 0.6–2.0	
Dysthymia	1.9 1.2–3.0	0.9 0.5–1.5					
Any mood disorder[a]	5.8 4.6–7.3	1.6 1.0–2.4	3.7 2.3–5.9	1.1 0.2–2.3	7.0 5.3–8.7	1.9 1.1–3.0	1.87** 1.10–3.17
Any anxiety disorder W1–2[b]	16.1 13.9–18.4	8.3 6.8–9.7	5.9 4.0–8.2	2.9 1.5–4.7	21.6 18.6–24.6	11.2 9.0–13.2	3.63*** 2.46–5.35
Any anxiety disorder W1–2 excluding specific phobias[c]	6.5 5.2–8.0	2.6 1.8–3.7	2.6 1.3–4.3	0.9 0.2–1.9	8.5 6.7–10.7	3.5 2.4–5.0	
Specific phobias	12.3 10.3–14.3	6.5 5.2–7.9	4.1 2.4–6.1	2.2 1.0–3.9	16.8 14.1–19.5	8.8 6.9–10.8	
Panic disorder	2.1 1.4–3.0	0.5 0.2–1.1					
Agoraphobia without panic	1.2 0.6–1.9	0.6 0.2–1.2					
Social phobia	3.9 2.9–5.2	1.4 0.7–2.1					
GAD	1.5 0.9–2.2	0.5 0.2–0.9					
AUD	2.7 1.8–3.7	1.2 0.7–1.8	5.3 3.2–7.2	2.4 1.2–4.0	1.3 0.7–2.2	0.5 0.1–1.0	0.25** 0.12–0.50
Any mental disorder W1–2[d]	20.9 18.6–23.3	10.0 8.3–11.7	12.9 9.8–16.3	5.8 3.8–8.1	25.3 22.1–28.6	12.3 10.3–14.5	1.96*** 1.50–2.55
Any mental disorder W1–2 excluding specific phobias[e]	12.4 10.5–14.4	4.9 3.6–6.2	10.0 7.3–12.6	4.2 2.5–6.2	13.7 11.4–16.3	5.2 3.7–6.9	

Legends: ** $p < 0.01$, *** $p < 0.001$, *MDD* Major depressive disorder, *GAD* Generalized anxiety disorder, *AUD* Alcohol use disorders, i.e. alcohol dependence or alcohol abuse

CI Confidence interval. 95% CIs are based on standard errors obtained from bootstrapping (1000 replications), bias corrected for skewness in the bootstrap distribution and adjusted for cluster-effects among twins

[a]MDD and/or dysthymia

[b]Panic disorder, agoraphobia without panic, specific phobias, social phobia and/or GAD

[c]Panic disorder, agoraphobia without panic, social phobia and/or GAD

[d]Any mood disorder, Any anxiety disorder W1–2, AUD

[e]Any mood disorder, Any anxiety disorder W1–2 excluding specific phobias, AUD

difference showed that *Any mental disorder W1–2, Any anxiety disorder W1–2,* and *Any mood disorder* were more prevalent among women than men, while *AUD* was more prevalent among men than women (see Table 2).

In wave 2, the 12-month prevalence of *Any anxiety disorder W1–2* was 5.9% (95% CI = 4.0–8.2) for men and 21.6% (95% CI = 18.6–24.6) for women (see Table 3). Again, this was mainly due to the high prevalence of specific phobias (12-month prevalence was 4.1% with 95% CI = 2.4–6.1 for men and 16.8% with 95% CI = 14.1–19.5 for women). *Any mood disorder* was the second most prevalent group of disorders among women (12-month prevalence 7.0% with 95% CI = 5.3–8.7), and *AUD* was the second most common disorder among men (12-month prevalence = 5.3% with 95% CI = 3.2–7.2). *Any mental disorder W1–2, Any mood disorder,* and *Any anxiety disorder W1–2,* were more prevalent among women than men, and the reverse was true for *AUD* (see Table 3).

Stability

There was a reduction in *Any mental disorder W1–2,* Specific phobias, and *AUD* from wave 1 to wave 2 (95% CI for differences did not include zero). Estimates were stable for MDD and *Any anxiety disorder W1–2 excluding specific phobias* (95% CI for difference included zero).

Relative stability was measured with logistic regression, presented in Table 4. Having MDD, *Any anxiety disorder W1–2,* or *AUD* in the twenties, increased the risk of having these disorders ten years later. The results showed that *Any anxiety disorder W1–2* in wave 1 predicted MDD in wave 2, even controlled for MDD in wave 1.

Despite relative stability from wave 1 to wave 2, 82.4% of those who had MDD, 54.9% of those who had *Any anxiety disorder W1–2,* and 85.4% of those who had *AUD* in Wave 1 (12-mont prevalence), did not have the same disorder in wave 2.

Table 4 Relative stability in mental disorders from age 19–29 to age 30–42 estimated with logistic regression

	Disorder in W1 not adjusted for each other OR (95% CI)	MDD and Anxiety in W1 mutually adjusted for each other OR (95% CI)
MDD in wave 2		
MDD in wave 1	3.56*** (1.81–6.98)	2.60** (1.31–5.17)
Anxiety in wave 1	2.61*** (1.54–4.42)	2.18** (1.26–3.75)
Anxiety in wave 2		
MDD in wave 1	3.94*** (2.36–6.60)	1.77 (0.96–3.26)
Anxiety in wave 1	9.01*** (6.45–12.59)	8.33*** (5.90–11.78)
AUD in wave 2	8.10***	
AUD in wave 1	(3.69–17.76)	

Legends: *OR* Odds ratio, *CI* Confidence interval, *MDD* Major depressive disorder, Anxiety = *Any anxiety disorder W1-2 (*Panic disorder, agoraphobia without panic, specific phobias, social phobia and/or generalized anxiety disorder (GAD)). Standard errors were obtained from the robust estimator in Stata, accounting for cluster-effects among twins
Men and women were collapsed in the analyses to increase statistical power. All analyses were adjusted for age in wave 1

12-month versus 2-week prevalence estimates

The 12-month prevalence of MDD was significantly higher than the 2-week prevalence in both waves. The 12-month to two-week ratios for MDD was 4.8 (95% CI = 3.9–7.5) in wave 1 and 4.6 (95% CI = 3.1–8.6) in wave 2. For *Any anxiety disorder W1–2* the ratios were 1.3 (95% CI = 1.3–1.4) in wave 1 and 1.9 (95% CI = 1.7–2.2) in wave 2, indicating a more episodic nature of MDD than anxiety disorders.

Comorbidity

Tetrachoric correlations between 12-month MDD, *Any anxiety disorder W1–2,* and *AUD* within each wave are presented in Table 5. There was a strong association between MDD and *Any anxiety disorder W1–2* in both waves.

Comorbidity was also examined by calculating how many of those who had one disorder, also had another disorder. The results are presented in Table 6. The comorbidity numbers for *AUD* should be interpreted with caution in wave 2, as few people had this diagnosis. Figure 2 shows the number of people with pure versus comorbid MDD, *Any anxiety disorder W1–2,* and *AUD* in hypothetical samples of 100 men and 100 women in the twenties and in the thirties/forties.

Table 5 Tetrachoric correlations between different disorders at wave 1 (age 19–29) and wave 2 (age 30–42)

		Wave 1			Wave 2		
		MDD	Anxiety W1–2[a]	AUD	MDD	Anxiety W1–2[a]	AUD
Wave 1	MDD		0.45***	0.00	0.31**	0.38***	0.16
	Anxiety W1–2[a]			0.10	0.26**	0.65***	0.02
	AUD				0.07	0.07	0.49***
Wave 2	MDD					0.54***	0.12
	Anxiety W1–2[a]						0.03
	AUD						

Legends: [a]Panic disorder, agoraphobia without panic, specific phobias, social phobia and/or generalized anxiety disorder (GAD)
MDD Major depressive disorder. *AUD* Alcohol use disorders, i.e. alcohol dependence or alcohol abuse. Standard errors were obtained from the jackknife estimator, accounting for cluster-effects among twins. $^{**}p < 0.01$, $^{***}p < 0.001$. Men and women were collapsed to increase statistical power

Table 6 Comorbidity wave 1 (age 19–29) and wave 2 (age 30–42)

	Men			Women		
	% with comorbid MDD	% with comorbid Anxiety W1–2 [a]	% with comorbid AUD	% with comorbid MDD	% with comorbid Anxiety W1–2[a]	% with comorbid AUD
Wave 1						
MDD		34.6 17.6–55.6	3.8 0–14.3		66.2 54.8–76.8	6.8 1.5–13.7
Anxiety W1–2[a]	15.8 7.3–26.8		17.5 8.5–27.3	17.4 13.1–21.9		5.9 3.6–9.0
AUD	1.9 0–7.1	17.5 8.5–27.3		11.1 3.4–21.1	35.6 22.2–50.0	
Wave 2						
MDD		33.3 13.0–53.6	16.7 3.7–31.8		57.0 46.5–67.0	2.0 0.0–5.4
Anxiety W1–2[a]	17.4 8.3–31.1		8.7 2.0–18.0	19.5 14.8–24.3		1.7 0.3–3.4
AUD	11.4 2.9–23.3	11.8 3.0–23.5		14.3 0.0–37.5	7.1 0.0–25.0	

Legends: *MDD* Major depressive disorder, *AUD* Alcohol use disorders, i.e. alcohol dependence or alcohol abuse
[a]Panic disorder, agoraphobia without panic, specific phobias, social phobia and/or generalized anxiety disorder (GAD)

Sensitivity analyses of concordance between twins

As mentioned in the methods section, the use of twins may have affected results, and sensitivity analyses were therefore performed. If one twin did not have any mental disorder during the last 12 months in wave 1, the co-twin's risk of having a mental disorder was 21.7% (compared to 27.8% in the full sample). When one twin had a mental disorder, the co-twin's risk was 43.7%. This concordance between twins was expressed in an intra-class correlation of 0.21. Prevalence of MDD, *Any anxiety disorders W1*, *AUD*, and *Any mental disorder W1* were estimated for a sub-sample where one twin was randomly chosen from each pair (see Table 7). The estimates were quite similar to estimates from both twins. The ratio of the results (estimates from the entire sample/estimates from only one twin) varied between 1.00 and 1.04.

Discussion

MDD, anxiety disorders, and AUD were highly prevalent at age 19–29. The prevalence of mental disorders was lower at age 30–42, and this was mainly due to decrease

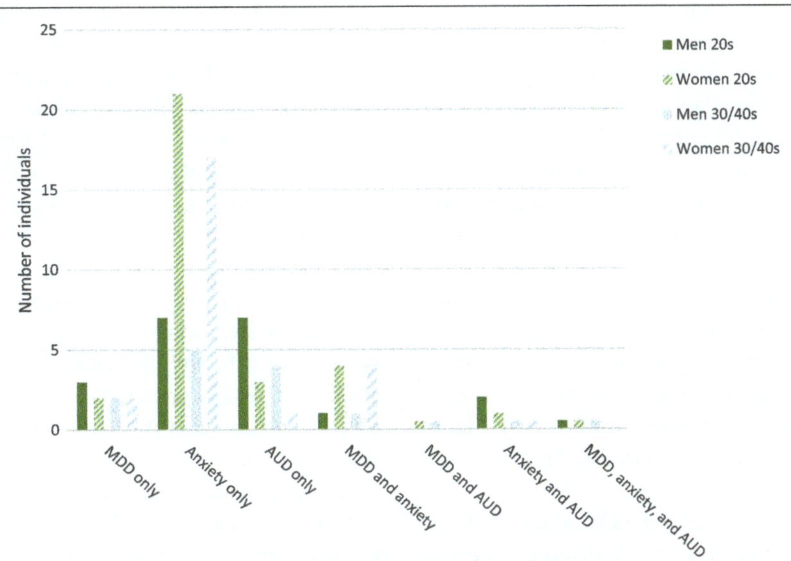

Fig. 2 Combinations of disorders in hypothetical groups of 100 men and 100 women at different ages. Legend: MDD = major depressive disorder, Anxiety = Any anxiety disorder W1–2 (Panic disorder, agoraphobia without panic, specific phobias, social phobia and/or generalized anxiety disorder (GAD)), AUD = alcohol use disorder (i.e. alcohol dependence and alcohol abuse)

Table 7 Prevalence estimates in wave 1 when using both twins versus one twin in each pair

	12-month prevalence estimate using both twins 95% CI[c]	12-month prevalence estimate only including one twin from each pair 95% C.I.	Ratio Entire sample estimate/ Estimate using one twin from each pair
MDD	6.2 5.0–7.4	6.2 4.5–8.0	1.00
Any anxiety disorder W1[a]	20.4 18.3–22.7	19.6 17.2–22.5	1.04
AUD	6.0 4.8–7.3	5.8 4.4–7.5	1.03
Any mental disorder W1[b]	27.8 25.4–30.3	27.8 24.7–31.0	1.00

Legends: *CI* Confidence interval, *MDD* Major depressive disorder
[a]Panic disorder, agoraphobia without panic, specific phobias, social phobia, generalized anxiety disorder (GAD), obsessive-compulsive disorder (OCD), and/or post--traumatic stress disorder (PTSD)
AUD Alcohol use disorders, i.e. alcohol dependence or alcohol abuse
[b]Any mental disorder W1 = Any mood disorder, Any anxiety disorder W1, AUD
[c]95% CIs are based on standard errors obtained from bootstrapping (1000 replications), bias corrected for skewness in the bootstrap distribution, and adjusted for cluster-effects among twins

in AUD and specific phobias. Prevalence estimates of MDD and anxiety disorders excluding specific phobias were stable in this period. Individuals who had MDD, an anxiety disorder, or AUD in the twenties were of increased risk of having these disorders in the thirties/forties compared to those who did not have these diagnoses in the twenties.

Prevalence estimates

The 12-month prevalence of depressive disorders in people in the twenties was lower in the current study compared to young adults in the CICS [16], the Dunedin study, NZMHS, NCS, and NCS-R [21, 23], but similar to the prevalence among 26-year-olds in the Simmons longitudinal study [24]. The current findings were very similar to results from these other studies with regard to prevalence of anxiety disorders in the twenties. In the Dunedin study, alcohol dependence among people aged 18 to 32 years was more prevalent than the broader category of AUD in both waves in the current study [21]. Likewise, the narrower category alcohol abuse was more prevalent in TRAILS and NCS-R than AUD in the current sample [22, 23]. In the Simmons longitudinal study, the prevalence of AUD was similar to the current results [24].

Our findings are in line with previous studies showing that anxiety disorders tend to be the most prevalent group of disorders, both in the general adult population and among young adults [21, 52]. The current results are in line with previous Norwegian findings of higher prevalence of specific phobias compared to international studies [6, 53].

The most prevalent groups of disorders were mood disorders and AUD among men and mood disorders among women when specific phobias were excluded. Such phobias are very common, but by definiton highly situation-specific. The current results allowed differentiating between this very circumscrbied disorder and mental disorders that affect people in more complex ways across different situations (e.g. MDD, GAD, and AUD).

Stability

Mental disorders became less prevalent as participants went from the twenties to the thirties/forties. Our results converge with findings from the Simmons Longitudinal study regarding a decrease in specific phobias and AUD [24]. Other anxiety disorders did not become less prevalent in the current study. Findings from the Dunedin study showed a marked decrease in acohol dependence, and quite stable prevalence of MDD and anxiety disorders (including specific phobias, GAD, panic disorder, agoraphobia, OCD, and PTSD) from age 21 to age 32 [21]. Decrease in AUD across young adulthood may reflect the circumstances of people in the twenties, who often do not have responsibility for children, and many are students.

Results from a previous study indicate that a third of those who met diagnostic criteria for AUD in late adolescence, also met criteria for AUD at age 26 [54]. In the current study, only about 15% of those who met diagnostic criteria for AUD in the twenties also had AUD in the thirties/forties. Hence, the course of AUD seems to be less chronic from the twenties to the thirties/forties than from late adolescence to age 26. Nevertheless, the current results showed that those who had AUD in the twenties, had increased risk of having AUD in the thirties/forties compared to those who did not have AUD in the twenties.

Previous studies have found that the majority of individuals with anxiety and depressive disorders at one time point are free from these disorders after three to 11 years [25–27, 55]. This was also the case in the current study. However, those who had MDD or anxiety disorders in the twenties, had increased risk of having these disorders in the thirties/forties compared to those who did not have the disorders in the twenties. This is in line with previous findings from a wider age group of adults (age 18 to 65 at baseline) [56].

Anxiety disorders in the twenties strongly predicted MDD ten years later, even controlling for MDD in the twenties, in line with findings of stable and unspecific genetic risk of mental disorders [34, 35, 57]. The association between MDD in the twenties and anxiety disorders in the thirties/forties, controlled for anxiety disorders in the twenties, was not statistically significant, which may be due to low statistical power. However, others have reported similar results by showing that baseline GAD predicted persistence of MDD, but not the other way around among adolescents and young adults in the NCS-2 [31]. This is also in line with other longitudinal findings from the general adult population, showing that anxiety at one time point predicted depression at a later time to a stronger degree than the reverse [58]. In the Netherlands Mental Health Survey and Incidence Study (NEMESIS), mood disorder at follow-up was predicted by anxiety disorders three years earlier, and incident anxiety disorder was predicted by previous mood disorders [59]. In the US National Epidemiological Survey on Alcohol and Related Conditions (NESARC), there was reciprocal longitudinal associations between incidence of MDD and GAD [60]. The Finnish Health 2011 study reported that baseline anxiety disorder predicted new-onset MDD at 11-year follow-up [61]. Hence, anxiety disorders and MDD seem to have common risk factors, but it is unclear whether anxiety is a more robust predictor of later MDD than the reverse.

MDD seemed to be more episodic in its nature than anxiety disorders, in line with previous studies [22, 55]. There was no change toward a more or less chronic course of any of these disorders when the participants got older.

Comorbidity

There was substantial comorbidity between disorders within each wave, in line with previous research [4, 7, 32, 37], and no evidence of increased or decreased comorbidity between MDD and anxiety disorders from the twenties to the thirties/forties. In both waves, more than half of women and about one third of men with MDD, also had an anxiety disorder. Among those who had an anxiety disorder, one in five or fewer, also had MDD. Young people with vulnerability of both MDD and anxiety, may at any time point have higher risk of experiencing a current anxiety disorder than current MDD because the latter disorder tends to be more episodic.

Implications for policy makers

Previous research has shown that most people with mental disorders go untreated [62, 63]. The current results highlight the need to make adequate treatment easily available for young adults, to help them cope with their developmental tasks (e.g. attain education and work experience). Easily available treatment is important because of the high prevalence of mental disorders in the twenties and the thirties/forties, and because these disorders were long lasting and/or recurrent across ten years for a substantial number of young adults.

The high prevalence of AUD between age 19 and 29 suggests that it is important to implement alcohol interventions particularly tailored to fit this age group and their often-changing life circumstances. Specific phobias may impose functional impairment only in particular situations, but may be serious if those situations are difficult to avoid. There seems to be a particularly high need for efficient treatment of specific phobias for people in the twenties.

Other anxiety disorders and MDD did not become less prevalent with age. Anxiety disorders and MDD did not become more episodic from the twenties to the thirties/forties, and comorbidity between them did not change during this period. Hence, mental health needs for other disorders than AUD and specific phobias are stable from the twenties to the thirties/forties, and many young adults will need treatment for more than one mental disorder.

As noted by Schaefer and colleagues, public knowledge about the very common nature of mental disorders may contribute to reduced stigma [64]. In line with this, public information about the current findings of high prevalence of mental disorders among young adults may contribute to reduced stigma in this age group.

Strengths and limitations

The major strength of the present study is the large population-based sample, which has been assessed twice across 10 years for DSM-IV disorders by structured interviews. However, some limitations warrant consideration. First, the results may not be generalizable to other age groups. Second, there may be bias in the results due to selection in recruitment and attrition at follow-up. People with mental health problems tend to be underrepresented in survey studies [65]. However, as discussed above, mental health variables did not predict participation in either of the interview waves [41, 42], and bias due to selective response may thus not be substantial.

Third, the results are based on a sample of twins, which may reduce generalizability to the general population. A study from the US compared self-reported symptoms of depression, panic-phobia, somatization, and insomnia between twins and their non-twin relatives, and found that twins had significantly, but modestly, higher scores on the panic-phobia factor, but reported similar levels of psychiatric symptoms as their non-twin relatives on the other factors [66]. The authors concluded that *"twins are typical for the general non-twin population in their risk for psychiatric symptoms and syndromes."* (p. 590). Nevertheless, the current findings may be affected by the fact that two individuals from each family were recruited to the study. There was substantial concordance between two twins in a pair regarding mental disorders. Sensitivity analyses were performed with only one twin from each pair included, and results were very similar to the results from both twins.

Conclusion

Mental disorders are common among young people in the twenties and the thirties/forties, but AUD and specific phobias seem to become less prevalent over this age period. Nevertheless, some people are at enduring increased risk of impaired functioning due to mental disorders in consecutive developmental periods. Policy makers should ensure that mental health interventions are available and tailored for young people to help them master their developmental tasks.

Abbreviations

AUD: Alcohol use disorders; CI: Confidence interval; CICS: Children in Community Study; DSM-IV: Diagnostic and Statistical Manual of Mental Disorders, Fourth Edition; GAD: Generalized anxiety disorder; GBD: Global Burden of Disease; M-CIDI: Munich Composite International Diagnostic Interview; MDD: Major depressive disorder; NCS: US National Comorbidity Survey; NCS-2: US National Comorbidity Survey follow-up; NCS-R: US National Comorbidity Survey Replication; NEMESIS: Netherlands Mental Helath Survey and Incidence Study; NESARC: National Epidemiological Survey on Alcohol and Related Conditions; NIPHTP: Norwegian Institute of Public Health Twin Panel; NZMHS: New Zealand Mental Health Survey; OCD: Obsessive-compulsive disorder; PTSD: Post-traumatic stress disorder; Q1: Questionnaire 1 in 1992; Q2: Questionnaire 2 in 1998; TRAILS: Tracking Adolescents' Individual Lives Survey; YLD: Years lived with disability

Acknowledgements

Not applicable.

Funding

Supported by Research Council of Norway grant 196148/V50. Previous collection and analysis of twin data from this project was in part supported by grant MH-068643 from the National Institutes of Health and grants from the Norwegian Research Council, the Norwegian Foundation for Health and Rehabilitation, the Norwegian Council for Mental Health, the Borderline Foundation, and the European Commission. The funding bodies did not have any role in the design of the study, the collection, analysis, or interpretation of data, or in writing the manuscript.

Authors' contributions

KG: Contributed to the design of the study, conducted the analyses and interpreted the results, authored the manuscript and approved of the final manuscript as submitted. AKK: Contributed to the design of the study, interpretation of results, authored the manuscript and approved of the final manuscript as submitted. RN: Contributed to the design of the study, interpretation of results, authored the manuscript and approved of the final manuscript as submitted. GPK: Contributed to the design of the study, the data collection, interpretation of results, reviewed and revised the manuscript, and approved of the final manuscript as submitted. SEV: Contributed to the design of the study, interpretation of results, reviewed and revised the manuscript, and approved of the final manuscript as submitted. TR-K: Contributed to the design of the study, the data collection, the interpretation of results, reviewed and revised the manuscript and approved of the final manuscript as submitted.

Consent for publication

Not applicable.

Competing interests

The authors declare that they have no competing interests.

Author details

[1]Department of mental disorders, Norwegian Institute of Public Health, Oslo, Norway. [2]Centre for Disease Burden, Norwegian Institute of Public Health, Bergen, Norway. [3]Department of Psychosocial Science, University of Bergen, Bergen, Norway. [4]Nydalen DPS, Division of Mental Health and Addiction, Oslo University Hospital, Oslo, Norway. [5]Department of Psychology, University of Oslo, Oslo, Norway. [6]Health Data and Digitalisation, Norwegian Institute of Public Health, Oslo, Norway. [7]Institute of Clinical Medicine, University of Oslo, Oslo, Norway.

References

1. Wang PS, Aguilar-Gaxiola S, Alonso J, Angermeyer MC, Borges G, Bromet EJ, Bruffaerts R, de Girolamo G, de Graaf R, Gureje O, et al. Use of mental health services for anxiety, mood, and substance disorders in 17 countries in the WHO world mental health surveys. Lancet. 2007;370(9590):841–50.
2. GBD 2015 Disease and Injury Incidence and Prevalence Collaborators. Global, regional, and national incidence, prevalence, and years lived with disability for 310 diseases and injuries, 1990–2015: a systematic analysis for the global burden of disease study 2015. Lancet. 2016;388(10053):1545–602.
3. Alonso J, Angermeyer MC, Bernert S, Bruffaerts R, Brugha TS, Bryson H, de Girolamo G, Graaf R, Demyttenaere K, Gasquet I, et al. Prevalence of mental disorders in Europe: results from the European study of the epidemiology of mental disorders (ESEMeD) project. Acta Psychiatr Scand Suppl. 2004;420:21–7.
4. Kessler RC, Chiu WT, Demler O, Merikangas KR, Walters EE. Prevalence, severity, and comorbidity of 12-month DSM-IV disorders in the National Comorbidity Survey Replication. Arch Gen Psychiatry. 2005;62(6):617–27.
5. Kringlen E, Torgersen S, Cramer V. Mental illness in a rural area: a Norwegian psychiatric epidemiological study. Soc Psychiatry Psychiatr Epidemiol. 2006; 41(9):713–9.
6. Kringlen E, Torgersen S, Cramer V. A Norwegian psychiatric epidemiological study. Am J Psychiatr. 2001;158(7):1091–8.
7. Jacobi F, Hofler M, Strehle J, Mack S, Gerschler A, Scholl L, Busch MA, Hapke U, Maske U, Seiffert I, et al. Twelve-months prevalence of mental disorders in the German health interview and examination survey for adults - mental health module (DEGS1-MH): a methodological addendum and correction. Int J Methods Psychiatr Res. 2015;24(4):305–13.
8. de Graaf R, ten Have M, van Gool C, van Dorsselaer S. Prevalence of mental disorders and trends from 1996 to 2009. Results from the Netherlands mental health survey and incidence Study-2. Soc Psychiatry Psychiatr Epidemiol. 2012;47(2):203–13.
9. Arnett JJ, Zukauskiene R, Sugimura K. The new life stage of emerging adulthood at ages 18-29 years: implications for mental health. Lancet Psychiatry. 2014;1(7):569–76.
10. Arnett JJ. Emerging adulthood. A theory of development from the late teens through the twenties. Am Psychol. 2000;55(5):469–80.
11. Vander Stoep A, Beresford SAA, Weiss NS, McKnight B, Cauce AM, Cohen P. Community-based study of the transition to adulthood for adolescents with psychiatric disorder. Am J Epidemiol. 2000;152(4):352–62.
12. Kessler RC, Merikangas KR, Berglund P, Eaton WW, Koretz DS, Walters EE. Mild disorders should not be eliminated from the DSM-V. Arch Gen Psychiatry. 2003;60(11):1117–22.
13. Mojtabai R, Stuart EA, Hwang I, Eaton WW, Sampson N, Kessler RC. Long-term effects of mental disorders on marital outcomes in the National

Comorbidity Survey ten-year follow-up. Soc Psychiatry Psychiatr Epidemiol. 2017;52(10):1217–26.
14. Mojtabai R, Stuart EA, Hwang I, Susukida R, Eaton WW, Sampson N, Kessler RC. Long-term effects of mental disorders on employment in the National Comorbidity Survey ten-year follow-up. Soc Psychiatry Psychiatr Epidemiol. 2015;50(11):1657–68.
15. Mojtabai R, Stuart EA, Hwang I, Eaton WW, Sampson N, Kessler RC. Long-term effects of mental disorders on educational attainment in the National Comorbidity Survey ten-year follow-up. Soc Psychiatry Psychiatr Epidemiol. 2015;50(10):1577–91.
16. Crawford TN, Cohen P, First MB, Skodol AE, Johnson JG, Kasen S. Comorbid Axis I and Axis II disorders in early adolescence: outcomes 20 years later. Arch Gen Psychiatry. 2008;65(6):641–8.
17. Ormel J, Oerlemans AM, Raven D, Laceulle OM, Hartman CA, Veenstra R, Verhulst FC, Vollebergh W, Rosmalen JG, Reijneveld SA, et al. Functional outcomes of child and adolescent mental disorders. Current disorder most important but psychiatric history matters as well. Psychol Med. 2017;47(7): 1271–82.
18. Veldman K, Reijneveld SA, Ortiz JA, Verhulst FC, Bultmann U. Mental health trajectories from childhood to young adulthood affect the educational and employment status of young adults: results from the TRAILS study. J Epidemiol Community Health. 2015;69(6):588–93.
19. Vander Stoep A, Weiss NS, Kuo ES, Cheney D, Cohen P. What proportion of failure to complete secondary school in the US population is attributable to adolescent psychiatric disorder? J Behav Health Serv Res. 2003;30(1):119–24.
20. Johnson JG, Cohen P, Kasen S, Smailes E, Brook JS. Association of maladaptive parental behavior with psychiatric disorder among parents and their offspring. Arch Gen Psychiatry. 2001;58(5):453–60.
21. Moffitt TE, Caspi A, Taylor A, Kokaua J, Milne BJ, Polanczyk G, Poulton R. How common are common mental disorders? Evidence that lifetime prevalence rates are doubled by prospective versus retrospective ascertainment. Psychol Med. 2010;40(6):899–909.
22. Ormel J, Raven D, van Oort F, Hartman CA, Reijneveld SA, Veenstra R, Vollebergh WA, Buitelaar J, Verhulst FC, Oldehinkel AJ. Mental health in Dutch adolescents: a TRAILS report on prevalence, severity, age of onset, continuity and co-morbidity of DSM disorders. Psychol Med. 2015;45(2):345–60.
23. National Comorbidity Survey (NCS) [https://www.hcp.med.harvard.edu/ncs/ftpdir/NCS-R_12-month_Prevalence_Estimates.pdf].
24. Tanner JL, Reinherz HZ, Beardslee WR, Fitzmaurice GM, Leis JA, Berger SR. Change in prevalence of psychiatric disorders from ages 21 to 30 in a community sample. J Nerv Ment Dis. 2007;195(4):298–306.
25. Lamers F, Beekman AT, van Hemert AM, Schoevers RA, Penninx BW. Six-year longitudinal course and outcomes of subtypes of depression. Br J Psychiatry. 2016;208(1):62–8.
26. Markkula N, Harkanen T, Nieminen T, Pena S, Mattila AK, Koskinen S, Saarni SI, Suvisaari J. Prognosis of depressive disorders in the general population- results from the longitudinal Finnish health 2011 study. J Affect Disord. 2016;190:687–96.
27. Rhebergen D, Batelaan NM, de Graaf R, Nolen WA, Spijker J, Beekman AT, Penninx BW. The 7-year course of depression and anxiety in the general population. Acta Psychiatr Scand. 2011;123(4):297–306.
28. Copeland WE, Adair CE, Smetanin P, Stiff D, Briante C, Colman I, Fergusson D, Horwood J, Poulton R, Costello EJ, et al. Diagnostic transitions from childhood to adolescence to early adulthood. J child Psychol Psychiatry. 2013;54(7):791–9.
29. Costello EJ, Copeland W, Angold A. The great Smoky Mountains study: developmental epidemiology in the southeastern United States. Soc Psychiatry Psychiatr Epidemiol. 2016;51(5):639–46.
30. Johnson JG, Cohen P, Kasen S. Minor depression during adolescence and mental health outcomes during adulthood. Br J Psychiatry. 2009;195(3):264–5.
31. Kessler RC, Gruber M, Hettema JM, Hwang I, Sampson N, Yonkers KA. Co-morbid major depression and generalized anxiety disorders in the National Comorbidity Survey follow-up. Psychol Med. 2008;38(3):365–74.
32. Alonso J, Angermeyer MC, Bernert S, Bruffaerts R, Brugha TS, Bryson H, de Girolamo G, Graaf R, Demyttenaere K, Gasquet I, et al. 12-month comorbidity patterns and associated factors in Europe: results from the European study of the epidemiology of mental disorders (ESEMeD) project. Acta Psychiatr Scand Suppl. 2004;420:28–37.
33. Newman DL, Moffitt TE, Caspi A, Magdol L, Silva PA, Stanton WR. Psychiatric disorder in a birth cohort of young adults: prevalence, comorbidity, clinical significance, and new case incidence from ages 11 to 21. J Consult Clin Psychol. 1996;64(3):552–62.
34. Krueger RF, Markon KE. Reinterpreting comorbidity: a model-based approach to understanding and classifying psychopathology. Annu Rev Clin Psychol. 2006;2:111–33.
35. Kendler KS, Aggen SH, Knudsen GP, Roysamb E, Neale MC, Reichborn-Kjennerud T. The structure of genetic and environmental risk factors for Syndromal and Subsyndromal common DSM-IV Axis I and all Axis II disorders. Am J Psychiatr. 2011;168(1):29–39.
36. Lamers F, van Oppen P, Comijs HC, Smit JH, Spinhoven P, van Balkom AJ, Nolen WA, Zitman FG, Beekman AT, Penninx BW. Comorbidity patterns of anxiety and depressive disorders in a large cohort study: the Netherlands study of depression and anxiety (NESDA). J Clin Psychiatry. 2011;72(3):341–8.
37. Merikangas KR, Zhang HP, Avenevoli S, Acharyya S, Neuenschwander M, Angst J. Longitudinal trajectories of depression and anxiety in a prospective community study - the Zurich cohort study. Arch Gen Psychiatry. 2003; 60(10):993–1000.
38. Zlomke K, Davis TE 3rd. One-session treatment of specific phobias: a detailed description and review of treatment efficacy. Behav Ther. 2008;39(3):207–23.
39. Grant BF, Compton WM, Crowley TJ, Hasin DS, Helzer JE, Li TK, Rounsaville BJ, Volkow ND, Woody GE. Errors in assessing DSM-IV substance use disorders. Arch Gen Psychiatry. 2007;64(3):379–80. author reply 381-372
40. Nilsen TS, Knudsen GP, Gervin K, Brandt I, Roysamb E, Tambs K, Orstavik R, Lyle R, Reichborn-Kjennerud T, Magnus P, et al. The Norwegian twin registry from a public health perspective: a research update. Twin Res Hum Genet. 2013;16(1):285–95.
41. Reichborn-Kjennerud T, Czajkowski N, Ystrom E, Orstavik R, Aggen SH, Tambs K, Torgersen S, Neale MC, Roysamb E, Krueger RF, et al. A longitudinal twin study of borderline and antisocial personality disorder traits in early to middle adulthood. Psychol Med. 2015;45:1–11.
42. Tambs K, Ronning T, Prescott CA, Kendler KS, Reichborn-Kjennerud T, Torgersen S, Harris JR. The Norwegian Institute of Public Health Twin Study of mental health: examining recruitment and attrition Bias. Twin Res Hum Genet. 2009;12(2):158–68.
43. Nilsen TS, Brandt I, Magnus P, Harris JR. The Norwegian twin registry. Twin Res Hum Genet. 2012;15(6):775–80.
44. Harris JR, Magnus P, Tambs K. The Norwegian Institute of Public Health twin program of research: an update. Twin Res Hum Genet. 2006;9(6):858–64.
45. Wittchen HU, Pfister H. DIA-X interviews (M-CIDI): manual fur screening-Verfahren und interview. Frankfurt: Swets & Zeitlinger; 1997.
46. American Psychiatric Association. Diagnostic and statistical manual of mental disorders. 5th ed. Washington: American Psychiatric Association; 2013.
47. Copeland W, Shanahan L, Costello EJ, Angold A. Cumulative prevalence of psychiatric disorders by young adulthood: a prospective cohort analysis from the great Smoky Mountains study. J Am Acad Child Adolesc Psychiatry. 2011;50(3):252–61.
48. Roberts BW, Wood D, Caspi A: The development of personality traits in adulthood. In: Handbook of personality theory and research. Third edn. Edited by John OP, Robins RW, Pervin LA. New York: Guilford; 2008: 375–398.
49. Efron B, Tibshirani R. Bootstrap methods for standard errors, confidence intervals, and other measures of statistical accuracy. Stat Sci. 1986;1(1):54–75.
50. Singh K, Xie M. Bootstrap: a statistical method. In: Peterson P, Baker E, McGaw B, editors. International encyclopedia of education. Edn: Amsterdam: Rutgers University NJ: Elsevier Science; 2010.
51. Fitzmaurice GM, Laird NM, Ware JH. Applied longitudinal analysis. New Jersey: Wiley-interscience; 2004.
52. Kessler RC, Aguilar-Gaxiola S, Alonso J, Chatterji S, Lee S, Ormel J, Ustun TB, Wang PS. The global burden of mental disorders: an update from the WHO world mental health (WMH) surveys. Epidemiol Psichiatr Soc. 2009; 18(1):23–33.
53. Sandanger I, Nygard JF, Ingebrigtsen G, Sorensen T, Dalgard OS. Prevalence, incidence and age at onset of psychiatric disorders in Norway. Soc Psychiatry Psychiatr Epidemiol. 1999;34(11):570–9.
54. Copeland WE, Angold A, Shanahan L, Dreyfuss J, Dlamini I, Costello EJ. Predicting persistent alcohol problems: a prospective analysis from the great Smoky Mountain study. Psychol Med. 2012;42(9):1925–35.
55. Penninx BW, Nolen WA, Lamers F, Zitman FG, Smit JH, Spinhoven P, Cuijpers P, de Jong PJ, van Marwijk HW, van der Meer K, et al. Two-year course of depressive and anxiety disorders: results from the Netherlands study of depression and anxiety (NESDA). J Affect Disord. 2011; 133(1–2):76–85.

56. Lahey BB, Zald DH, Hakes JK, Krueger RF, Rathouz PJ. Patterns of heterotypic continuity associated with the cross-sectional correlational structure of prevalent mental disorders in adults. JAMA psychiatry. 2014;71(9):989–96.
57. Gillespie NA, Kirk KM, Evans DM, Heath AC, Hickie IB, Martin NG. Do the genetic or environmental determinants of anxiety and depression change with age? A longitudinal study of Australian twins. Twin Res. 2004; 7(1):39–53.
58. Fichter MM, Quadflieg N, Fischer UC, Kohlboeck G. Twenty-five-year course and outcome in anxiety and depression in the upper Bavarian longitudinal community study. Acta Psychiatr Scand. 2010;122(1):75–85.
59. de Graaf R, ten Have M, Tuithof M, van Dorsselaer S. First-incidence of DSM-IV mood, anxiety and substance use disorders and its determinants: results from the Netherlands mental health survey and incidence Study-2. J Affect Disord. 2013;149(1–3):100–7.
60. Grant BF, Goldstein RB, Chou SP, Huang B, Stinson FS, Dawson DA, Saha TD, Smith SM, Pulay AJ, Pickering RP, et al. Sociodemographic and psychopathologic predictors of first incidence of DSM-IV substance use, mood and anxiety disorders: results from the wave 2 National Epidemiologic Survey on alcohol and related conditions. Mol Psychiatry. 2009;14(11):1051–66.
61. Markkula N, Marola N, Nieminen T, Koskinen S, Saarni SI, Harkanen T, Suvisaari J. Predictors of new-onset depressive disorders - results from the longitudinal Finnish health 2011 study. J Affect Disord. 2017;208:255–64.
62. Torvik FA, Ystrom E, Gustavson K, Rosenstrom TH, Bramness JG, Gillespie N, Aggen SH, Kendler KS, Reichborn-Kjennerud T. Diagnostic and genetic overlap of three common mental disorders in structured interviews and health registries. Acta Psychiatr Scand. 2018;137(1):54–64.
63. Wang PS, Lane M, Olfson M, Pincus HA, Wells KB, Kessler RC. Twelve-month use of mental health services in the United States: results from the National Comorbidity Survey Replication. Arch Gen Psychiatry. 2005;62(6):629–40.
64. Schaefer JD, Caspi A, Belsky DW, Harrington H, Houts R, Horwood LJ, Hussong A, Ramrakha S, Poulton R, Moffitt TE. Enduring mental health: prevalence and prediction. J Abnorm Psychol. 2016;126:212–24.
65. Torvik FA, Rognmo K, Tambs K. Alcohol use and mental distress as predictors of non-response in a general population health survey: the HUNT study. Soc Psychiatry Psychiatr Epidemiol. 2012;47(5):805–16.
66. Kendler KS, Martin NG, Heath AC, Eaves LJ. Self-report psychiatric symptoms in twins and their nontwin relatives: are twins different? Am J Med Genet. 1995;60(6):588–91.

Characteristics, motivations and experiences of volunteer befrienders for people with mental illness

Sarah Toner[1], Lauren M. Hickling[1], Mariana Pinto da Costa[1,2], Megan Cassidy[1] and Stefan Priebe[1*]

Abstract

Background: The literature suggests that many people in the general population tend to distance themselves from those with mental illness. However, there are volunteers that behave differently, spending their free time with people with mental illness and providing direct input in the form of befriending. Whilst there are a range of befriending programmes, little is known about who these volunteer befrienders are, and a previous review of different forms of volunteering in mental health care found data on only 63 befrienders.

Methods: We conducted a systematic electronic search of databases (BNI, CNIL, EMBASE, MEDLINE, PsycINFO, Cochrane Registers, Web of Science) to detect all papers reporting characteristics of befriending volunteers in mental health care published between 2011 and April 2018. The articles retrieved were combined with previous papers identified in an earlier review and with relevant papers identified by experts in the field. The articles that met the inclusion criteria were extracted and narratively synthesised.

Results: Nine studies met the inclusion criteria for this review, reporting characteristics of a total of 577 volunteer befrienders. The most often reported characteristics were age and gender, motivations to volunteer and experience of the role. Whilst characteristics vary greatly, most volunteers are female, and the average age is 50 years. Motivations generally fit into the categories of "giving" and "getting" and experiences are mixed.

Conclusion: Published research on volunteer befrienders has increased in the last eight years, but is still limited. The range of characteristics suggests that there is a potential for encouraging a variety of people to volunteer as befrienders for people with mental illness. Understanding the characteristics and motivations of volunteers may help refine programmes and improve the experience of the volunteer befrienders.

Keywords: Review, Befriending, Characteristics, Mental illness, Volunteering, Motivation, Experience

Background

People with mental illness can often face negative stereotypes, discriminatory behaviour and sometimes even self-stigma [1], and the literature suggests that some people in the general population have a tendency to distance themselves from those with mental illness [2]. Despite this, some people seek direct contact and offer their free time as volunteers to support individuals with mental illness.

A particular form of volunteering in mental health care is befriending [3, 4], where volunteers usually provide repeated, one-to-one and face-to-face contact to develop social relationships with people with mental illness. Some studies reported a reduction of depressive symptoms [5, 6] and social isolation [7] in people supported by befrienders. The literature suggests that volunteer befrienders can reap benefits as well, even outside mental health, such as being able to help others, gain experience, or develop a sense of satisfaction from befriending [8, 9].

Yet, research on befriending is limited, and little is known about the characteristics of those who volunteer

* Correspondence: s.priebe@qmul.ac.uk
[1]Unit for Social and Community Psychiatry (WHO Collaborating Centre for Mental Health Service Development), Queen Mary University of London, London, UK
Full list of author information is available at the end of the article

to become befrienders [5]. Such information is crucial for befriending programmes as it is imperative to find, recruit and retain the necessary volunteers.

Motivations of volunteers have been explored previously, for example, as illustrated in the 'Octagon Model' [10], which covers the dimensions of 'giving' versus 'getting', 'distance' versus 'proximity', 'thought' versus 'action', and 'continuity' versus 'newness' of experience.

In 2012, Hallett et al. [11] published a systematic review of volunteers in mental health care, addressing their characteristics, reasons for volunteering, and experience in the volunteering role (based on a search in November 2010). However, Hallett et al.'s [11] review included all types of volunteering, such as, helping in groups, providing training in educational programmes, and one-off support for events. It found information on a total of 540 volunteers but only 63 of these were befrienders. Hallett et al. [11] identified a generally mixed demographic; however, a large proportion of befrienders were female. Additionally, experiences of befriending were mostly positive, and the motivations of "giving" something to others or "getting" something from the experience were cited commonly for volunteer befrienders.

Against this background, our aim has been to conduct a systematic review to identify the characteristics of volunteer befrienders and to describe their motivations and experiences. We assumed that the literature since the Hallett et al. [11] review would provide more data on which to draw conclusions about who volunteers to befriend people with mental illness.

Methods

A systematic literature review, in accordance with the Preferred Reporting Items for Systematic Reviews and Meta-analyses (PRISMA) guidelines [12], was used to identify the characteristics of befriender volunteers in mental health. This was combined with a narrative synthesis grounded on the guidelines developed by Popay et al. [13] to describe their motivations and experiences in volunteering.

Search strategy

We searched the following databases: BNI, CNIL, EMBASE, MEDLINE, PsycINFO, Cochrane Registers, Web of Science (Psychiatry) and grey literature databases. The following search terms were used: volunteer descriptors (Group 1), mental health descriptors (Group 2) and outcome descriptors (Group 3) (Full list of search terms is available as Additional file 1). The results from this search conducted on 11 April 2018 were included.

A secondary hand search was performed in relevant psychiatric journals, grey literature and references, and experts were contacted to identify additional relevant papers in the field.

Eligibility criteria

The review included primary studies reporting data on volunteer befrienders. Eligibility criteria were: i) participants were unpaid lay/nonprofessional volunteers, ii) the volunteer activity was a regular commitment (e.g. not a 'one-off') with an adult mental health population, iii) the volunteering activity involved only one-to-one, face-to-face contacts.

Texts were excluded if they reported information about: i) volunteers that were currently peers, peer workers, family members, paid carers, paid lay workers, mental health professionals or already known friends, ii) the volunteer activity was not specific to a population with severe mental illness (e.g. dementia/substance abuse/HIV/refugees/cancer volunteering), iii) the volunteering had other formats beyond one-to-one (e.g. groups), face-to-face contact (e.g. telephone helpline/online volunteering), iv) volunteering was part of a course requirement, v) volunteering was a one-off activity (e.g. helping after a natural disaster), vi) the literature was in an inappropriate extraction material (e.g. charity advertising booklet or report).

Data extraction and analysis

Following the search, all potential studies were exported into EndNote version X5 bibliographic software and duplicates removed. Titles and abstracts were screened for inclusion with a random selection of 20% of the abstracts being screened by a second assessor. If there was any ambiguity about the study, the full paper was obtained and reviewed by two assessors. Inter-reviewer agreement at the screening stage was 94%. There were no discrepancies relating to those papers selected for inclusion in the full-text search. Data extraction was completed by two assessors. Disagreements regarding full-texts were addressed by discussion and input from a third reviewer.

The following quantitative and qualitative data of the studies were extracted: i) about the studies: year, country, setting, aims, and methods; ii) about volunteers: number, age, gender, education level, employment status, religion, ethnicity, relationship status, living arrangements, motivations, previous experience in mental health volunteering, previous connection to organisation, previous experience as a patient in mental health care, volunteer role, volunteer activities, length of commitment, positive and negative experiences; iii) about the volunteering organisation: type, patient group supported, benefits to people with a mental illness, method of recruiting volunteers, volunteer selection criteria, matching process, volunteer training and supervision.

Narrative synthesis was used to analyse the motivations and experiences of the volunteers. MPC independently conducted the preliminary synthesis based on the extracted findings. By deductively conducting the narrative synthesis, preliminary themes were developed based on the hypothetic-deductive approach featured in the literature, with motivations categorised either as 'giving' (doing something for others) or 'getting', (doing something for themselves); and experiences as 'positive' or 'negative'.

These overarching categories were discussed with all members of the team through an iterative process of continuous discussion, critical reflection, reference to the extracted data and feedback, to ensure a range and depth of the materials. Similar concepts were grouped into the most suitable overarching category, and sub-categories were created where relevant. Tabulation and grouping data was used, selecting suitable illustrative quotations.

Results

The searches yielded a total of 24,655 papers which were then screened. Of these, two met the eligibility criteria. Results were combined with the studies identified in the earlier review [11], and one paper identified by experts that was unpublished at the time, but has been published since. A total of nine studies reporting volunteer befriender characteristics were included. The results of the searches and reasons for exclusion are detailed in Fig. 1.

Overview of the papers

As shown in Table 1, papers identified in the current review came from five different countries: five from the UK [14–18], and one each from Austria [19], Germany [20], Ireland [21] and the USA [22] and included a variety of study designs. Two papers did not state how many volunteers were included, and three provided data on fewer than 30 volunteers [18, 20, 22]. Not including the volunteers in the papers where no numbers were provided, we obtained information on a total of 577 volunteers. Texts were written in English or German.

Volunteering programmes

The majority of befriending programmes were run by third sector, non-profit organisations [14–20, 22], and one was specifically set up for a randomised controlled trial (RCT) run by an Irish university [21]. Many studies stated that the aim of befriending was to reduce social isolation and promote social activities and inclusion [14, 16, 18].

Six papers mentioned the duration of the befriending relationship. For most programmes, the intended average duration was 12 months with large variations of the actual relationship length [14, 16–18, 22]. One programme requested a nine month commitment from befrienders [21].

Three studies referred to matching befrienders and befriending recipients (hereafter, referred to as befriendees). Sheridan et al. [21] reported that their volunteer befriender cohort completed a profile of demographic characteristics, social life and leisure preferences. This was used to match

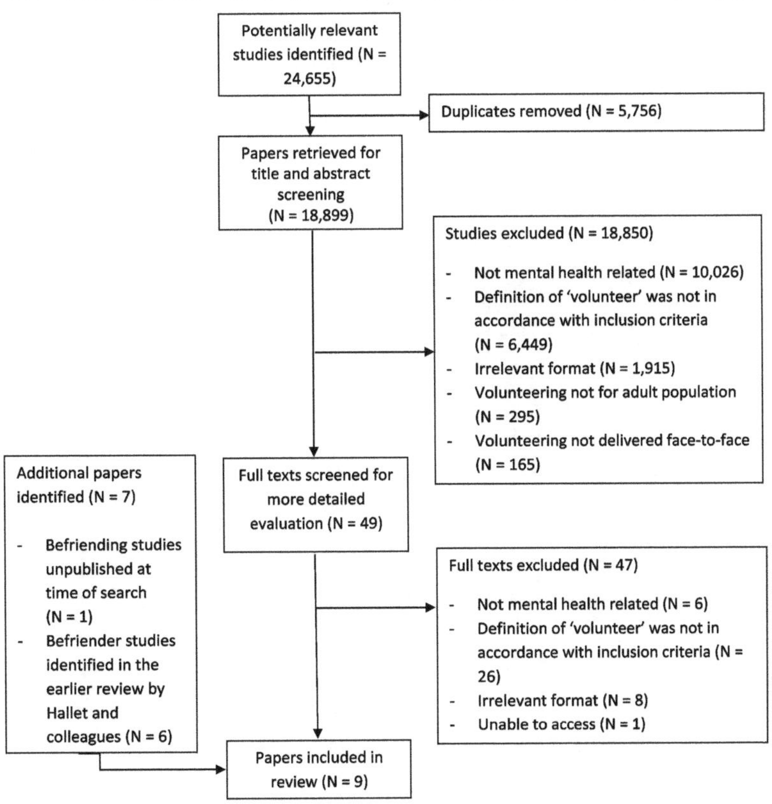

Fig. 1 PRISMA Diagram

Table 1 Summary of papers included in the systematic review

Country	Year	Study design	Number of volunteers interviewed	Volunteer age (mean and age range)	Volunteer gender (% female)	Mental disorders of patients[b]
Austria [19]	2018	Survey of volunteers across 5 of the 8 regions in Austria	360	54.5	78.8	Adults with Serious Mental Illness (SMI)
[a]Germany [20]	1990	Small questionnaire study	13	21–27	"Mostly female"	Chronically mentally ill
Ireland [21]	2015	Prospective RCT of befriending	73	Not stated	Not stated	Adults with SMI
UK [14]	2013	Service evaluation (questionnaire and qualitative interviews with volunteers)	80, 14 of whom took part in qualitative interviews	20–60 years-old	Not stated	Mothers with post-natal depression and complex needs
[a]UK [15]	1989	Naturalistic study, description of service	31	18–59	73.3	Isolated and lonely users of outpatient psychiatric services. Diagnoses: schizophrenia, manic depressive psychosis, depressive neurosis, anxiety states, dependent personality disorder.
[a]UK [16]	2003	Naturalistic study, profile of service	No detail	No detail	No detail	Socially isolated outpatients experiencing long standing mental health problems. 36% have depression, 10% dual diagnosis, 54% other (schizophrenia, manic-depression, anxiety, and long-term mental health problems).
[a]UK [17]	2003	Naturalistic study, profile of service	No detail	University students	Not stated ('Problems recruiting enough male volunteers')	People with enduring or severe/complex mental health problems. 70% of the 450 had schizophrenia.
[a]UK [18]	2011	Small questionnaire study	8	50 (29–65)	25	Adults (outpatients) with difficulties to form and sustain friendships due to moderate/severe mental health problems.
[a]USA [22]	2009	Naturalistic study, service evaluation	12	Unclear. All but one estimated to be over 30, some of retirement age	66.7	People with severe mental illness (outpatients). Specific psychiatric diagnosis not obtained.

[a]Papers taken from review conducted by Hallett et al. [11]
[b]Using the terminology of the original publications
Total befrienders (N) = 577 (360 + 13 + 73 + 80 + 31 + 8 + 12)

participants based on shared interests. Similar approaches were taken in the remaining two studies [17, 18].

Training and supervision of befrienders were outlined in six papers, in which both were described as compulsory [14–18, 22]. This ranged from a one-day programme [21] to six days of training delivered by the project co-ordinator, covering anticipated roles and responsibilities [14]. In another programme befrienders received support during the programme when needed but no initial training [20].

The processes of recruiting befrienders were described in three papers. Sheridan et al. [21] recruited them for their RCT through an "extensive strategy" across a wide range of groups and organisations in the community. Among the remaining studies [16, 17], newspaper advertisements were most often used followed by poster displays, word of mouth, local radio adverts, leaflets and student enquiries.

Selection processes for choosing befrienders were discussed by two papers. For the RCT [21], befrienders were selected for participation through an interview process, completion of a police vetting process and two character references for each application. The other study recruited "current psychology undergraduates or graduates who have expressed a desire to do clinical psychology training" [17].

Characteristics of volunteers

Age

As shown in Table 1, seven papers provided some information on the age of volunteers. Befrienders had a mean of 50 years-old with a very wide range between 18 and 65 years old [14, 15, 18–20, 22].

Gender

Six of the papers reported the gender of the befrienders. In most papers, the majority of befrienders were female [15, 17, 19, 20, 22]. Only one study [18] reported a sample with more males (75%) than females.

Employment status

Two papers indicated the employment status of the volunteers. One reported that half of volunteers were retired [18] with the remainder either unemployed or in full-time education. Another study reported that all volunteer befrienders were university students [17].

Ethnicity

The ethnicity of the volunteers was reported in one paper from the United Kingdom. The sample was described as 'mainly White British' [14].

Relationship status

The relationship status was included in three papers. Two of these found that the majority of volunteers were married or in civil partnerships [14, 19]. In contrast, the majority (10/13) of volunteers described by Brackhane and colleagues [20] were living alone.

Past psychiatric history

Two papers gave information about the volunteers' past psychiatric history, reporting that approximately one third of befrienders had personal experience of mental health care [18, 22].

Motivations for volunteering

Four papers [14, 15, 17, 19] reported the motivations of the befrienders in the study (Table 2). Motivations to volunteer were studied by Klug and colleagues [19], using a list of nineteen predefined motivations.

Table 2 *Motivations of volunteer befrienders*

Getting	
Tombs et al., 2003 [17]	*"undergraduates and graduates enquiring about shadowing or unpaid placements in order to gain experience for clinical training"*
	"to gain assistant and research assistant post"
Klug et al., 2018 [19]	*"Curious to find out if I am suitable for the role"*
	"Test out career aspirations"
	"Enhance my awareness of mental health issues"
	"Befriending looks good on my CV"
	"To gain psychologically relevant experience (for my career)"
	"Acquire new skills"
	"Meet new people"
	"Find explanations for my own behaviour"
	"Have close contact with others"
	"To feel like a better person"
	"To feel needed and acknowledged"
	"To be accepted and liked"
Giving	
Kingdon et al., 1989 [15]	*"a practical way of giving something back after being helped"*
Coe et al., 2013 [14]	*"I wanted to give something back to the community really and I feel that I have done that. Um. It's kind of made me feel accepted in a way"*
Klug et al., 2018 [19]	*"I have received voluntary help in the past, and wanted to give something back"*
	"Feel responsibility to help others"
	"Helping others is part of my philosophy of life"
	"Helping others is part of my religious belief"
	"I wanted to do something useful with my spare time"

The different reasons and motivations of volunteers were categorised in two main themes, "getting" and "giving", as illustrated in Table 2.

"Giving" These motivations were expressed in four studies [14–16, 19], where volunteers shared a desire to give something back through the programme. Kingdon et al. [15] stated that their befrienders wanted to take part in a befriending programme to give back to the service that they had used previously. Similarly, many volunteers working with mothers with post-natal depression had experienced post-natal depression themselves, and described this as a motivation for volunteering [14]. McGowan et al. [16] reported that volunteer befrienders wanted to "give" something of themselves during their time, although they did not describe more specific examples.

"Getting" Five studies described "getting" as a motivation for volunteers [14, 16, 17, 19, 20]. Still, what volunteers wanted to get was quite varied, and ranged from: i) 'getting involved with the community' [14], ii) testing out their own suitability for befriending role, iii) finding explanations for their own behaviours [16, 20], iv) testing out potential career aspirations [16, 17], v) learning more about local mental health services, vi) acquiring new skills or vii) meeting new people [16].

Experiences of volunteering

Volunteers' experiences in the role were discussed in five of the ten papers [14, 17, 18, 20, 22]. The experiences described by the volunteer befrienders were quite varied, at times positive (Table 3) and on other occasions negative (Table 4).

Positive experiences Qualitative interviews from Coe and Barlow [14] portrayed positive experiences of volunteer befrienders, describing ways in which they supported the befriendee, feeling rewarded for contributing to the befriendee's recovery. The positive experience of feeling good about helping someone else was also expressed by eight of 12 volunteers interviewed by McCorkle and colleagues [22]. Some described ways in which volunteering contributed to them personally, such as increasing their self-esteem, confidence and acceptance [14]. Many volunteers felt that with time they gained a genuine friend themselves, wanting to continue the relationship as friends, with many expressing that the benefits of one-to-one volunteering far outweighed the cost in time, money and energy [22].

A positive impact from volunteering on attitudes toward mental illness was discussed in three papers [18, 20, 22]. The experience of volunteering made befrienders reevaluate their preconceptions surrounding mental illness, which they considered a valuable growth opportunity [22]. In some cases this changed previously negative attitudes toward people with mental illness; some lost their initial concerns about the unreliability of people with a mental illness, and found them "surprisingly normal" [20]. For others with personal experience of mental illness, volunteering offered a new perspective on their own problems [18], learning and reflecting about themselves, and instilled a sense that they had benefitted from befriending as much as the befriendee [22].

Negative experiences Negative experiences were described in relation to the behavior of the befriendee in three papers [18, 20, 22]. Some befrienders were left feeling unappreciated [22] when the befriendee did not maintain communication, was often late, or appeared to use the befriender "as a taxicab". Other volunteers expressed difficulties in dealing with confidentiality and privacy, balancing their personal feelings with a sense of professionalism when sensitive information was disclosed by the befriendee [18]. Another matter which was disliked was the recruitment process [17, 21], the bureaucracy (police checks) and waiting (lengthy delays) experiences once recruited, making befrienders drop out of the programme before they had even begun.

Discussion

Main findings

This review provided data on 577 volunteer befrienders from nine studies, around nine times as many befrienders as summarised in a previous review. Yet, more than half of the total number of included befrienders derived from one large study in Austria [19].

The findings suggest that the mean age of befrienders is 50 years-old, but with a very broad range, that they are predominantly female, and that many have experience of psychiatric treatment either themselves or through a close friend or family member. Overall, there was a substantial variation in the socio-demographic characteristics of befrienders between, and also within, studies.

In terms of motivations for befriending, both "giving" something to the befriendee community or in general, and "getting" something out of the programme for themselves appear important.

Positive experiences generally centre around the impact of befriending on the befriendee and own changes in attitudes toward mental illness, while negative experiences related to feeling unappreciated by the befriendee or bad experiences with the befriending organisation. Volunteers had mixed feelings about their relationship with paid mental health professionals and tend to perceive a lack of clarity surrounding their role as a befriender.

Table 3 *Positive experiences of the volunteer befrienders*

1.Satisfaction with the relationship with the befriendee	
1.1.Spending nice time together	
McCorkle et al., 2009 [22]	*"meeting each other's families, dining in each other's homes, celebrating holidays together."*
	"He enjoys getting together. We enjoy each other, getting together and talking, and I've decided that that's of value to me."
1.2.Trusting each other	
Mitchell & Pistrang, 2011 [18]	*"She seems to be able to talk to me about all sorts of things. Sometimes really personal things… it's a confidential situation, it's not going any further than us. So maybe that's what gives her the freedom to talk."*
	"While I'm talking to him I'm not constantly thinking of the roles that I'm the befriender and he is the befriendee, we're two people having a chat."
	"I'm just myself and he's just himself, we just happen to be doing this particular thing, in this particular relationship, in this particular way. .. It's more important for us just to be ourselves."
McCorkle et al., 2009 [22]	"We're there for each other."
1.3. Wanting to continue the relationship as friends	
McCorkle et al., 2009 [22]	*"If [the befriending scheme] ended, he and I would probably still be friends 10 years hence, still doing some stuff together"*
	"in this movement from 'helper/helpee' to true friends"
2. Good experience with the volunteering scheme	
2.1.Access to support/supervision	
Tombs et al. 2003 [17]	*"the most useful aspect being the provision of supervision by clinical psychologists and advice about writing application forms"*
Mitchell & Pistrang, 2011 [18]	*"When she was cutting it was really difficult and I was really distressed about it, so I called [befriending scheme coordinator] to see how to handle it…so it was like dealing with it together. It's not like I'm alone dealing with the situation."*
2.2.Usefulness of sharing experiences with other volunteers	
McCorkle et al., 2009 [22]	*"It's so nice because other volunteers who've already gone through it and have found out what works have helped me a lot."*
3. Personal gains with the relationship	
3.1. Feeling good to provide new experiences to the befriendee	
Mitchell & Pistrang, 2011 [18]	*"to get out and visit places and do things that otherwise [befriendee] wouldn't have done naturally on his own, and that's an exposure to a whole load of different things…it's opening that window of things out there."*
	"about creating opportunities for [befriendee] to go where perhaps he wouldn't have gone before in relationships."
3.2. Filling their own free time	
McCorkle et al., 2009 [22]	"filling the gap created by retirement."
3.3. Feeling rewarded for contributing to the befriendee's recovery	
McCorkle et al., 2009 [22]	*"No matter how much time, or lost sleep, or stress you feel the investment requires, the satisfaction of being intimately involved with another life in recovery is just extraordinarily self-enhancing, reinforcing."*
	"I feel good about myself that I've been able to do something for him."
Coe et al., 2013 [14]	*"But I remember this particular girl the first time I met her she just … I could tell by her eyes what pain she was in. She just had … she sort of glared at me. And now she does actually look happy again and there is that sparkle in her eyes."*
	"It's just really … I just found it really rewarding. I wanted to give something back to the community really and I feel that I have done that. Um. It's kind of made me feel accepted in a way."
3.4. Being supported by the befriendee	
McCorkle et al., 2009 [22]	*"I like it that she's been there even for me, when I needed someone to lean on, that I could talk to her."*
3.5. Learning/reflecting about themselves	
McCorkle et al., 2009 [22]	*"required dealing with one's own negative preconceptions about mental illness."*
Mitchell & Pistrang, 2011 [18]	*"…it's part of that looking at whatever the situation is, from a lot of different perspectives…You look at it in a balanced type of way, rather than in one fixed way."*
	"It makes me think about me, who I am…you do have to say to yourself, 'Am I happy with where I am?', and if there are things that are getting to me where is that layer occurring and you know, because I do become more conscious."
	"It helps you reassess some of the things that have happened to yourself, and how other people may have reacted or looked at it."
3.6. Changing attitudes towards people with mental disorders	
Mitchell & Pistrang, 2011 [18]	*"… It's nice to sort of confirm that what you read in the papers isn't representative of the mental health."*
4. Professional gains with the experience	
4.1. Having contact with people with mental disorders	
Mitchell & Pistrang, 2011 [18]	*"I don't know anyone with a diagnosed mental disorder so I had no idea what someone like that would be like."*
4.2. Helping to clarify their career path	
Tombs et al., 2003 [17]	*"it has also been useful in clarifying whether clinical psychology is the career."*
4.3. Helping to build the CV	
Tombs et al., 2003 [17]	*"[helped with the] demand for relevant voluntary experience whilst competition for assistants' posts remains high and most posts require some previous client experience."*

Strengths and limitations

To our knowledge, this is the first systematic review focusing on the characteristics, motivations and experiences of befrienders in mental health care. It provides a

Table 4 *Negative experiences of the volunteer befrienders*

1. Bad experience with the volunteering schemes	
1.1.Bureaucracy/waiting when recruited	
Tombs et al., 2003 [17]	*"the increase in delays in registering befrienders might well have a negative impact on recruitment as volunteers may need to wait for up to six months before being allocated a client."*
	"waiting three months for clearance to proceed and, regrettably … may have to wait several months more."
1.2.The costs linked with the activities	
Tombs et al., 2003 [17]	*"volunteers are expected to pay for their own refreshments and entertainment."*
McCorkle et al., 2009 [22]	*"insisted on full equality of financial contribution and decision making so that the [befriending] relationship did not encourage passivity and dependency."*
1.3. Feeling pressured with the commitment to meet	
Brackhane et al., 1990 [20]	*"tension between free voluntary input and a sense of duty or obligation"*
McCorkle et al., 2009 [22]	*"after a rough day at work, meeting could feel more like a commitment than like fun."*
2.Dissatisfaction with the relationship with their befriendee	
2.1.Expectations of their befriendee not being met	
McCorkle et al., 2009 [22]	*"expected a client who was much younger, physically active, and interested in going places and doing things, but ended up with a middle-aged client without those interests."*
2.2.Disliking their befriendee	
Tombs et al., 2003 [17]	*"Declined befriending … because they did not like the potential befrienders on offer"*
McCorkle et al., 2009 [22]	*"Then I got to thinking, not every match is going to succeed and go off and go to college."*
2.3.Difficult to empathise with the befriendee	
Mitchell & Pistrang, 2011 [18]	*"Some of it I can empathise with and some of it I've absolutely no idea at all…I don't think you will ever get a hundred percent fit with other people… And if you did have that hundred percent fit, it might be ideally the wrong person for them because they'll just wallow in it with them."*
3. Challenges in the relationship	
3.1.Difficulties in adopting an attentive/supportive role as a volunteer	
Brackhane et al., 1990 [20]	*"avoided emotional talks because of anxiety to get too much worked up about it"*
Mitchell & Pistrang, 2011 [18]	*"I'd say the hardest thing is not giving a true reaction to the things she says, and biting my lip rather than making or voicing my judgments or opinions…"*
	"I'm keeping a watchful eye, but not making it obvious"
3.2.Difficulties in setting boundaries	
Mitchell & Pistrang, 2011 [18]	*"It's more to do with where I'm putting my boundaries… It's kind of making sure that the whole conversation isn't about me…The unequal-ness of the relationship is that one. It's not about me."*
3.3.Difficulties in dealing with confidentiality/privacy	
McCorkle et al., 2009 [22]	*"the awkwardness of running into a friend or business acquaintance when with one's match."*
3.4.Difficulties in tolerating the befriendee's behaviour	
McCorkle et al., 2009 [22]	"[tolerating] heavy smoking and coffee consumption, occasional outbursts of anger."
3.5.Feeling exploited by the befriendee	
McCorkle et al., 2009 [22]	*"There was no joy in it for me by going and picking her up and taking her to whatever store she wanted to go to. I knew I wouldn't last like that. So I started setting limits and explaining to her that that's not what friends do. They do that occasionally, maybe, but that isn't what a friend does."*
	"feeling treated as a taxicab was an unpleasant experience."
3.6.Difficulties in ending the relationship	
McCorkle et al., 2009 [22]	*"…He's as far as he's gonna be, I think, but I still can't leave him, 'cause I feel like we've just developed a bond!"*
	"I can't imagine not having my [befriendee] friend in my life. I really can't"
	"worried about what would happen if life changes (such as moving elsewhere for graduate school) prevented continuation of the relationship."
Mitchell & Pistrang, 2011 [18]	*"I feel like it's slightly kind of a bit like a taboo subject [the end of the relationship]. Um, I think I would be scared of saying the wrong thing, if it came up."*

summary of the different motivations and experiences of befriender volunteers that appear plausible and are in line with previous literature on volunteering. It covers a significant number of befrienders, but also a range of countries, and languages (English and German) exceeding those in a previous wider review on different types of volunteering in mental health care [11]. A further strength is that to reduce the publication bias, unpublished literature and hand searches of relevant journals were performed to maximise the search. In addition, the themes of the narrative synthesis were identified across a diversity of papers and were discussed within the multidisciplinary team of the co-authors to reduce bias of findings.

The study, however, has several limitations. First, whilst the total number of 577 included befrienders may allow more general conclusions than previously possible, it is still small in the light of the wide use of befriending schemes in some countries, particularly considering that data on 360 befrienders were from only one large survey [19]. Secondly, all papers are from a limited number of high-income countries, and there remains a lack of information about what types of befriending programmes, if any, exist in other countries and what the characteristics of the befrienders in those programmes are. Thirdly, although it was possible to extract some qualitative data about the motivations and experiences of volunteers, papers included only a few quotations, and hence the available data was limited to conduct the narrative synthesis. Fourthly, the quantitative data extracted for this review were not consistently reported, which makes it difficult to synthesise the data and compare studies. Finally, with respect to experiences, one may assume that most studies were biased through the selection of interviewees. Befrienders with very negative experiences are more likely to end their befriending sooner and avoid participation in research interviews than those who liked their befriending role and did it for longer.

Comparison with the literature

Whilst the earlier wider review [11] identified details on only 63 volunteer befrienders, this review found reports on an additional 514 befrienders. Given that the previous review covered the whole period of time since the inception of the included databases and this one added only eight years, the increase of research data on befrienders may reflect a rising research interest in befriending programmes.

The findings here are consistent with those reported by Hallett and colleagues [11]. This is in regards to the predominance of women among befrienders, the otherwise wide range of socio-demographic characteristics, the mix of motivations of "giving" and "getting" for volunteer befrienders, and the mostly positive but still mixed experiences of befrienders.

The categorisation of motivations into "giving" and "getting" reflects one of the four dimensions of the 'Octagon Model' which has been used to describe the motivations of volunteers in general [10]. Klug and colleagues [19] applied such categorisations in their assessment of volunteer motivations. They identified four subgroups of befrienders based on their characteristics (age, gender, marital status and employment status), which were associated with different motivations to engage in befriending. The largest subgroup included married, retired females (median age = 64), which were largely motivated by their responsibility to help others. This motivation was also predominant in two other subgroups, comprised of married retired males (median age = 58), and married females in full-time employment (median age = 51). The final subgroup consisted of single females in full-time employment (median age = 44). The most frequent motivations in the four groups were similar and included aspects of both 'giving' and 'getting'. Only the fourth and youngest group differed in some aspects from the other groups and stated more often the wish to acquire new skills and career aspirations as motivations. It remains unclear to what extent different subgroups of befrienders may respond to different recruitment strategies and benefit from different types of programmes and supervision.

Implications

The fact that there is a wide variation in the characteristics of volunteer befrienders, including employment and relationship status, suggests that a typical volunteer befriender does not exist and that there is a potential to recruit volunteers for befriending programmes from very different groups in the population. The majority of befrienders being female might reflect gender differences in attitudes, social roles or both. The motivations of different groups and their potentials to engage in specific befriending programmes are likely to vary, and more research is required to tailor recruitment strategies and programmes for people with different backgrounds, interests and social situations. In particular, additional qualitative research should be conducted to further explore the motivations and experiences of different volunteers. Studies with sufficiently large samples should allow the exploration of potentially relevant subgroups, of which only one study has been able to do so far [19].

Allowing volunteering opportunities that are consistent with volunteers' motivations may improve volunteers' satisfaction and retention in these programmes. Equally, exploring the experiences in more detail may help with designing programmes that maximise the satisfaction of befrienders and encourage them to stay in programmes or volunteer again if they had engaged previously and since ceased participating.

Whilst this review summarised data of research publications, this is still limited and inconsistently reported. Therefore, in the future, data about volunteers should be routinely collected and published on a large scale to map out and further develop befriending programmes. This is currently hindered by a number of factors, one of which being that many programmes are run outside mainstream health services with less developed data documentation systems.

Conclusions

The results reported in this review suggest an increased attention to befriending programmes in research over the last eight years. Apart from most befrienders being female, the variability of characteristics of befrienders suggests that generalised conclusions are difficult. At the same time, it may underline the wide potential to establish more befriending programmes in different contexts, whilst the different motivations and experiences of befrienders point to possibilities for refining and specifying programmes for different types of befrienders.

Abbreviations

NHS: National Health Service; NIHR: National Institute of Health Research; PRISMA: Preferred Reporting Items for Systematic Reviews and Meta-Analyses; RCT: Randomised Controlled Trial; SMI: Serious Mental Illness

Acknowledgements

The authors wish to acknowledge the researchers at the Unit for Social and Community Psychiatry, who provided feedback on an early draft of this paper.

Funding
This paper presents independent research funded by the National Institute for Health Research (NIHR) under its Programme Grants for Applied Research Programme (Reference Number RP-PG-0611-20002). The funding body was not involved in, and did not influence, the design of the study, data collection, analysis or interpretation of the data. The views expressed are those of the author(s) and not necessarily those of the National Health Service (NHS), the NIHR or the Department of Health.

Authors' contributions
SP developed the study idea and designed the study. ST completed the full search and data extraction. LH and MC completed a check and extraction from a proportion of the search results. SP reviewed any discrepancies. MPC conducted the narrative synthesis. ST, SP, LH, MC and MPC drafted the manuscript; all authors commented on and agreed to the final manuscript.

Consent for publication
Not applicable.

Competing interests
The authors declare that they have no competing interests.

Author details
[1]Unit for Social and Community Psychiatry (WHO Collaborating Centre for Mental Health Service Development), Queen Mary University of London, London, UK. [2]Institute of Biomedical Sciences Abel Salazar (ICBAS), University of Porto, Porto, Portugal.

References
1. Livingstone J, Boyd J. Correlates and consequences of internalized stigma for people living with mental illness: a systematic review and meta-analysis. Soc Sci Med. 2010;71(12):2150–61.
2. Angermeyer M, Dietrich S. Public beliefs about and attitudes towards people with mental illness: a review of population studies. Acta Psychiatra Scand. 2006;113(3):163–79.
3. Thompson R, Valenti E, Siette J, Priebe S. To befriend or to be a friend: a systematic review of the meaning and practice of "befriending" in mental health care. J Ment Health. 2015;25:71–7.
4. Priebe S, Pavlickova H, Eldridge S, Golden E, McCrone P, Ockenden N, et al. Effectiveness of one-to-one volunteer support for patients with psychosis: protocol of a randomised controlled trial. BMJ Open. 2016;6(8):e011582.
5. Mead N, Lester H, Chew-Graham C, Gask L, Bower P. Effects of befriending on depressive symptoms and distress: systematic review and meta-analysis. Br J Psychiatry. 2010;196(2):96–101.
6. Siette J, Cassidy M. S P. effectiveness of befriending interventions: a systematic review and meta-analysis. BMJ Open. 2017;7:e014304.
7. Mulvihill J. The unique and valuable support provided by mentoring and befriending. Work with Older People. 2011;15(1):34–7.
8. Greenwood D, Gordon C, Pavlou C, Bolton J. Paradoxical and powerful: volunteers' experiences of befriending people with dementia. Dementia. 2018;17(7):821–39.
9. Heslop P, Robinson C. Befriending-more than just finding friends; 2004.
10. Yeung A. The octagon model of volunteer motivation: results of a phenomenological analysis. Volunt Int J Volunt Nonprofit Organ. 2004;15(1):21–46.
11. Hallett C, Klug G, Lauber C, Priebe S. Volunteering in the care of people with severe mental illness:a systematic review. BMC Psychiatry. 2012;12:226.
12. Moher D, Liberati A, Tetzlaff J, Altman D, Group P. Preferred reporting items for systematic reviews and meta-analyses: the PRISMA statement. PLoS Med. 2009;6:e1000097.
13. Popay J, Roberts H, Snowden A, Petticrew M, Arai L, Rodgers M, et al. Guidance on the conduct of narrative synthesis in systematic reviews. A product from the ESRC methods Programme. Lancaster: Lancaster University; 2006.
14. Coe C, Barlow J. Supporting women with perinatal mental health problems: the role of the voluntary sector. Community Pract. 2013;86(2):23–7.
15. Kingdon D, Turkington D, Collis J, Judd M. Befriending: cost-effective community care. Psychiatr Bull. 1989;13(7):350–1.
16. McGowan B, Jowett C. Promoting positive mental health through befriending. Int J Ment Heal Promot. 2003;5(2):12–24.
17. Tombs D, Stowers C, Fairbank S, Arkill T. A befriending service for individuals with complex, enduring mental health problems. Clin Psychol, BPS Mon Div. 2003;28:33–6.
18. Mitchell G, Pistrang N. Befriending for mental health problems: processes of helping. Psychol Psychother Theory Res Pr. 2011;84(2):151–69.
19. Klug G, Toner S, Fabisch K, Priebe S. Characteristics and motivations of volunteers providing one-to-one support for people with mental illness: a survey in Austria. Soc Psychiatry Psychiatr Epidemiol; 2018:53:841–7.
20. Brackhane R, Strehl C, Wurzer I. Lay help in rehabilitation of psychiatrically handicapped patients–report of two comparative empirical studies. Rehabil. 1990;29(4):254–60.
21. Sheridan A, Drennan J, Coughlan B, O'Keeffe D, Frazer K, Kemple M, et al. Improving social functioning and reducing social isolation and loneliness among people with enduring mental illness: report of a randomised controlled trial of supported socialisation. Int J Soc Psychiatry. 2015;61(3):241–50.
22. McCorkle B, Dunn E, Yu Mui W, Gagne C. Compeer friends: a qualitative study of a volunteer friendship programme for people with serious mental illness. Int J Soc Psychiatr. 2009;55(4):291–305.

Preferences for befriending schemes: a survey of patients with severe mental illness

Sarah Toner[1], Megan Cassidy[1], Agnes Chevalier[1], Aida Farreny[1], Monica Leverton[1], Mariana Pinto da Costa[1,2,3] and Stefan Priebe[1*]

Abstract

Background: Befriending has become a widely used method for tackling social isolation in individuals with severe mental illness (SMI), and evidence exists to support its effectiveness. However, patient preferences for befriending remain unclear. We aimed to determine whether patients with SMI want a volunteer befriender and, if so, the volunteer characteristics and character of the relationship they would prefer.

Methods: A survey of outpatients was conducted across London-based community mental health teams, for individuals diagnosed with affective or psychotic disorders. Questions consisted of measures of demographic characteristics, befriending preferences and social context, including measures of time spent in activities, number of social contacts, loneliness and subjective quality of life (SQOL). Binary logistic regressions were used to investigate potential predictors of willingness to participate in befriending.

Results: The sample comprised of 201 participants with a mean age of 43 years. The majority (58%) of the sample indicated willingness to participate in befriending. In univariable analyses this was associated with less time spent in activities in the previous week, higher level of loneliness and lower SQOL. When all three variables were tested as predictors in a multivariable analysis, only lower SQOL remained significantly associated with willingness to take part in befriending.

Relative to other options presented, large proportions of participants indicated preference for weekly (44%), 1-hour (39%) meetings with a befriender, with no limits on the relationship duration (53%). Otherwise, patient preferences exhibited great variability in relation to other characteristics of befriending schemes.

Conclusions: A substantial number of patients with SMI appear willing to take part in a befriending scheme. Patients with lower SQOL are more likely to accept befriending, so that befriending schemes may be a realistic option to help patients with particularly low SQOL. The large variability in preferences for different types of befriending suggests that there is no one-size-fits-all formula and that schemes may have to be flexible and accommodate different individual preferences.

Keywords: Befriending, Preference, Mental illness, Loneliness, Social isolation, Social contacts, Quality of life

* Correspondence: s.priebe@qmul.ac.uk
[1]Unit for Social and Community Psychiatry (WHO Collaborating Centre for Mental Health Service Development), Newham Centre for Mental Health, Queen Mary University of London, London, UK
Full list of author information is available at the end of the article

Background

Individuals with severe mental illness (SMI) reportedly experience higher levels of social isolation and loneliness than the general population, which is linked with low levels of social support [1, 2]. Isolation and loneliness negatively impact on both physical and mental health [3], and potentially exacerbate pre-existing mental health problems. Such patterns may be seen in patients with schizophrenia; negative symptoms may include social withdrawal and blunted emotional responses, which persist even in stable patients [4]. Such symptoms may both increase the likelihood and worsen the impact of social isolation.

Social isolation experienced by individuals with SMI can be tackled through interventions from volunteering organisations, representing an important resource for health services when utilised efficiently [5]. Volunteers often provide support and help to build closer relationships with both services and communities [6]. One example of this is a type of volunteering termed 'befriending'. This denotes a one-to-one companionship facilitated by a volunteering organisation or a health or social service to foster a supportive relationship between a volunteer and an individual with a physical or mental disorder.

Befriending remains poorly understood and under researched with regard to the extent and nature of its impact on patient outcomes [7, 8]. Systematic reviews show a shortage of high quality studies [2, 9]. Based on existing studies, the reviews report a tangible benefit of befriending on depressive symptoms [2] and for both physical and mental health disorders [9]. Siette and colleagues [9] highlighted existing limitations within befriending practices, including the need to better define appropriate populations for befriending schemes. The authors assert that greater efficacy may be achieved through balancing the frequency, length and modality of befriending. This process may be enriched by input from patients, which is currently lacking. This is particularly relevant given that patients with SMI experiencing negative symptoms may be particularly hard to reach through befriending schemes.

Although befriending can be used to support patients with SMI, little is known about their preferences with regard to the aim of befriending, structure of the scheme and its activities, or the nature of the befriender-patient relationship. This conflicts with the growing focus on patient perspectives in informing their care, which has been sought-after and encouraged in health services [10, 11]. Identifying and addressing the preferences of those patients who are particularly challenging to recruit into social interventions, such as those with pronounced negative symptoms, particularly relevant if these schemes are to be successful in targeting social isolation.

Through a survey of current patients with SMI, we firstly aimed to determine if patients would like to take part in a befriending scheme. We secondly wanted to ascertain whether their willingness to become a befriendee can be predicted by patient characteristics or measures of social context relating to isolation and social activity. Thirdly, we aimed to explore what type of befriending scheme patients would prefer, if one was offered. In doing so, we intended to provide guidance for the development of future befriending schemes and help to improve the effectiveness of existing schemes.

Method

This study aimed to determine whether patients with SMI want to participate in a befriending scheme and, if so, what volunteer and relationship characteristics they prefer.

This was a cross-sectional survey study conducted in patients from nine community mental health teams across East London. We collected data from patients about their sociodemographic characteristics, befriending preferences and social context. A favourable opinion was given by the NHS Research Ethics Committee (Ref 14/SW/1011).

Eligibility criteria

To be deemed eligible, patients were required to meet the following criteria: (1) Aged over 18 years; (2) under the care of secondary mental health services; (3) diagnosed with a psychotic (F20-F29) or an affective disorder (F30-F39) according to the International Statistical Classification of Diseases and Related Health Problems - Tenth Revision (ICD-10), 5th edition [12]; (4) sufficient proficiency in spoken English to understand the consent process and answer the questionnaire items. Patients were excluded if deemed by their clinician to have insufficient capacity to consent at the time of assessment, or if the patient was participating in a befriending research trial, which was ongoing at the time of the assessments.

Procedure

The research team identified eligible patients in nine community mental health teams in East London. Eligible patients were then approached on the day of their appointment with a clinician to explain the study's aims, provide more information if requested and obtain informed written consent prior to assessment. All interviewers were trained researchers.

Instruments

The questionnaire obtained data on patients' sociodemographic characteristics including age, gender, years since first diagnosis of mental illness, weekly hours in employment, and monthly income of patients. This was followed by a brief description of befriending and questions relating to preferences for such schemes. Participants were first asked whether they had heard of befriending prior to the questionnaire and if they would take part in befriending if a scheme were advertised. The participants who expressed willingness were then asked a series of multiple-choice questions regarding their preferences for the characteristics of a volunteer befriender, as well as the type of befriending relationship (e.g. meeting frequency, meeting and relationship duration, and potential activities). In an open-ended question, patients who indicated that they would not like to take part in befriending were asked to give a reason for their answer.

Measures of social context assessed time spent in leisure activities (time use), social contacts, loneliness and quality of life. Time use was measured using an adapted version of the United Kingdom Time Use Survey [13], which listed potential activities and asked patients how many times the interviewee had engaged in the activity in the week prior to assessment, how long was spent doing the activity and whether this was with another person or alone [14]. Social contacts were measured using the Social Contacts Assessment [15] which asks participants to list anyone with whom they have had a social contact in the previous week, excluding people they live with or health professionals. Loneliness was rated on an item from the World Health Organization Quality of Life Assessment [16] asking "How lonely do you feel in your life?" with response options ranging from 1 (not at all) to 5 (extremely). Finally, subjective quality of life (SQOL) was assessed using the Manchester Short Assessment of Quality of Life (MANSA) [17], which asks participants to rate satisfaction with 12 life domains on a scale from 1 (couldn't be worse) to 7 (couldn't be better). The mean score of those 12 items is used to reflect SQOL.

Sample size and data entry

The sample size in this exploratory study was based on an estimate for a between-group comparison of two groups. Comparing two groups with a sample size of 100 provides 80% power to detect an effect size of 0.30 at a 5% significance level. Therefore, we aimed to recruit a total sample of 200 patients.

Data were entered into SPSS (version 24) for analysis [18]. Further, 20% of the data were randomly selected, stratified according to the researcher who originally entered the data, re-entered and compared against the database to increase reliability of the data entry procedure.

Analysis

Characteristics of the whole sample and the befriending preferences of those patients who expressed a willingness to take part in befriending were represented by descriptive outputs. Open questions were analysed using content analysis.

A univariable binary logistic regression was used to explore whether the following patient characteristics were related to the dependent variable, i.e. willingness to engage in a befriending scheme: age, gender, familiarity with befriending schemes, diagnostic group (F2 or F3), years since diagnosis, weekly hours spent in employment, monthly income, weekly time use, social contacts in the past week, loneliness and SQOL. Variables with a significant association with the willingness to take part in befriending ($p < 0.1$) were then entered in a multivariable binary logistic regression model. Patients with missing data for any variables presented in the results were excluded from the relevant analysis.

Results

Of the 898 patients screened, 201 were included in the final analysis. The selection process is detailed in Fig. 1.

Sample characteristics

Sample characteristics are shown in Table 1. Approximately three quarters of the sample had been diagnosed with schizophrenia or related disorder (75%, $N = 151$) and the remainder were diagnosed with an affective disorder.

Willingness to participate in a befriending scheme

Overall 116 (58%) participants indicated a willingness to take part in a befriending scheme. Of these, 51 had never heard of befriending prior to the assessment, from a total of 85 who had no prior knowledge of befriending (42% of the sample).

Of the 84 unwilling individuals, reasons for not wanting to take part fell into the following categories: befriending is not relevant to their social needs (47%, $N = 34$); lack of interest or time (26%, $N = 19$); aversion to the label of mental illness (19%, $N = 14$); and general interest but only under different personal circumstances (e.g. if mental health deteriorated) (8%, $N = 6$).

Predicting willingness

The univariable regression models for willingness to participate in befriending are shown in Table 2. Loneliness, number of social contacts and SQOL were significantly associated with willingness to take part in befriending. In the multivariable regression only SQOL remained significant at the 5% level, with lower SQOL indicating greater inclination to take part in a befriending scheme.

Befriending preferences

Almost two-thirds of the 116 participants indicating willingness to take part in befriending stated that their main aim would be to make a new friend (62%, $N = 71$) rather than the alternative option presented (to do more activities).

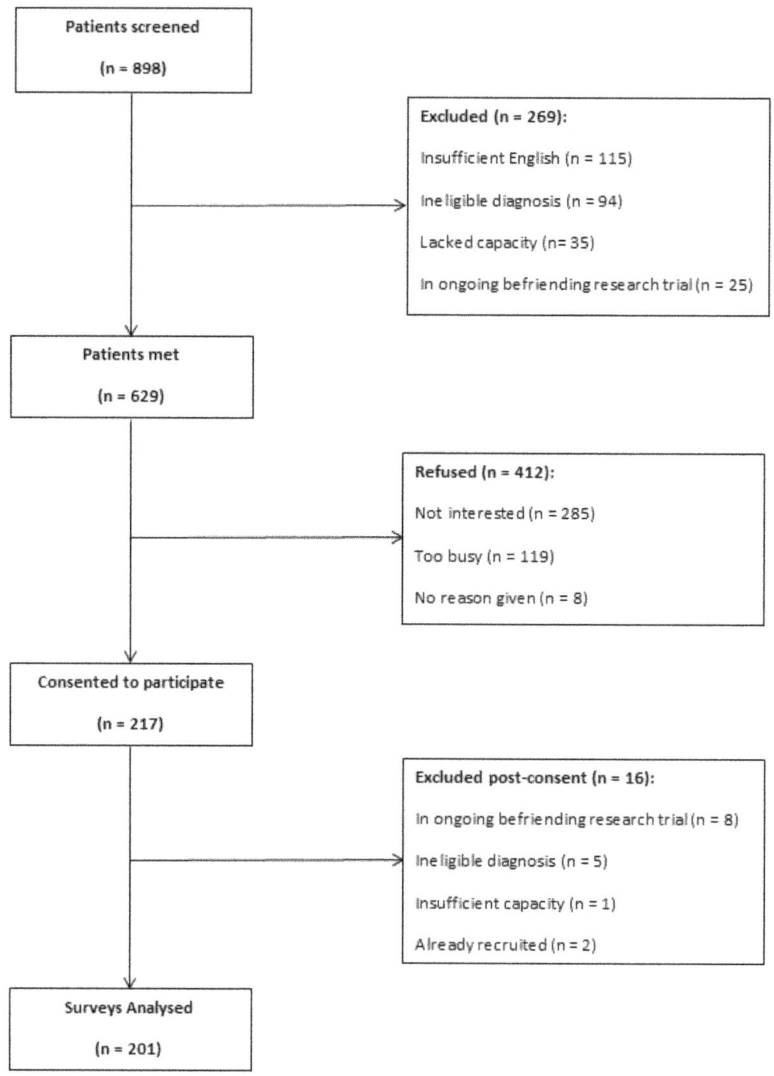

Fig. 1 CONSORT diagram of patients approached to participate

Characteristics of volunteer befriender

Approximately one-third of patients had no preference (34%, $N = 39$) while 29% ($N = 33$) wanted someone similar to them and 29% ($N = 33$) would prefer a psychology or counselling student. Only 9% ($N = 10$) of respondents would prefer being matched with someone different to them.

Further, 70% ($N = 81$) of patients would want the volunteer befriender to be in contact with their mental health care team. A majority (62%, $N = 72$) also reported that they would prefer a befriender with lived experience as a patient in mental health care, while 21% ($N = 24$) of individuals had no preference, and 17% ($N = 20$) explicitly said they would not want a befriender with lived experience.

Type of the relationship with the befriender

The preferred relationship with a volunteer befriender was most frequently to have 'a real friendship' (32%, $N = 37$), followed by 'someone who talks with me and listens' (30%, $N = 35$), 'someone who does activities with me' (20%, $N = 23$), 'someone to spend time with' (11%, $N = 13$) and 'no preference' (7%, $N = 8$).

When offered a list of potential activities to do with a befriender more than half of participants asked selected the following, regardless of their primary aim for taking part: eating in a café or restaurant (70%, $N = 81$), just getting out of the house (61%, $N = 70$), going to the cinema or theatre (57%, $N = 66$), gym/playing sports (64%, $N = 73$), going for walks (72%, $N = 83$) and shopping (58%, $N = 67$). Further, 42% ($N = 47$) felt the scheme

Table 1 Demographic characteristics, SQOL, loneliness and time use of sample

Characteristic	Sample (N = 201)
Age, M (SD)	43.4 (10.7)
Gender (Male), N (%)	132 (65.7)
Years since diagnosis, M (SD)	15.3 (9.7)
Ethnicity, N (%)	
White	55 (27.4)
Black African	36 (17.9)
Black Caribbean	28 (13.9)
Bangladeshi	20 (10.0)
Black Other	15 (7.5)
Pakistani	10 (5.0)
Indian	6 (3.0)
Chinese	2 (1.0)
Other	29 (14.4)
Employment, N (%)	
Unemployed	167 (83.5)
Paid employment	16 (8.0)
Training/education	5 (2.5)
Retired	6 (3.0)
Other	6 (3.0)
Hours spent in employment (weekly), M (SD)	2.2 (7.7)
Monthly Income (£), M (SD)	776.9 (516.7)
Time Use (Hours)[a], M (SD)	3.1 (3.7)
Social Contacts[b], M (SD)	2.0 (2.2)
Loneliness[c], M (SD)	2.6 (1.4)
Subjective Quality of Life (MANSA)[d], M (SD)	4.4 (1.1)

[a]Time spent doing activities over the week prior to interview
[b]Number of social contacts in week prior to assessment, either face-to-face or via technology
[c]Scored from 1 (Not at all) to 5 (Extremely)
[d]Satisfaction ratings range from 1 (couldn't be worse) to 7 (couldn't be better)

should cover the costs of these activities, while 32% (N = 35) stated the scheme should make a partial contribution, and the remaining 26% (N = 29) were prepared to cover their own costs.

Patients more often favoured weekly meetings (44%, N = 50) than the other options presented: more than once per week (25%, N = 29), fortnightly (12%, N = 14), monthly or less (15%, N = 17) or no preference (4%, N = 5). Similarly, 39% (N = 45) of patients preferred hour-long meetings rather than alternative options: less than half an hour (3%, N = 3), half an hour (16%, N = 19), 2 hours (18%, N = 21), more than 2 hours (19%, N = 22) and no preference (5%, N = 6).

With respect to duration of the relationship, the majority felt that it should be open-ended (53%, N = 62). Others selected 6 months as a preferred duration (16%, N = 18) with less than 10% selecting each of the remaining options available: no preference (N = 11), 1 month (N = 3), 3 months (N = 4), 9 months (N = 3), 12 months (N = 10) and more than 12 months (N = 5).

Discussion

Main findings

Reported preferences for befriending schemes showed that a substantial number of patients with SMI would like to take part in a befriending scheme if one were advertised. Patients with lower SQOL were more likely to express a willingness to become a befriendee.

Of those patients willing to take part, approximately 40% preferred weekly, 1-hour long meetings, and 53% would like the relationship to be open ended rather than having a specified duration. However, consensus on the exact type of the preferred befriending was limited, and for most characteristics of both the befriender and the type of relationship there was a considerable variation in responses.

Table 2 Univariable logistic regression model for willingness to engage in befriending

Variables	Univariable analysis			Multivariable analysis		
	OR	(95% CI)	P-value	OR	(95% CI)	P-value
Age	1.000	(0.974 to 1.026)	.983	–	–	–
Gender (male)	0.835	(0.461 to 1.512)	.551	–	–	–
Heard of befriending (Y)	1.213	(0.685 to 2.147)	.508			
Diagnostic Group (F3)	1.000	(0.523 to 1.913)	1.00			
Years since diagnosis	1.003	(0.974 to 1.033)	.852	–	–	–
Weekly working hours	0.977	(0.942 to 1.014)	.229	–	–	–
Monthly Income	1.000	(0.999 to 1.001)	.512	–	–	–
Time use (hours)	0.998	(0.924 to 1.077)	.951	–	–	–
Social Contacts	0.876	(0.770 to 0.998)	.046	0.884	(0.774 to 1.011)	.072
Loneliness	1.387	(1.112 to 1.729)	.004	1.220	(0.945 to 1.577)	.128
SQOL	0.627	(0.469 to 0.838)	.002	0.707	(0.506 to 0.990)	.043

Strengths and limitations

The present study is, to the authors' knowledge, the first to explicitly focus on patient preferences for befriending, in keeping with the growing focus on patient perspectives [10, 11]. The sample size offered sufficient statistical power to detect major differences between groups either willing or unwilling to take part in befriending. Further, patients were assessed by experienced, trained researchers through face-to-face meetings, thus contributing to the reliability of the data.

The main limitation of the study relates to the selective nature of the recruitment procedure. The sample was exclusively recruited in East London, and the interviewed patients represent only 32% of those screened and eligible. It is therefore unclear to what extent the findings are generalizable to other populations with SMI.

Similarly, the diagnostic codes used to assess eligibility may have resulted in some participants being included without a SMI. Mild depression, for instance, falls within the diagnostic groups included. However, the low likelihood of such diagnoses being found in CMHT settings and the high proportion of individuals with a psychotic or related disorder lends itself to justifying the overall sample being considered severe. The decision to include a variable sample also allows for greater applicability of the findings to psychiatric populations, which is further supported by the lack of statistical relationship between diagnostic group and willingness to participate in befriending.

The eligibility criteria may have impacted the findings due to exclusion of individuals involved in an ongoing befriending trial. While the overall impact is presumably negligible due to the small number excluded, it is possible that the proportion of people with SMI willing to participate in befriending would have been increased if these individuals had been included. However, the criterion was in place to maintain separation of the samples such that the research findings of the present study and the present trial could contribute to the existing literature independently and inform one another.

A further limitation relates to the potential recall bias for some of the measures used. The Social Contacts Assessment and time use survey necessitate memory of the week prior to the assessment. However, this may have been aided by the presence of a skilled researcher rather than self-administration of the questionnaire.

Comparison with literature

The present findings for patients' SQOL [19], loneliness and number of social contacts [15] are consistent with previous studies of similar diagnostic groups, thus suggesting that the results may be applicable beyond the present sample. However, existing literature on befriending schemes is limited to volunteer experiences and organisational features of befriending, as these are typically the limiting factor to expanding such services [20]. As such, little is available for comparison with the present findings with regard to patient preference.

Systematic reviews of existing befriending schemes offer insight into the character of befriending relationships from the perspective of the organisation running the scheme [2, 9]. Through their systematic search, Siette and colleagues [9] found 14 befriending trials. All involved one-to-one interactions between the volunteer befriender and patients. The median frequency and duration of each session was approximately weekly, for 1 hour, and lasted around 3 months (the maximum allowed was 12 months). These figures would generally indicate agreement with preferences expressed by the current sample. Similarly, Hallet and colleagues [21] noted that many schemes they reviewed required a minimum time commitment from volunteers (typically 12 months). However, the real-life duration exhibited great variation, reflecting patient preferences for open-ended relationships. This variation appears to reflect deviation from the prescribed model by the befriender pair, rather than flexibility of the schemes. The frequency of contact, too, varied largely between organisations and befriender pairs within those organisations, with some meeting for 5 hours per week and others only 4 hours per month. While the apparent variability between schemes may cater to the varied patient preferences reported here, it is unclear whether patients have sufficient access to their preferred befriending scheme, or if existing schemes offer the flexibility to adapt to individual preferences.

Consideration should also be given to the role of befriending in relation to peer support. Two-thirds of the current sample would like a befriender with experience as a patient in mental health care. While this points to an overlap between the services in terms of patient preferences, the similarities may not extend to volunteer characteristics and motivations, or the overall aim of the services. However, a recent survey of volunteer befrienders has provided data on volunteer befriender characteristics (Klug, Toner, Fabisch & Priebe, unpublished observations). Around one-third of the volunteer sample had experience of psychiatric treatment, thereby suggesting that volunteer befriender characteristics may be consistent with patient preferences. Further, the preferences expressed by patients may be applicable to and provide insight for other community-based schemes akin to befriending.

Implications

Whilst socio-demographic characteristics of patients were not significantly linked with the willingness to participate in befriending schemes, lower SQOL may be a relevant factor when considering patients' likelihood to take part in befriending schemes. As such, it appears that patients with greater inclination to seek out a befriender may also be those who are most in need for such interventions, and perhaps garner the greatest benefit as a result (e.g. improvement in overall SQOL). Similarly, almost half of those expressing unwillingness to participate did so because they felt the scheme was not relevant to their social needs. While it is possible that this lack of desired social interaction is reflective of the negative symptoms of schizophrenia, the results suggest that subjective quality of life remains higher in this unwilling group despite the potential for negative symptoms influencing responses. Although it appears that this group remains difficult to reach through social interventions such as befriending, they represent only a small proportion of the present sample with SMI. Thus, befriending schemes are likely to be taken up by those patients for whom they have been designed, which may be seen as reassuring and encouraging. Future research should establish to what extent befriending schemes can be effective in improving the SQOL of people with SMI.

While patient preferences are variable, they highlight an important consideration for befriending schemes: rigid prescriptive structures for the relationship between a volunteer and patient may be inappropriate or unhelpful. As such, schemes should aim to develop a sufficiently flexible structure to accommodate individual preferences. A useful default structure, potentially for those unsure about these schemes or requiring some initial guidance would be the more commonly selected weekly, 1-hour sessions outside their home.

Finally, the low proportion of patients with prior knowledge of befriending should be considered in the interpretation of the findings. Although patients were given a brief description of befriending before completing the survey, it is unclear whether a more comprehensive understanding and wider familiarity with such schemes would impact upon the expressed willingness to take part.

Conclusion

The findings suggest that a significant proportion of patients with SMI are interested in befriending. In particular, those with lower SQOL were more likely to want a befriender. The findings therefore highlight that patients with the greatest need for befriending may also be those most likely to take it up and potentially benefit from it. Further, the variability in patient preferences for befriending suggests that if befriending schemes are to successfully relieve social isolation in mental health populations, a flexible design may be more appropriate than a one-size-fits-all approach.

Abbreviations

MANSA: Manchester short assessment of quality of life; SMI: Severe mental illness; SQOL: Subjective quality of life

Acknowledgements

We would like to thank the staff in the following community mental health teams for their help with recruitment to the study: Stepney and Wapping CMHT, Bethnal Green and Globe Town CMHT, Isle of Dogs CMHT, Newham North Recovery Team, Newham South Recovery Team, Bow and Poplar CMHT, South Hackney CMHT, North Hackney CMHT, Stockwood CMHT, Newham Centre for Mental Health, Newham Early Intervention Service, Balaam Street Clozapine Clinic and Old Montague Street Clozapine Clinic with particular mention to Laura Pisaneschi.

We would also like to acknowledge the research team in the Unit for Social and Community Psychiatry (Queen Mary University of London) for their support and feedback of the manuscript, as well as members of the research team who helped with data collection –Elizabeth Worswick, Rawda El-Nagib, Gonca Ramjaun, Husnara Khanom and Neelam Laxhman.

Funding

This paper presents independent research funded by the National Institute for Health Research (NIHR) under its Programme Grants for Applied Research Programme (Reference Number RP-PG-0611-20002). The funding body was not involved in, and did not influence, the design of the study, data collection, analysis or interpretation of the data. The views expressed are those of the author(s) and not necessarily those of the NHS, the NIHR or the Department of Health.

Authors' contributions

SP designed the study; MC and AC were responsible for supervision of the research group; ST, MC, AC, ML, AF and MPC contributed to the collection and collation of data; ST conducted data analysis; ST and SP drafted the manuscript; all authors commented on and agreed to the final manuscript. All authors read and approved the final manuscript.

Authors' information

ST, MC, AC and ML are researchers with a psychology background. AF is a post-doctoral researcher. MPC is a clinical psychiatrist and PhD candidate. SP is clinical-academic psychiatrist.

Consent for publication

Not applicable.

Competing interests

The authors declare that they have no competing interests.

Author details

[1]Unit for Social and Community Psychiatry (WHO Collaborating Centre for Mental Health Service Development), Newham Centre for Mental Health, Queen Mary University of London, London, UK. [2]Hospital de Magalhães Lemos, Porto, Portugal. [3]Institute of Biomedical Sciences Abel Salazar (ICBAS), University of Porto, Porto, Portugal.

References

1. Bronowski P, Załuska M. Social support of chronically mentally ill patients. Arch Psychiatry Psychother. 2008;10:2.
2. Mead N, Lester H, Chew-Graham C, Gask L, Bower P. Effects of befriending on depressive symptoms and distress: systematic review and meta-analysis. Br J Psychiatry. 2010;196(2):96–101.
3. Windle K, Francis J, Coomber C. Preventing loneliness and social isolation: interventions and outcomes. London: Social Care Institute for Excellence; 2011. p. 1–16.

4. Buchanan RW. Persistent negative symptoms in schizophrenia: an overview. Schizophr Bull. 2006;33(4):1013–22.
5. Skills for Health: The 'hidden' workforce: volunteers in the health sector in England. The Mackinnon partnership and skills for health. 2009. http://www.skillsforhealth.org.uk. Accessed 13 Nov 2017.
6. McCorkle BH, Dunn EC, Yu Mui W, Gagne C. Compeer friends: a qualitative study of a volunteer friendship programme for people with serious mental illness. Int J Soc Psychiatry. 2009;55(4):291–305.
7. McGowan B, Jowett C. Promoting positive mental health through befriending. Int J Ment Health Promot. 2003;5(2):12–24.
8. Philip K, Spratt J. A synthesis of published research on mentoring and befriending: The Mentoring and Befriending Foundation; 2007. http://www.mandbf.org/wp-content/uploads/2011/03/Research-synthesis-executive-summary.pdf. Accessed 13 Nov 2017
9. Siette J, Cassidy M, Priebe S. Effectiveness of befriending interventions: a systematic review and meta-analysis. BMJ Open. 2017;7(4):e014304.
10. Chaplin R, Quirk A. How patient-centred are you. Shared decision-making in psychiatric practice (learning module): Royal College of Psychiatrists CPD Online (http://www.psychiatrycpd.co.uk/learningmodules/howpatient-centredareyous.aspx; 2012. Accessed 13 Nov 2017
11. National Institute for Clinical Excellence. Patient experience in adult NHS services: improving the experience of care for people using adult NHS services: NICE clinical guideline; 2012. https://www.nice.org.uk/guidance/cg138. p. 138. Accessed 13 Nov 2017
12. World Health Organization. International classification of diseases and related health problems, 10th revision. 5th ed. Geneva: World Health Organization; 2016.
13. Sullivan O, Gershuny J. Speed-up society? Evidence from the UK 2000 and 2015 time use diary surveys. Sociology. 2017; https://doi.org/10.5255/UKDA-SN-8128-1.
14. Priebe S, Savill M, Wykes T, Bentall RP, Reininghaus U, Lauber C, Bremner S, Eldridge S, Röhricht F. Effectiveness of group body psychotherapy for negative symptoms of schizophrenia: multicentre randomised controlled trial. Br J Psychiatry. 2016;209(1):54–61.
15. Giacco D, Palumbo C, Strappelli N, Catapano F, Priebe S. Social contacts and loneliness in people with psychotic and mood disorders. Compr Psychiatry. 2016;66:59–66.
16. World Health Organisation. The World Health Organization quality of life assessment (WHOQOL): position paper from the World Health Organization. Soc Sci Med. 1995;41:1403–9.
17. Priebe S, Huxley P, Knight S, Evans S. Application and results of the Manchester Short Assessment of quality of life (MANSA). Int J Soc Psychiatry. 1999;45(1):7–12.
18. Corp IBM. IBM SPSS statistics for windows, version 24.0. Armonk: IBM Corp; 2016.
19. Laxhman N, Greenberg L, Priebe S. Satisfaction with sex life among patients with schizophrenia. Schizophr Res. 2017;190:63–7.
20. Dean J, Goodlad R. Befriending and community care: 'nobody today has any time, have they?'. Housing Care Support. 1999;1(4):4–7.
21. Hallett C, Klug G, Lauber C, Priebe S. Volunteering in the care of people with severe mental illness: a systematic review. BMC Psychiatry. 2012;12(1):226.

22

Perceptions of free will in obsessive-compulsive disorder

Lucas J. B. van Oudheusden[1*], Stasja Draisma[1], Sandra van der Salm[2,3], Danielle Cath[4], Patricia van Oppen[1], Anton J. L. M. van Balkom[1] and Gerben Meynen[5,6,7]

Abstract

Background: The aim of this study was to explore perceptions of free will in the repetitive behaviors of patients with obsessive-compulsive disorder (OCD) and to explore their relation with core clinical characteristics.

Methods: Experiences of free will were assessed with the Symptomatology And Perceived Free will rating scale (SAPF) in 295 subjects with a lifetime diagnosis of OCD. Patients' scores on the SAPF were subjected to an explorative principal axis factor analysis (PAF). Factor scores were regressed on five OCD symptom dimensions and on seven clinical variables: illness duration, severity of OCD, insight, anxiety and depression, suicidal ideation and quality of life.

Results: The PAF revealed three factors: the perceived ability to control and change one's course of action when faced with an obsession or compulsion (the "alternative possibilities" factor); the experience of obsessions or compulsions as intentional (the "intentionality" factor); and the experience of being the source or owner of the obsessions or compulsions (the "ownership" factor). Lower scores on the "alternative possibilities" factor were associated with lower scores on the washing dimension ($\beta = 0.237$, $p = 0.004$) and higher scores on the precision dimension ($\beta = -0.190$, $p = 0.025$) and independently associated with longer illness duration ($\beta = -0.134$, $p = 0.039$), higher illness severity ($\beta = -0.298$, $p < 0.001$) and lower quality of life ($\beta = 0.172$, $p = 0.046$). Lower scores on the "intentionality" factor were independently associated with lower quality of life ($\beta = 0.233$, $p = 0.027$). Higher scores on the "ownership" factor were associated with higher scores on the precision dimension ($\beta = 0.207$, $p = 0.023$) and independently associated with poorer insight ($\beta = 0.170$, $p = 0.045$).

Conclusions: The most notable finding of this study is that a diminished experience of free will in OCD is associated with core clinical characteristics: illness duration and severity, insight and quality of life.

Keywords: Obsessive-compulsive disorder, Perceptions of free will, Phenomenology, Insight, Quality of life

Background

Obsessive-compulsive disorder (OCD) is a psychiatric disorder that is characterized by the presence of obsessions and/or compulsions. In the Diagnostic and Statistical Manual of Mental Disorders (DSM), obsessions are defined as recurrent and persistent thoughts, urges, or images that are experienced as intrusive and unwanted; compulsions are defined as repetitive behaviors or mental acts that an individual feels driven to perform in response to an obsession or according to rules that must be applied rigidly [1]. The definitional terms "intrusive", "unwanted", "driven" and "must" suggest that the notion of free will plays a central role in the phenomenology of OCD. More specifically, they suggest that, in OCD, the experience of free will and the capacity to act freely are somehow affected. Indeed, OCD patients are often painfully aware of the sharp contrast between the unex pected and unwanted intrusion of obsessional thou ghts or urges and the performance of compulsive rituals on the one hand, and their normal experience of having "free" thoughts or urges and performing "free" acts on the other hand. The experience of a significant loss of freedom and control over one's thoughts

* Correspondence: l.oudheusden@ggzingeest.nl
[1]Department of Psychiatry, Amsterdam Public Health, Amsterdam UMC, Vrije Universiteit Amsterdam, GGZ inGeest, Oldenaller 1, 1081, HJ, Amsterdam, The Netherlands
Full list of author information is available at the end of the article

and actions lies at the heart of the suffering of OCD patients [2].

The concept of free will has been studied and debated extensively by philosophers for the past two millennia [3]. Although these studies have given rise to many different perspectives, Walter [4] discerns three main aspects of free will in the contemporary philosophical debate. According to his interpretation, acting out of free will can be conceived of in the following ways: 1. having the ability to act otherwise, that is, having alternative possibilities open to one; 2. acting or choosing for (understandable) reasons, which implies intentional behavior; 3. being the owner or (causal) source of one's actions [5].

When discussing conditions of diminished freedom, philosophers often invoke mental disorders – and OCD specifically – as examples. Regarding OCD, Levy [6] writes:

> *We understand that a person suffering from obsessive-compulsive disorder, spending all day washing his hands and checking dozens of times that he remembered to lock the front door, cannot be thought of as having free will. His actions are mechanically dictated by stereotyped scripts, from which he cannot escape. Thus, obsessive-compulsive disorder is a malady of free will.*

Given the importance of the experience of (diminished) free will in OCD phenomenology, it is surprising that the topic has received little attention in empirical research. The present study is designed to address this gap in the literature. Thus, our main aim is to shed new light on what it means to be obsessed and to be compelled in the context of OCD, by exploring perceptions of free will in patients with OCD using insights derived from the philosophy of free will. Having a clearer view on these perceptions might encourage professionals to explore the experiential realm of their patients with them, in addition to the more standard diagnostic approach of assessing symptoms, illness severity, symptom subtypes and comorbidity. The second aim of our study is to explore the clinical significance of free will experience in OCD. Because OCD is a heterogeneous disorder with respect to its thematic content, we first investigated the association between different OCD symptom dimensions and experiences of free will. Furthermore, we assessed the association between experiences of free will and seven clinical variables that were selected based on the a priori hypothesis that they might influence, or be influenced by, experiences of free will: illness duration, OCD severity, insight, severity of comorbid anxiety and depression, severity of suicidal ideation and quality of life.

Methods

Design and setting

The present study is embedded within the Netherlands Obsessive Compulsive Disorder Association (NOCDA) study, a multicenter naturalistic cohort study designed to investigate the long-term course and outcome in OCD. The study design and baseline characteristics of the study sample are described in detail elsewhere [7]. In short, at baseline, we included 419 patients with a lifetime diagnosis of OCD, as determined by the administration of the Structured Clinical Interview for DSM-IV Axis I Disorders (SCID-I) [8]. Baseline measurements took place between 2005 and 2009 and included validated semi-structured interviews and self-report questionnaires to gather information on a broad range of variables related to (amongst others) OCD, comorbidity and psychosocial consequences. All included participants were contacted at 2-, 4- and 6-year follow-up, irrespective of their treatment status. The rating scale used to assess free will experience (see below) was administered during the 4-year follow-up wave, in which 295 subjects participated. The study was approved by the Medical Ethical committee of the VU Medical Centre, Amsterdam.

Questionnaire

The Symptomatology And Perceived Free will rating scale (SAPF) is a self-report questionnaire that operationalizes and applies insights from the philosophy of free will as captured in the conceptual framework by Walter [see introduction] to the study of psychopathology. It was originally developed by Van der Salm et al. to study perceptions of free will in a range of movement disorders, including tic disorder [9]. The fifteen items that make up the questionnaire all capture different aspects of free will experience. Because tic disorder and OCD share several important features with regard to phenomenology, comorbidity, underlying neurobiology and treatment strategies [10, 11], the SAPF was considered to be a suitable starting point for the exploration of free will perceptions with regard to obsessive-compulsive behavior. For this study, the wording of the fifteen items was adapted to enable specific application to obsessions and compulsions, without altering any further content. The questionnaire starts by asking the patient whether he or she suffers the most from obsessions or from compulsions. The patient is then requested to fill in the questionnaire with his or her most prominent symptom in mind. Answers to all but one of the questions are given on a Visual Analogue Scale, ranging from 0 ("not at all") to 100 ("completely"). For the present analysis, we excluded one question that was dichotomous in nature and three questions that dealt with general perceptions of free will and not with symptom-specific experiences, leaving 11 items. See Fig. 1 for the individual items.

Clinical characteristics

The Padua Inventory-Revised (PI-R) [12, 13] was used to assess the presence and severity of five OCD symptom dimensions: (I) impulses, (II) washing, (III) checking, (IV) rumination and (V) precision. Illness duration was defined as the interval between the age at interview and the reported age at onset of OCD as assessed with the SCID-1 [8]. Severity of obsessive-compulsive symptoms was measured with the Yale-Brown Obsessive-Compulsive Severity Scale (Y-BOCS; Range 0–40; Cronbach's α for this sample: 0.926) [14]. The degree of insight into OCD symptoms was assessed with the Overvalued Ideas Scale (OVIS; Range 0–10; Cronbach's α: 0.663) [15]. The Beck Anxiety Inventory (BAI; Range: 0–63; Cronbach's α: 0.933) and Beck Depression Inventory (BDI; Range: 0–63; Cronbach's α: 0.912) were used to assess severity of comorbid anxiety and depressive symptoms respectively [16, 17]. Severity of suicidal ideation was measured with the Beck Scale for Suicidal Ideation (BSS; Range: 0–38; Cronbach's α: 0.872) [18]. Quality of life was assessed with the EQ-5D, yielding a utility score ranging from – 0.59 to 1.00 [19].

Statistical analyses

Scores on the 11 items of the SAPF for the whole study sample were explored with descriptive statistics. Differences in the mean scores on the 11 items between the group of patients who suffered most from obsessions and the group of patients who suffered most from compulsions were assessed with independent-samples t-tests.

To investigate the interrelatedness of the 11 items of the SAPF, the individual item scores were statistically modelled as the expression of one or more latent factors. To extract the factor structure, an exploratory principal axis factor analysis (PAF) was performed. A preliminary analysis revealed that the Kaiser-Meyer-Olkin (KMO) measure of sampling adequacy was acceptable (0.722). Bartlett's test was significant and the determinant of the correlation matrix was 0.062, indicating that the matrix was suitable for PAF. To facilitate interpretation, the scores on item 1 and item 6 were recoded, so that a score of "0" signifies "no freedom/control" and a score of "100" signifies "maximum freedom/control", similar to the other nine items. Missing data were dealt with through listwise deletion: 35 subjects had missings on all SAPF items, and an additional nine subjects had missings on one or more (but not all) SAPF items, leaving a final study sample of 251 subjects. The decision regarding the number of factors to retain was based on the factor eigenvalues (using Kaiser's criterion of > 1) and the scree plot. To facilitate interpretation, oblique rotation (direct oblimin) was applied. Given the sample size, factor loadings of 0.32 and larger were considered to be significant [20]. Items were allocated to a factor based on their highest loading. The internal consistency of the factors was assessed

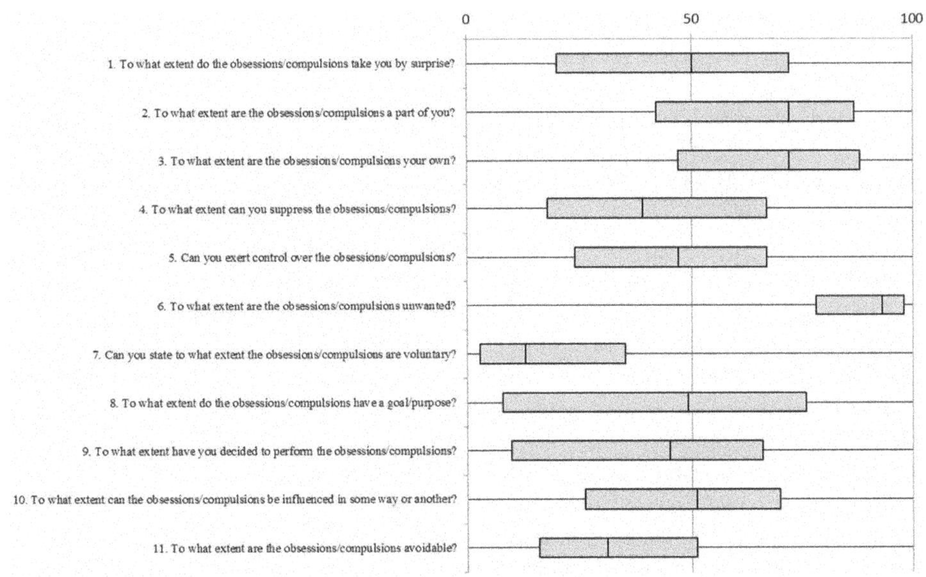

Fig. 1 Answers to the 11 questions of the SAPF for the whole study sample. The bars are boxplots, with the central line representing the median score, the edges of the boxes representing the first and third quartile, respectively, and the whiskers extending to the minimum and maximum values. A score of "0" means "not at all", and a score of "100" means "completely". Note that for most questions a score of "0" implies minimal freedom, whereas for questions 1 and 6, a score of "0" implies maximal freedom

with Cronbach's alpha. Subject-specific factor scores for each of the factors were calculated using the regression method.

The association between experiences of free will and OCD symptom dimensions was assessed by regressing the factor scores for the different PAF-derived factors on the five PI-R dimensional scores, using simple regression analyses, each time correcting for the PI-R total score. To investigate how experiences of free will are related to other important clinical aspects in OCD, the PAF-derived factor scores were regressed on the seven clinical characteristics mentioned above, with multiple regression analyses. In the multiple regression analyses, a forced entry method was used for entering the predictors into the model. *P*-values ≤0.05 were considered to indicate statistical significance. All analyses were performed with SPSS version 22.

Results

Sample characteristics

The mean age of the 295 participants was 38.4 years (SD 15.6). 53.9% of the participants were female. The mean age at onset was 18.5 years (SD 9.8), the mean illness duration was 20.5 years (SD 15.7), and the mean current illness severity as measured with the Y-BOCS was 15.4 (SD 9.2), reflecting a moderate illness severity. The mean score on the OVIS was 4.4 (SD 1.3), reflecting an average level of fair insight into the obsessive-compulsive symptoms. The mean score on the BAI was 13.6 (SD 10.9), reflecting mild to moderate levels of comorbid anxiety. The mean score on the BDI was 11.6 (SD 9.8), reflecting low levels of comorbid depression. The level of suicidal ideation, as assessed with the BSS, was minimal (mean score: 1.7 (SD 5.1)). One hundred and thirty subjects (44.1%) reported that their most prominent symptom was an obsession, whereas 67 subjects (22.7%) reported that their most prominent symptom was a compulsion. The remaining 98 subjects (33.2%) did not report a most prominent symptom.

Perceptions of free will in OCD patients according to the SAPF

The answers to the 11 questions for the whole sample are presented in Fig. 1. Here we highlight several findings. The answers for each of the items ranged from "0" to "100", indicating that for each question, very diverse perceptions exist within the study sample. Compared to all other items, subjects appeared to be most outspoken and in agreement about the items that assess whether the obsessions or compulsions are unwanted (item 6) and voluntary (item 7). The relatively high median of item 6 and the relatively low median of item 7 and the relatively small distribution of both items indicate that subjects generally experienced their symptoms as highly unwanted and involuntary. The majority of the subjects had scores between 50 and 100 on items 2 and 3, indicating that they tended to experience the obsessions or compulsions as a part of themselves (item 2) and as their own (item 3).

A comparison of subjects whose most prominent symptom was an obsession with those subjects whose most prominent symptom was a compulsion revealed several significant, albeit small, differences. Subjects with predominant obsessions experienced their symptoms as more of a surprise than subjects with compulsions (item 1) (mean obs.: 52.7 vs. mean comp. 40.1, $t = 3.00$, $p = 0.003$). Subjects with predominant compulsions experienced their symptoms more as the result of a decision (item 9) (mean obs.: 34.2 vs. mean comp. 48.4, $t = -3.10$, $p = 0.002$) and at the same time as more difficult to suppress (item 4) (mean obs.: 44.4 vs. mean comp. 34.7, $t = 2.50$, $p = 0.012$) than subjects with predominant obsessions. There were no significant differences in scores on the other eight items between the two groups.

Factor structure of the SAPF

Based on the eigenvalues and the scree plot resulting from the PAF, three factors were retained for subsequent analysis (eigenvalues were 3.07, 2.04 and 1.13, respectively). Factor 1 explained 27.9% of the variance, factor 2 explained 18.5%, and factor 3 explained 10.3%. The item loadings per factor are presented in Table 1. Factor 1 is characterized by a high loading of the items concerning the ability to suppress, control, influence, and avoid the obsessions or compulsions (items 4, 5, 10 and 11). These items all focus on the perceived ability of the patient to control and change his or her course of action when faced with an obsession or compulsion. In other words, the items reflect the perceived presence of behavioral alternatives to giving in to the obsessions or compulsions. It therefore seems appropriate to label this factor as the "alternative possibilities" factor. Factor 2 is characterized by a high loading of the items that assess whether the obsessions or compulsions are (in)voluntary, (un)-wanted, (non-)purposeful and the result of a decision (items 6, 7, 8 and 9). These items deal with the intentional aspects of obsessive-compulsive behavior, and the factor can therefore be best labeled as the "intentionality" factor. Factor 3 is characterized by a high loading of the items that assess the extent to which the obsessions or compulsions are owned by the person and part of one's self (items 2 and 3). These items deal with matters of ownership and it therefore seems appropriate to label this factor as the "ownership" factor. The internal consistency and reliability, as measured with Cronbach's alpha, were good for factor 1 (0.809), limited for factor 2 (0.590) and

Table 1 Principal axis factor analysis on 11 SAPF items with item loadings per factor

	Factor 1 "Alternative possibilities"	Factor 2 "Intentionality"	Factor 3 "Ownership"
	Expl. variance: 27.9% Cronbach's α: 0.809	Expl. variance: 18.5% Cronbach's α: 0.590	Expl. variance: 10.3% Cronbach's α: 0.692
4. To what extent can you suppress the obsessions/compulsions?	**0.998**	−0.191	0.166
5. Can you exert control over the obsessions/compulsions?	**0.735**	0.032	0.001
10. To what extent can the obsessions/compulsions be influenced in some way or another?	**0.616**	0.077	−0.081
11. To what extent are the obsessions/compulsions avoidable?	**0.448**	0.094	−0.208
1. To what extent do the obsessions/compulsions take you by surprise?[a]	0.224	0.135	− 0.122
7. Can you state to what extent the obsessions/compulsions are voluntary?	0.217	**0.702**	0.011
6. To what extent are the obsessions/compulsions unwanted?[a]	0.163	**0.609**	− 0.007
8. To what extent do the obsessions/compulsions have a goal/purpose?	−0.179	**0.440**	0.073
9. To what extent have you decided to perform the obsessions/compulsions?	−0.054	**0.436**	0.040
3. To what extent are the obsessions/compulsions your own?	0.060	0.040	**0.785**
2. To what extent are the obsessions/compulsions a part of you?	−0.024	0.101	**0.630**

[a]*recoded*
bold: given the sample size, factor loadings of 0.32 and larger were considered to be significant [20]

acceptable for factor 3 (0.692). A closer look at the correlations between the items that constitute factor 2 showed that the cohesion within this factor was mainly driven by the correlation between item 6 ("unwanted") and item 7 ("voluntary"). Correlations between the three factors were positive for factors 1 and 2 and factors 2 and 3, but negative for factors 1 and 3 (corr (1, 2): 0.151; corr (1, 3): − 0.415; corr (2, 3): 0.115).

Association with clinical characteristics

A higher score on the washing subscale of the PI-R was associated with a higher score on the "alternative possibilities" factor ($\beta = 0.237$, $p = 0.004$). Conversely, a higher score on the precision subscale of the PI-R was associated with lower score on the "alternative possibilities" factor ($\beta = -0.190$, $p = 0.025$) and a higher score on the "ownership" factor ($\beta = 0.207$, $p = 0.023$). The other OCD symptom dimensions were not associated with any of the SAPF-derived factors.

Associations between the three factors of the SAPF and the seven other clinical characteristics are presented in Table 2. Lower scores on the "alternative possibilities" factor were independently associated with longer illness duration ($\beta = -0.134$, $p = 0.039$), higher illness severity ($\beta = -0.298$, $p < 0.001$) and lower quality of life ($\beta = 0.172$, $p = 0.025$). Lower sco res on the "intentionality factor" were independently associated with lower quality of life ($\beta = 0.233$, $p = 0.027$). Higher scores on the ownership factor were

Table 2 Multiple regression of the three aspects of free will experience on clinical characteristics

	Factor 1 "Alternative possibilities"		Factor 2 "Intentionality"		Factor 3 "Ownership"	
	Beta[a]	p	Beta	p	Beta	p
Illness duration	−0.134	0.039*	0.045	0.563	0.130	0.085
Y-BOCS severity	−0.298	0.000*	0.013	0.893	0.015	0.873
Beck Anxiety Index	−0.039	0.663	0.028	0.793	0.024	0.813
Beck Depression Inventory	−0.087	0.418	0.024	0.854	0.155	0.216
Beck Suicide Scale	−0.023	0.772	0.010	0.915	−0.001	0.994
EQ-5D	0.172	0.046*	0.233	0.027*	− 0.015	0.882
OVIS	− 0.076	0.297	0.042	0.630	0.170	0.045*

Abbreviations: Y-BOCS: Yale-Brown Obsessive Compulsive Scale; EQ-5D: EuroQol – 5 Dimensions; OVIS: Overvalued Ideas Scale
[a]*Beta values represent standardized coefficients*
*: *significant at* $p \leq 0.05$

independently associated with poorer insight ($\beta = 0.170$, $p = 0.045$).

Discussion

To our knowledge, this is the first study to investigate perceptions of free will in patients with OCD using a questionnaire that allows for quantitative analysis. Our results suggest that the SAPF discerns three aspects of free will experience in OCD: 1. the perceived ability to change one's course of action when faced with an obsession or compulsion (the "alternative possibilities" factor); 2. the degree to which patients experience that their obsessions and compulsions occur for a reason or as the result of deliberate intent (the "intentionality" factor) 3. the degree to which patients experience that they are the owner or originator of their obsessions or compulsions (the "ownership" factor). The three-factor structure of the SAPF as revealed by the exploratory factor analysis maps fairly well onto Walter's theoretical framework described in the introduction of this article. The distinct nature of these three aspects is underscored by the fact that they differ in their associations with core clinical aspects of the disorder (see below).

The first aspect of free will experience in OCD is the perceived ability to control and change one's course of action when faced with an obsession or compulsion. The scores on the SAPF items that load on the "alternative possibilities" factor (items 4, 5, 10 and 11: see Fig. 1) suggest that as a group, OCD patients experience very little freedom to pursue a different course of action when faced with their symptoms. In a recent review on psychosurgery and free will, De Ridder et al. [21] identify behavioral inflexibility as the core problem in OCD and suggest that successful psychosurgery for OCD can "*increase the behavioral options, thereby increasing fle xible decision making and free will.*" The importance of behavioral inflexibility in OCD is also reflected in the standard psychotherapeutic approach to OCD; the primary goal of exposure and response prevention is to increase the amount of behavioral options the patient can choose from when he or she is faced with obsessional anxiety [22].

An interesting finding is that the perceived ability to control and change one's course of action when faced with an obsession or compulsion diminishes as illness duration increases. This is in line with recent studies that suggest that illness development in OCD is associated with a shift away from consciously controlled behavior towards habit formation [for a comprehensive overview, see [23]]. Our results also suggest that patients who experience their obsessive thinking or compulsive acting as the *only* behavioral option instead of one of several behavioral alternatives, tend to have a higher severity of OCD and a lower quality of life (see Table 2). It is likely that the association with OCD severity is at least in part the result of conceptual overlap between the SAPF items that load on factor 1 and several items of the Y-BOCS. The association with quality of life is of interest in light of previous studies that have shown that OCD has a significant impact on the quality of life of patients and that this impact is mainly driven by illness severity and presence of comorbidity [24]. The fact that patients with a diminished experience of having alternative possibilities had a lower quality of life, regardless of their illness severity and comorbidity burden, suggests that free will experience plays an independent role in the way OCD patients perceive their well-being.

The second aspect of free will experience in OCD is the degree to which patients experience that their obsessions and compulsions occur for a reason or as the result of deliberate intent. The group scores on the related SAPF items show that although patients generally perceive their obsessions and compulsions as highly unwanted (item 6) and involuntary (item 7), there is large within-group variation in the extent to which they perceive their behavior as goal-directed (item 8) and as the result of a decision (item 9). A part of the variation in item 9 could be explained by the focus of the questionnaire: compulsions were experienced more as the result of a decision than obsessions. Interestingly, a perceived lack of intent or reason underlying the obsessive-compulsive symptoms was associated with a lower quality of life. The association between OCD and a diminished quality of life has been firmly established in previous research [25]. A consistent finding is that the presence of comorbid depressive symptoms plays an important mediating role [24]. There is also evidence that the presence of compulsions has a stronger negative effect on quality of life than the presence of obsessions [26]. Of note, the association between a perceived lack of intent or reason underlying the obsessive-compulsive symptoms and a lower quality of life was adjusted for the severity of comorbid depression and general illness severity. A tentative interpretation of this association could be that a prolonged experience of being forced to perform empty, pointless rituals has a negative impact on one's sense of purpose and meaning in life. However, it should also be noted that the limited psychometric quality of factor 2 (see Results section) puts the validity of this association into question.

The third aspect of free will experience in OCD is the degree to which patients experience that they are the owner of their obsessions or compulsions. The group scores on the related SAPF items show that patients exhibit a strong sense of ownership or belonging with regard to their symptoms (items 2 and 3: see Fig. 1). The experience of self-ownership is indeed recognized as a core phenomenological feature of OCD [27]. As a sense of ownership can be seen as a prerequisite for mastery over one's actions (and therefore also one's symptoms), we have so far considered it as an indicator of free will. In this context, the finding that patients with poorer insight tend to have a heightened experience of being the owner of their symptoms is of interest. It might be that this factor of the SAPF actually measures the degree of egosyntonicity, that is, the degree to which a patient has incorporated his or her symptoms into his or her self-image or identity. Clinical experience suggests that rather than *increasing* free will, egosyntonicity actually makes it harder for patients to distance themselves from their symptoms and thereby can lead to a *decrease* in mastery and free will. The fact that a *heightened* experience of being the source of the symptoms is associated with a *diminished* experience of having alternative possibilities also questions the assertion that a sense of ownership indicates free will in the context of OCD. The finding that a higher score on the precision subscale of the PI-R was associated with a heightened experience of being the source of the obsessions or compulsions fits with the empirical finding that patients with prominent precision symptoms often have a comorbid obsessive-compulsive personality disorder [11] and experience their symptoms as egosyntonic.

The conceptual distinction presented in this study might have several clinical implications.

First of all, a more nuanced understanding of what it means to be obsessed and compelled in the context of OCD may help healthcare professionals to better empathize with the challenges that OCD patients face. This could improve the quality of the therapeutic re lationship, as many patients with OCD experience significant shame and confusion with regard to their own symptoms. Secondly, the incorporation of these concepts in the clinical discourse might enrich the practice of cognitive behavioral therapy. Exploring experiences that are at the core of the patient's distress might help them to let go of long held dysfunctional beliefs and increase motivation to engage in behavioral experiments. Finally, the inclusion of these concepts in follow-up consultations might expand the ways in which professionals and patients track cha nges during treatment, above and beyond measuring scores on an illness severity rating scale.

Strengths of this study include the large sample size and the detailed characterization of the cohort. Several limitations have to be addressed. The fact that this is the first study to apply the SAPF to a population of OCD patients warrants caution when interpreting the results. Future studies are needed to further assess the validity of the questionnaire for this specific population. In addition, the reliability analysis shows that the psychometric quality of the SAPF could benefit from adjustments to the items that constitute the "intentionality factor" (factor 2).

In our opinion, two directions for future research seem particularly promising. First, a more detailed analysis of differences in perceptions of free will between obsessions and compulsions would be very informative. In the current design of the study, subjects are asked to rate free will perceptions for either their main obsession or their main compulsion, which limits the comparison of free will perceptions regarding obsessions versus compulsions to between-person differences. An interesting future modification to the design of the SAPF might be to ask subjects to rate free will perceptions with regard to both their main obsession and their main compulsive behavior. This would result in within-person differences in free will perceptions, that can then be compared across the entire sample. Such a comparison could shed new light on the longstanding debate about the functional nature of compulsive behavior. Traditionally, compulsive behavior is distinguished from other types of stereotyped or repetitive behaviors by referring to the functional nature of compulsive behavior (in contrast to the random nature of other repetitive behaviors). Compulsive behavior is seen as a goal-directed effort on the part of the patient to reduce the anxiety or distress that is evoked by obsessions [28]. It is for this reason that in previous editions of the DSM, OCD was classified as an anxiety disorder. Current perspectives on compulsive behavior tend to de-emphasize its anxiety-driven character [29, 30], which is reflected in the decision to remove OCD from the group of anxiety disorders in the latest edition of the DSM [1]. By distinguishing free will perceptions with regard to obsessions and compulsions within the same subject, one could test the hypothesis (along more traditional lines) that patients who report more obsessional anxiety also have a stronger experience of reason or intent underlying their compulsive behavior. Furthermore, as the washing and checking symptom dimension is thought to be more anxiety-driven than other OCD symptom dimensions [31], one could test the hypothesis that subjects who score high on these dimensions also have a strong experience of intent underlying their compulsive behavior.

A second interesting direction for future research would be to track within-person changes in free will perceptions over time. Repeated assessments in a naturalistic context could shed more light on the effect of prolonged illness duration on perceptions of intent and ownership accompanying compulsive behavior. Repeated assessments in a treatment context could shed light on the role these (changing) free will perceptions play in the improvement of quality of life that usually accompanies successful treatment.

Conclusions

To conclude, the present study sheds new light on what it means to be obsessed and to be compelled in the context of OCD by distinguishing three aspects in the experience of free will in this disorder; namely, the perceived ability to change one's course of action when faced with an obsession or compulsion; the experience of obsessions or compulsions as intentional; and the experience of being the source or origin of the obsessions or compulsions. The most notable finding of this study is that a diminished experience of free will in OCD is associated with important clinical parameters; in particular illness duration and severity, insight and quality of life. The clinical relevance of the conceptual distinction presented in this study lies in the positive impact it might have on the therapeutic relationship between professional and patient and the enrichment it might offer to the practice of cognitive behavioral therapy and the process of tracking changes during treatment. Future studies could focus in more detail on differences in free will perceptions between obsessions and compulsive behaviors, and longitudinal assessment of changes in free will perceptions during treatment. The results of the present study suggest that the experience of free will in OCD is a clinically relevant avenue for future investigations.

Abbreviations

BAI: Beck anxiety inventory; BDI: Beck depression inventory; BSS: Beck scale for suicidal ideation; DSM: Diagnostic and statistical manual of mental disorders; EQ-5D: EuroQol – 5 dimensions; KMO: Kaiser-meyer-olkin measure of sampling adequacy; NOCDA: Netherlands obsessive compulsive disorder association; OCD: Obsessive-compulsive disorder; OVIS: Overvalued ideas scale; PAF: Principal axis factor analysis; PI-R: Padua inventory-revised; SAPF: Symptomatology and perceived free will rating scale; SCID-1: Structured clinical interview for DSM-IV Axis I disorders; Y-BOCS: Yale-brown obsessive-compulsive severity scale

Acknowledgments

Not applicable

Funding

The research infrastructure needed to complete the baseline measurements (including personnel and materials) was financed almost exclusively by the participating organizations (Academic department of Psychiatry, VU Medical Center/GGZ inGeest, Amsterdam; Marina de Wolf Centre for Anxiety Research, Ermelo; Centre for Anxiety Disorders 'Overwaal', Lent; Dimence, GGZ Overijssel; Department of Psychiatry, Leiden University Medical Center, Leiden; Mental Health Care Centre Noord- en Midden-Limburg, Venray; Academic Anxiety Centre, PsyQ Maastricht, Maastricht University, Division Mental Health and Neuroscience). The fieldwork coordinator was financed for one year by a research grant from the Stichting Steun VCVGZ. The funding bodies mentioned above had no role in the design of the study nor the collection, analysis and interpretation of the data.

Authors' contributions

Conception and design / analysis and interpretation of data: LvO SD SvdS DC PvO AvB GM. Drafting / revising article: LvO SD SvdS DC PvO AvB GM. Final approval: LvO SD SvdS DC PvO AvB GM. All authors read and approved the final manuscript.

Consent for publication

Not applicable

Competing interests

The authors declare that they have no competing interests.

Author details

[1]Department of Psychiatry, Amsterdam Public Health, Amsterdam UMC, Vrije Universiteit Amsterdam, GGZ inGeest, Oldenaller 1, 1081, HJ, Amsterdam, The Netherlands. [2]Brain Center Rudolf Magnus, Department of Neurology and Neurosurgery, University Medical Center Utrecht, Utrecht, The Netherlands. [3]Stichting Epilepsie Instellingen Nederland (SEIN), Zwolle, The Netherlands. [4]Department of Clinical and Health psychology, Altrecht Academic Anxiety Centre, Utrecht University, Utrecht, The Netherlands. [5]Faculty of Humanities, Vrije Universiteit Amsterdam, Amsterdam, The Netherlands. [6]GGZ inGeest, Amsterdam, The Netherlands. [7]Willem Pompe Institute for Criminal Law and Criminology, Utrecht University, Utrecht, The Netherlands.

References

1. American Psychiatric Association. Diagnostic and statistical manual of mental disorders. Washington, DC; 2013.
2. Denys D. Obsessionality & compulsivity: a phenomenology of obsessive-compulsive disorder. Philos Ethics Humanit Med 2011;6:3. https://doi.org/10.1186/1747-5341-6-3.
3. Kane R, editor. The Oxford handbook of free will: second edition. New York: Oxford University Press; 2011.
4. Walter H. Neurophilosophy of free will. From libertarian illusions to a concept of natural autonomy. Cambridge, MA: MIT Press; 2001.
5. Meynen G. Free will and mental disorder: exploring the relationship. Theor Med Bioeth. 2010;31:429–43.
6. Levy DA. Neural holism and free will. Philos Psychol. 2003;16:205–28. https://doi.org/10.1080/09515080320103337.
7. Schuurmans J, van Balkom AJLM, van Megen HJGM, Smit JH, Eikelenboom M, Cath DC, et al. The Netherlands obsessive compulsive disorder association (NOCDA) study: design and rationale of a longitudinal naturalistic study of the course of OCD and clinical characteristics of the sample at baseline. Int J Methods Psychiatr Res. 2012;21:273–85. https://doi.org/10.1002/mpr.1372.
8. First MB, Spitzer RL, Gibbon M, Williams JBW. Structured Clinical Interview for DSM-IV Axis I Disorders – Patient Edition (Scid-I/P, Version 2.0). Lisse: Swets & Zeitlinger; 1999.
9. van der Salm SM, Cath DC, van RA-F, Koelman JH, de Haan RJ, Tijssen MA, et al. Clinician and patient perceptions of free will in movement disorders: mind the gap. J Neurol Neurosurg Psychiatry. 2017;88:532–3. https://doi.org/10.1136/jnnp-2016-315152.
10. Ferrão YA, Miguel EC, Stein DJ. Tourette's syndrome, trichotillomania, and obsessive-compulsive disorder: how closely are they related? Psychiatry Res. 2009;170:32–42. https://doi.org/10.1016/j.psychres.2008.06.008.
11. Leckman JF, Denys D, Simpson HB, Mataix-Cols D, Hollander E, Saxena S, et al. Obsessive–compulsive disorder: a review of the diagnostic criteria and possible subtypes and dimensional specifiers for DSM-v. Depress Anxiety. 2010;27:507–27.
12. Sanavio E. Obsessions and compulsions: the Padua inventory. Behav Res Ther. 1988;26:169–77. https://doi.org/10.1016/0005-7967(88)90116-7. Accessed 8 Dec 2017.
13. Van Oppen P, Hoekstra RJ, Emmelkamp PM. The structure of obsessive-compulsive symptoms. Behav Res Ther. 1995;33:15–23. https://doi.org/10.1016/0005-7967(94)E0010-G. Accessed 8 Dec 2017.
14. Goodman WK, Price LH, Rasmussen SA, Mazure C, Fleischmann RL, Hill CL, et al. The Yale-Brown obsessive compulsive scale. I Development, use, and reliability. Arch Gen Psychiatry. 1989;46:1006–11 http://www.ncbi.nlm.nih.gov/pubmed/2684084. Accessed 10 Mar 2017.
15. Neziroglu F, McKay D, Yaryura-Tobias JA, Stevens KP, Todaro J. The overvalued ideas scale: development, reliability and validity in obsessive-compulsive disorder. Behav Res Ther. 1999;37:881–90. https://doi.org/10.1016/S0005-7967(98)00191-0. Accessed 12 Jan 2017.
16. Beck AT, Epstein N, Brown G, Steer RA. An inventory for measuring clinical

anxiety: psychometric properties. J Consult Clin Psychol. 1988;56:893–7 http://dx.doi.org/10.1037/0022-006X.56.6.893. Accessed 3 Oct 2016.
17. Beck AT, Ward CH, Mendelson M, Mock J, Erbaugh J. An inventory for measuring depression. Arch Gen Psychiatry. 1961;4:561–71.
18. Beck AT, Kovacs M, Weissman A. Assessment of suicidal intention: the scale for suicide ideation. J Consult Clin Psychol. 1979;47:343–52.
19. EuroQol Group. EuroQol--a new facility for the measurement of health-related quality of life. Health Policy. 1990;16:199–208. https://doi.org/10.1016/0168-8510(90)90421-9. Accessed 10 Mar 2017.
20. Stevens JP. Applied multivariate statistics for the social sciences. 4th ed. Hillsdale, NJ: Erlbaum; 2002.
21. De Ridder D, Vanneste S, Gillett G, Manning P, Glue P, Langguth B. Psychosurgery reduces uncertainty and increases free will? A review. Neuromodulation. 2016;19:239–48. https://doi.org/10.1111/ner.12405.
22. Meynen G. Obsessive-compulsive disorder, free will, and control. Philos Psychiatry Psychol. 2012;19:323–32.
23. Gillan CM, Robbins TW, Sahakian BJ, van den Heuvel OA, van Wingen G. The role of habit in compulsivity. Eur Neuropsychopharmacol. 2016;26:828–40. https://doi.org/10.1016/j.euroneuro.2015.12.033.
24. Eisen JL, Mancebo MA, Pinto A, Coles ME, Pagano ME, Stout RL, et al. Impact of obsessive-compulsive disorder on quality of life. Compr Psychiatry. 47:270–5. https://doi.org/10.1016/j.comppsych.2005.11.006.
25. Subramaniam M, Soh P, Vaingankar JA, Picco L, Chong SA. Quality of life in obsessive-compulsive disorder: impact of the disorder and of treatment. CNS Drugs. 2013;27:367–83. https://doi.org/10.1007/s40263-013-0056-z.
26. Stengler-Wenzke K, Kroll M, Riedel-Heller S, Matschinger H, Angermeyer MC. Quality of life in obsessive-compulsive disorder: the different impact of obsessions and compulsions. Psychopathology. 2007;40:282–9. https://doi.org/10.1159/000104744.
27. Oulis P, Konstantakopoulos G, Lykouras L, Michalopoulou PG. Differential diagnosis of obsessive-compulsive symptoms from delusions in schizophrenia: a phenomenological approach. World J psychiatry. 2013;3:50–6. https://doi.org/10.5498/wjp.v3.i3.50.
28. Abramowitz JS, Deacon BJ. Obsessive-compulsive disorder: Essential phenomenology and overlap with other anxiety disorders. Concepts Controv Obs Disord. 2005;:119–149. https://doi.org/10.1007/0-387-23370-9_6.
29. Hollander E, Braun A, Simeon D. Should OCD leave the anxiety disorders in DSM-V? The case for obsessive compulsive-related disorders. Depress Anxiety. 2008;25:317–29.
30. Stein DJ, Fineberg NA, Bienvenu OJ, Denys D, Lochner C, Nestadt G, et al. Should OCD be classified as an anxiety disorder in DSM-V? Depress Anxiety. 2010;27:495–506.
31. Rozenman M, Peris T, Bergman RL, Chang S, O'Neill J, McCracken JT, et al. Distinguishing fear versus distress symptomatology in pediatric OCD. Child Psychiatry Hum Dev. 2017;48:63–72. https://doi.org/10.1007/s10578-016-0653-4

Permissions

All chapters in this book were first published in PSYCHIATRY, by BioMed Central; hereby published with permission under the Creative Commons Attribution License or equivalent. Every chapter published in this book has been scrutinized by our experts. Their significance has been extensively debated. The topics covered herein carry significant findings which will fuel the growth of the discipline. They may even be implemented as practical applications or may be referred to as a beginning point for another development.

The contributors of this book come from diverse backgrounds, making this book a truly international effort. This book will bring forth new frontiers with its revolutionizing research information and detailed analysis of the nascent developments around the world.

We would like to thank all the contributing authors for lending their expertise to make the book truly unique. They have played a crucial role in the development of this book. Without their invaluable contributions this book wouldn't have been possible. They have made vital efforts to compile up to date information on the varied aspects of this subject to make this book a valuable addition to the collection of many professionals and students.

This book was conceptualized with the vision of imparting up-to-date information and advanced data in this field. To ensure the same, a matchless editorial board was set up. Every individual on the board went through rigorous rounds of assessment to prove their worth. After which they invested a large part of their time researching and compiling the most relevant data for our readers.

The editorial board has been involved in producing this book since its inception. They have spent rigorous hours researching and exploring the diverse topics which have resulted in the successful publishing of this book. They have passed on their knowledge of decades through this book. To expedite this challenging task, the publisher supported the team at every step. A small team of assistant editors was also appointed to further simplify the editing procedure and attain best results for the readers.

Apart from the editorial board, the designing team has also invested a significant amount of their time in understanding the subject and creating the most relevant covers. They scrutinized every image to scout for the most suitable representation of the subject and create an appropriate cover for the book.

The publishing team has been an ardent support to the editorial, designing and production team. Their endless efforts to recruit the best for this project, has resulted in the accomplishment of this book. They are a veteran in the field of academics and their pool of knowledge is as vast as their experience in printing. Their expertise and guidance has proved useful at every step. Their uncompromising quality standards have made this book an exceptional effort. Their encouragement from time to time has been an inspiration for everyone.

The publisher and the editorial board hope that this book will prove to be a valuable piece of knowledge for researchers, students, practitioners and scholars across the globe.

List of Contributors

Yuanyuan Liu and Tao Zhang
Department of Epidemiology and Health Statistics, West China School of Public Health, Sichuan University, Chengdu, Sichuan, People's Republic of China

Weiwei Tang, Yaxi Li and Min Yang
Department of Epidemiology and Health Statistics, West China School of Public Health, Sichuan University, Chengdu, Sichuan, People's Republic of China
West China Research Center for Rural Health Development, Sichuan University, No.17 Section 3, South Renmin Road, Chengdu, Sichuan 610041, People's Republic of China

Xiang Liu
Department of Health and Social Behavior, West China School of Public Health, Sichuan University, Chengdu, Sichuan, People's Republic of China

Antti Tanskanen
Department of Clinical Neuroscience, Division of Psychiatry, Karolinska Institutet, Karolinska University Hospital, Stockholm, Sweden
National Institute for Health and Welfare, Helsinki, Finland

Miljana Vukadin, Frederieke G. Schaafsma and Johannes R. Anema
Department of Public and Occupational Health, Amsterdam Public Health research institute, VU University Medical Center, Van der Boechorststraat 7, 1081 BT Amsterdam, the Netherlands
Research Center for Insurance Medicine: collaboration between AMC- UMCG - UWV - VUmc, Amsterdam, the Netherlands

Marjan J. Westerman
Department of Health Sciences, Vrije Universiteit Amsterdam, De Boelelaan 1105, 1081 HV Amsterdam, the Netherlands

Harry W. C. Michon
Trimbos Institute, The Netherlands Institute of Mental Health and Addiction, Da Costakade 45, 3521 VS Utrecht, the Netherlands

Ulrike Stentzel, Neeltje van den Berg, Franziska Radicke and Wolfgang Hoffmann
Institute for Community Medicine, University Medicine Greifswald, Ellernholzstraße 1-2, 17487 Greifswald, Germany

Thea Schwaneberg
Institute for Community Medicine, University Medicine Greifswald, Ellernholzstraße 1-2, 17487 Greifswald, Germany
Department of Vascular Medicine, University Heart Center Hamburg, University Medical Center Hamburg-Eppendorf (UKE), Martinistraße 52, 20246 Hamburg, Germany

Lara N. Schulze and Hans-Jörgen Grabe
Department of Psychiatry and Psychotherapy, University Medicine Greifswald, Ellernholzstraße 1-2, 17487 Greifswald, Germany

Harald J. Freyberger
Department of Psychiatry and Psychotherapy, University Medicine Greifswald, Ellernholzstraße 1-2, 17487 Greifswald, Germany
HELIOS Hanseklinikum Stralsund, department for psychiatry and psychotherapy, Rostocker Chaussee 70, 18437 Stralsund, Germany

Jens M. Langosch
Bethanien Hospital for Psychiatry, Psychosomatics and Psychotherapy, Gützkower Landstraße 69, 17489 Greifswald, Germany

Farid Chakhssi
Scelta, GGNet, Apeldoorn, The Netherlands
Centre for eHealth and Well-being Research, Department of Psychology, Health, and Technology, University of Twente, 7500 AE Enschede, The Netherlands

Jannis T. Kraiss, Marion Sommers-Spijkerman and Ernst T. Bohlmeijer
Centre for eHealth and Well-being Research, Department of Psychology, Health, and Technology, University of Twente, 7500 AE Enschede, The Netherlands

Hayley McBain, Chris Flood and Mark Haddad
School of Health Sciences, City, University of London, Myddelton Street, London EC1V 0HB, UK

Kathleen Mulligan and Alan Simpson
School of Health Sciences, City, University of London, Myddelton Street, London EC1V 0HB, UK
East London NHS Foundation Trust, London, UK

Frederique Lamontagne-Godwin
School of Human and Social Sciences, University of West London, London, UK

Jacqui Chapman
Diabetes Specialist Nursing Service, East London NHS Foundation Trust, London, UK

Julia Jones
Centre for Research in Primary & Community Care (CRIPACC), University of Hertfordshire, Hatfield, Hertfordshire, UK

Anke Köbach, Martina Ruf-Leuschner and Thomas Elbert
Department of Clinical and Neuropsychology, University Konstanz, Universitätsstraße 10, 78457 Konstanz, Germany
Vivo international e.V., Postfach 5108, 78430 Konstanz, Germany

Yunge Fan and Ning Ma
Peking University Sixth Hospital; Peking University Institute of Mental Health; Key Laboratory of Mental Health, Ministry of Health (Peking University); National Clinical Research Center for Mental Disorders (Peking University Sixth Hospital), Beijing, China

Liang Ma and Wei Xu
Beijing Chaoyang District Mental Disease Prevention and Control Center, The Third Hospital of Chaoyang District, Beijing, China

J. Steven Lamberti and Eric D. Caine
Department of Psychiatry, University of Rochester Medical Center, Rochester, USA

Edwin de Beurs
Stichting Benchmark GGZ, Rembrandtlaan 46, 3723 BK Bilthoven, Netherlands
Leiden University, Wassenaarseweg 52, 2333 Leiden, AK, Netherlands

Matthijs Blankers
Arkin, Klaprozenweg 111, 1033 Amsterdam, NN, Netherlands
Trimbos Institute, Da Costakade 45, 3521 Utrecht, VS, Netherlands

Philippe Delespaul
Maastricht University, Minderbroedersberg 4-6, 6211 Maastricht, LK, Netherlands

Erik van Duijn
GGZ Delfland, Sint Jorisweg 2, 2612 Delft, GA, Netherlands

Yan-Mei Shen, Jian-Bo Liu, Xi-Long Cui, Yu-Qiong He, Yu-min Fang and Xue-Rong Luo
Department of Psychiatry, The Second Xiangya Hospital, Central South University, Changsha 410011, Hunan, China
Mental Health Institute of Central South University, China National Clinical Research Center on Mental Disorders (Xiangya), China National Technology Institute on Mental Disorders, Hunan Technology Institute of Psychiatry, Hunan Key Laboratory of Psychiatry and Mental Health, Changsha 410011, Hunan, China

Bella Siu Man Chan
The Department of Educational and Counselling Psychology, and Special Education, The University of British Columbia, Vancouver, Canada

Yuan-Yue Zhou
Mental Health Zhejiang University School of Medicine Hangzhou Seventh People's Hospital, Hangzhou 310013, China

Yu-Tao Xiang
Unit of Psychiatry, Faculty of Health Sciences, University of Macau, Macao SAR, China

Georgina Miguel Esponda and Sujit Rathod
Centre for Global Mental Health, Department of Population Health, Faculty of Epidemiology and Population Health, London School of Hygiene and Tropical Medicine, Keppel Street, London WC1E 7HT, UK

M. Scheffers and R. J. Bosscher
Windesheim University of Applied Sciences, School of Human Movement and Education, Campus 2-6, 8017 CA Zwolle, the Netherlands

Tessa Roberts
Centre for Global Mental Health, Department of Population Health, Faculty of Epidemiology and Population Health, London School of Hygiene and Tropical Medicine, Keppel Street, London WC1E 7HT, UK
Health Service and Population Research Department, Institute of Psychiatry, Psychology and Neuroscience, King's College London, London, UK

Dzmitry Krupchanka
Department of Social Psychiatry, National Institute of Mental Health, Prague, Czech Republic
Institute of Global Health, University of Geneva, Geneva, Switzerland

Rahul Shidhaye
Centre for Chronic Conditions and Injuries, Public Health Foundation of India, New Delhi, India
Care and Public Health Research Institute, Maastricht University, Maastricht, Netherlands

Vikram Patel
Department of Global Health and Social Medicine, Harvard Medical School, Boston, USA

Wei-Ting Tseng and Tiao-Lai Huang
Department of Psychiatry, Kaohsiung Chang Gung Memorial Hospital and Chang Gung University College of Medicine, No. 123, Dapi Road, Niaosong District, Kaohsiung City 833, Taiwan

H. Kalisvaart
Windesheim University of Applied Sciences, School of Human Movement and Education, Campus 2-6, 8017 CA Zwolle, the Netherlands
Altrecht Psychosomatic Medicine, Vrijbaan 2, 3705 WC Zeist, the Netherlands

J. T. van Busschbach
Windesheim University of Applied Sciences, School of Human Movement and Education, Campus 2-6, 8017 CA Zwolle, the Netherlands
Department of Psychiatry, University of Groningen, University Medical Center Groningen, CC72, 9700, RB Groningen, the Netherlands

S. A. M. van Broeckhuysen-Kloth
Altrecht Psychosomatic Medicine, Vrijbaan 2, 3705 WC Zeist, the Netherlands

R. Geenen
Altrecht Psychosomatic Medicine, Vrijbaan 2, 3705 WC Zeist, the Netherlands
Department of Psychology, Utrecht University, Heidelberglaan 1, 3584CS, Utrecht, the Netherlands

R. A. Schoevers
Department of Psychiatry, University of Groningen, University Medical Center Groningen, CC72, 9700, RB Groningen, the Netherlands
Research School of Behavioural and Cognitive Neurosciences (BCN), Interdisciplinary, Center for Psychopathology and Emotion regulation (ICPE), CC72, 9700, RB Groningen, the Netherlands

M. A. J. van Duijn
Department of Sociology, University of Groningen, Grote Rozenstraat, 31 9712 TG Groningen, the Netherlands

Ragnar Verbraeken
OPZ Geel, Geel, Belgium

Jurjen J. Luykx
Department Of Psychiatry, Rudolf Magnus Institute of Neuroscience, Utrecht University, Utrecht, The Netherlands
Department of Translational Neuroscience, Rudolf Magnus Institute of Neuroscience, Utrecht University, Utrecht, The Netherlands
SymforaMeander Hospital, Amersfoort, The Netherlands
Department of Psychiatry, ZNA Hospitals, Antwerp, Belgium

Katharina Piontek
Institute for Medical Psychology, University Medicine Greifswald, Greifswald, Germany
Department of Psychosomatic Medicine and Psychotherapy, University Medical Center Hamburg-Eppendorf, Hamburg, Germany

Meike C. Shedden-Mora, Maria Gladigau, Amina Kuby and Bernd Löwe
Department of Psychosomatic Medicine and Psychotherapy, University Medical Center Hamburg-Eppendorf, Hamburg, Germany

Juan Li, Meng-meng Zhang and Lin Zhao
The Second Affiliated Hospital of Xinxiang Medical University, 388# Jianshe Road, Muye, Xinxiang, China

Wen-qiang Li
The Second Affiliated Hospital of Xinxiang Medical University, 388# Jianshe Road, Muye, Xinxiang, China
Henan Key Laboratory of Biological Psychiatry (Xinxiang Medical University), 388# Jianshe Road, Muye, Xinxiang, China

Jun-lin Mu
The Second Affiliated Hospital of Xinxiang Medical University, 388# Jianshe Road, Muye, Xinxiang, China
Xinxiang Key Laboratory of Electrophysiology, 388# Jianshe Road, Muye, Xinxiang, China

Zhao-hui Zhang
The Second Affiliated Hospital of Xinxiang Medical University, 388# Jianshe Road, Muye, Xinxiang, China
Xinxiang Medical University, 601# Jinsui Road, Hongqi, Xinxiang, China
Henan Key Laboratory of Biological Psychiatry (Xinxiang Medical University), 388# Jianshe Road, Muye, Xinxiang, China
Xinxiang Key Laboratory of Electrophysiology, 388# Jianshe Road, Muye, Xinxiang, China

Rüdiger Zwerenz and Matthias Michal
Department of Psychosomatic Medicine and Psychotherapy, University Medical Center of the Johannes Gutenberg University Mainz, Untere Zahlbacher Str. 8, 55131 Mainz, Germany

Till Fabian Beutel
Department of Psychosomatic Medicine and Psychotherapy, University Medical Center of the Johannes Gutenberg University Mainz, Untere Zahlbacher Str. 8, 55131 Mainz, Germany
Institute of Occupational, Social and Environmental Medicine, University Medical Center of the Johannes Gutenberg University Mainz, Obere Zahlbacher Str. 67, 55131 Mainz, Germany

Sarah Toner, Lauren M. Hickling, Megan Cassidy and Stefan Priebe
Unit for Social and Community Psychiatry (WHO Collaborating Centre for Mental Health Service Development), Queen Mary University of London, London, UK

Danielle Cath
Department of Clinical and Health psychology, Altrecht Academic Anxiety Centre, Utrecht University, Utrecht, The Netherlands

Syed Rahman, Kristina Alexanderson and Ellenor Mittendorfer-Rutz
Department of Clinical Neuroscience, Division of Insurance Medicine, Karolinska Institutet, SE-171 77 Stockholm, Sweden

Michael Wiberg
Department of Clinical Neuroscience, Division of Insurance Medicine, Karolinska Institutet, SE-171 77 Stockholm, Sweden
Department of Analysis and Forecast, Swedish Social Insurance Agency, Stockholm, Sweden

Jussi Jokinen
Department of Clinical Neuroscience, Division of Psychiatry, Karolinska Institutet, Karolinska University Hospital, Stockholm, Sweden
Department of Clinical Sciences, Division of Psychiatry, Umeå University, Umeå, Sweden

Stein Emil Vollset
Centre for Disease Burden, Norwegian Institute of Public Health, Bergen, Norway

Ann Kristin Knudsen
Centre for Disease Burden, Norwegian Institute of Public Health, Bergen, Norway
Department of Psychosocial Science, University of Bergen, Bergen, Norway

Gun Peggy Knudsen
Health Data and Digitalisation, Norwegian Institute of Public Health, Oslo, Norway

Sarah Toner, Megan Cassidy, Agnes Chevalier, Aida Farreny, Monica Leverton and Stefan Priebe
Unit for Social and Community Psychiatry (WHO Collaborating Centre for Mental Health Service Development), Newham Centre for Mental Health, Queen Mary University of London, London, UK

Mariana Pinto da Costa
Unit for Social and Community Psychiatry (WHO Collaborating Centre for Mental Health Service Development), Newham Centre for Mental Health, Queen Mary University of London, London, UK
Hospital de Magalhães Lemos, Porto, Portugal
Institute of Biomedical Sciences Abel Salazar (ICBAS), University of Porto, Porto, Portugal

Hong Wen, Dan Wang and Xianmei Yang
Sichuan Provincial Mental Health Centre, Mianyang, Sichuan, People's Republic of China

Yasmin Gharavi
GGZ inGeest, Amsterdam, The Netherlands

Barbara Stringer
Research group Recovery and Rehabilitation, GGZ inGeest, Amsterdam, The Netherlands
The Mat Training & Education, Amsterdam, The Netherlands

Adriaan Hoogendoorn
Department of Psychiatry, Amsterdam Public Health research institute, VU University Medical Center, Amsterdam, The Netherlands

Berno Van Meijel
Department of Psychiatry, Amsterdam Public Health research institute, VU University Medical Center, Amsterdam, The Netherlands
Inholland University of Applied Sciences, Amsterdam, The Netherlands
Parnassia Psychiatric Institute, The Hague, The Netherlands
Academy for Masters in Advanced Nursing Practice, Utrecht, The Netherlands

Jan Boogaarts and Bas Van Raaij
The Mat Training & Education, Amsterdam, The Netherlands

Ragnar Nesvåg
Department of mental disorders, Norwegian Institute of Public Health, Oslo, Norway
Nydalen DPS, Division of Mental Health and Addiction, Oslo University Hospital, Oslo, Norway

Ted Reichborn-Kjennerud
Department of mental disorders, Norwegian Institute of Public Health, Oslo, Norway
Institute of Clinical Medicine, University of Oslo, Oslo, Norway

Kristin Gustavson
Department of mental disorders, Norwegian Institute of Public Health, Oslo, Norway
Department of Psychology, University of Oslo, Oslo, Norway

Lucas J. B. van Oudheusden, Stasja Draisma, Patricia van Oppen and Anton J. L. M. van Balkom
Department of Psychiatry, Amsterdam Public Health, Amsterdam UMC, Vrije Universiteit Amsterdam, GGZ inGeest, Oldenaller 1, 1081, HJ, Amsterdam, The Netherlands

Sandra van der Salm
Brain Center Rudolf Magnus, Department of Neurology and Neurosurgery, University Medical Center Utrecht, Utrecht, The Netherlands
Stichting Epilepsie Instellingen Nederland (SEIN), Zwolle, The Netherlands

Gerben Meynen
Faculty of Humanities, Vrije Universiteit Amsterdam, Amsterdam, The Netherlands
GGZ inGeest, Amsterdam, The Netherlands
Willem Pompe Institute for Criminal Law and Criminology, Utrecht University, Utrecht, The Netherlands

Index

A

Achenbach's Child Behavior Checklist, 151-152, 157

Andersen Behavioural Model, 124-125

Anxiety Disorder, 14-16, 18-21, 48, 53, 123, 125-127, 140, 151, 154-155, 157, 176, 185, 187-190, 194-198, 225, 227

Attention Deficit Hyperactivity Disorder, 151, 154, 157, 159

Auditory Hallucination, 73

Autism Spectrum Disorder, 157

B

Benzodiazepine, 73-74

Bipolar Disorders, 41, 65-66

Body Dysmorphic Disorder, 58

Bradyphrenia, 160-161, 163

C

Cardiac Arrest, 73, 75

Cardiovascular Disease, 35, 173-174, 182, 185

Chronic Obstructive Pulmonary Disease, 69, 71

Clozapine, 73-75, 217

Cognitive Behavioural Therapy, 48

Common Mental Disorders, 38, 47-48, 50-53, 55-56, 124-125, 139-141, 156, 186-188, 199-200

Conduct Disorder, 154-155, 157, 159

Corticosteroids, 69, 71-72

D

Defined Daily Dose, 47-48, 55

Delirium, 160, 162-164

Depressive Disorder, 14, 16, 18-19, 48, 55, 61, 105, 110, 122, 125, 140-141, 150, 154-155, 157, 175-176, 186, 189, 194-196, 198

Dialectical Behavior Therapy, 110, 123

Diazepam Intravenous Drip, 74

Dresden Body Image Questionnaire, 57-59, 61-64

Dual Antiplatelet Agents, 74-75

E

Epileptic Seizures, 160, 162-163

Excited Catatonia, 74-75

F

Female Genital Mutilation, 95, 101-102, 104-106

G

Generalized Anxiety Disorder, 15-16, 21, 123, 140, 151, 154-155, 157, 185, 187, 189, 194-196, 198

H

Hair Cortisol, 95-96, 100, 103-106

Health Service Utilization, 125, 140

Hopkins Symptom Checklist-25, 99, 105

Hyperarousal, 96

Hypothalamus-pituitary-adrenal (HPA) Axis, 96

I

Individual Placement and Support, 86-87, 93-94

Interaction-skills Training, 165-166, 171

L

Lithium, 74

Lorazepam, 73-75, 160-163

M

Major Depressive Disorder, 55, 122, 125, 140-141, 150, 154-155, 157, 186, 189, 194-196, 198

Meta-analysis, 13, 15, 21, 35, 84, 94, 105, 107-109, 115, 117-120, 122-123, 126, 136, 141, 154, 158, 171, 184, 210, 217-218

O

Obsessive-compulsive Disorder, 48, 125, 189, 196, 219- 220, 226-227

Occupational Therapy, 54

Oppositional Defiant Disorder, 151, 154-155, 157-159

P

Panic Disorder, 16, 20, 125-127, 189, 194-196

Perceived Stress Scale, 121, 183

Personal and Social Performance Scale, 78

Phobic Anxiety Disorder, 16, 48

Phonological Disorder, 155

Positive Predictive Value, 69, 71

Positive Psychology Interventions, 107, 117-120, 122-123

Postictum, 160

Primary Care Physicians, 14

Principal Axis Factor Analysis, 219, 221, 223, 226

Psychological Support, 22, 25, 28, 32-33

Psychoneuroendocrinological, 96

Psychosocial Stressors, 173-175, 177, 182, 185

Psychotic Disorders, 2, 13, 35, 41, 65-67, 77, 95, 99, 101, 108, 110, 160, 163, 211

Pulmonary Embolism, 73, 75

R

Reliable Change Index, 38, 40, 45

Risk Behavior, 1-12

Routine Outcome Monitoring, 37, 39, 45-46, 64

S

Schizoaffective Disorders, 66-67

Schizophrenia, 2, 7-10, 12-13, 16, 22-23, 25-26, 35, 65-67, 71-72, 74-75, 78-81, 94, 122, 144, 147, 150, 155, 163-164, 167, 171-172, 212-213, 217-218, 227

Serotonin Syndrome, 162

Severe Mental Illness, 9-10, 22, 32, 34-35, 37, 46, 76-77, 84, 86, 93-94, 150, 165-168, 171-172, 184, 202, 210-212, 217-218

Sinus Tachycardia, 74

Social Anxiety Disorder, 125

Social Phobia, 16, 155, 157, 189, 194-196

Somatic Disorders, 63, 107-110, 117-120

Somatoform Disorder, 14-21, 57-64, 176

Stigmatizing Attitudes, 143-144, 146-148

Suboptimal Antidepressant, 47

T

T-scores, 38-45

Theoretical Domains Framework, 22, 24, 29, 34-35

Trier Social Stress Test, 174, 183

Tucker Lewis Index, 60, 63

Type 2 Diabetes, 22-23, 35, 122

U

Urine Toxicology, 161

V

Venous Thromboembolism, 74-75

Visual Analogue Scale, 220

CPSIA information can be obtained
at www.ICGtesting.com
Printed in the USA
LVHW062013100122
708212LV00002B/206